Orbital
Disease

Orbital Disease

Present Status and Future Challenges

edited by
Jack Rootman

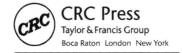

CRC Press
Taylor & Francis Group
Boca Raton London New York

CRC Press is an imprint of the
Taylor & Francis Group, an **informa** business

CRC Press
Taylor & Francis Group
6000 Broken Sound Parkway NW, Suite 300
Boca Raton, FL 33487-2742

First issued in paperback 2019

© 2011 by Taylor & Francis Group, LLC
CRC Press is an imprint of Taylor & Francis Group, an Informa business

No claim to original U.S. Government works

ISBN-13: 978-0-8247-4089-4 (hbk)
ISBN-13: 978-0-367-39308-3 (pbk)

A CIP record for this book is available from the British Library.

Library of Congress Cataloging-in-Publication Data available on application

Visit the Taylor & Francis Web site at
http://www.taylorandfrancis.com

and the CRC Press Web site at
http://www.crcpress.com

Contents

Introduction

The Vancouver Orbital Symposium represented an unusual opportunity to bring together many disciplines to review knowledge, interact, and assess challenges for the future. It also culminated and rewarded my tenure as chair of ophthalmology at the University of British Columbia and marks my return to full-time practice, teaching, and research.

The 47 faculty presentations, open submissions, and posters brought together experts from many disciplines including basic science, neuroimaging, radiotherapy, oncology, infectious disease, endocrinology, pathology, molecular biology, and surgery. We tackled major topics in orbital inflammatory disease, lymphoproliferative disorders, optic nerve, and meningeal lesions, problems in oncology, vascular disorders, and of course an extended look at the current status of thyroid orbitopathy.

This conference was anteceded by a two-day meeting of the Orbital Society, whose members became the core faculty of the symposium. I am grateful for the honor of their commitment to this endeavor and the plan to repeat this symposium under the auspices of the society every four to five years. The meeting was well attended throughout, and the discussions lively, intelligent, and enthusiastic. In short, this event was the highlight of my career and especially noteworthy by the participation of 27 of my fellows, to whom I am most grateful. Ultimately, it is the joy of lifelong learning and the challenge of patient care that set the tone of the symposium.

I look forward to the continued active endeavor.

Jack Rootman

Contributors

Hind M. Al-Katan   Department of Ophthalmology, Security
Forces Hospital, Riyadh, Saudi Arabia

Jugpal Arneja   The Faculty of Medicine, University of Manitoba,
Winnipeg, Manitoba, Canada

Stephen Baker   Department of Ophthalmology and Visual
Sciences, Eye Care Centre, Dalhousie University, Halifax,
Nova Scotia, Canada

Luigi Bartalena   Cattedra di Endocrinologia, Universita´
dell'Insubria, Varese, Italy

George B. Bartley   Mayo Clinic, Jacksonville, Florida, U.S.A.

Kenneth W. Berean   Department of Pathology, Vancouver
General Hospital, University of British Columbia, Vancouver,
British Columbia, Canada

Guilio Bonavolonta   Department of Ophthalmology, University
of Naples, Naples, Italy

Frank Buffam Department of Ophthalmology, University of British Columbia and the Vancouver General Hospital, Vancouver, British Columbia, Canada

Anthony W. Chow Division of Infectious Diseases, Department of Medicine, University of British Columbia and Vancouver Hospital Health Sciences Centre, Vancouver, British Columbia, Canada

Jonathan C. Choy Department of Pathology and Laboratory Medicine, St. Paul's Hospital, Providence Health Care, University of British Columbia, Vancouver, British Columbia, Canada

Kimberly P. Cockerham Department of Ophthalmology, Allegheny General Hospital, Pittsburgh, Pennsylvania, U.S.A.

Joseph M. Connors Division of Medical Oncology, University of British Columbia and British Columbia Cancer Agency, Vancouver, British Columbia, Canada

Peter J. Dolman Department of Ophthalmology and Visual Sciences, and Department of Pathology, University of British Columbia, Vancouver General Hospital, Vancouver, British Columbia, Canada

Jonathan J. Dutton University of North Carolina, Chapel Hill, North Carolina, U.S.A.

Ian Epstein Thyroid Research Laboratory, Dalhousie University, Halifax, Nova Scotia, Canada

Kenneth A. Feldman Department of Ophthalmology, Kaiser Permanente Medical Center, Harbor City, California, U.S.A.

Randy D. Gascoyne Department of Pathology, British Columbia Cancer Agency, Vancouver, British Columbia, Canada

Robert Alan Goldberg Jules Stein Eye Institute, UCLA School of Medicine, Los Angeles, California, U.S.A.

James H. Goldie University of British Columbia, Vancouver, British Columbia, Canada

Colum A. Gorman   Mayo Clinic, Rochester, Minnesota, U.S.A.

Douglas A. Graeb   Diagnostic and Therapeutic Neuroradiology, St. Michael's Hospital, University of Toronto, Toronto, Ontario, Canada

Gerald J. Harris   Section of Orbital and Oculoplastic Surgery, Department of Ophthalmology, Medical College of Wisconsin, Milwaukee, Wisconsin, U.S.A.

Thomas J. Joly   Department of Ophthalmology, Vancouver General Hospital, University of British Columbia, Vancouver, Canada

Steven E. Katz   William H. Havener Eye Center, The Ohio State University, Columbus, Ohio, U.S.A.

Michael Kazim   Columbia University, New York, New York, U.S.A.

John S. Kennerdell   Department of Ophthalmology, Allegheny General Hospital, Pittsburgh, Pennsylvania, U.S.A.

Dino D. Klisovic   William H. Havener Eye Center, The Ohio State University, Columbus, Ohio, U.S.A.

Marko I. Klisovic   William H. Havener Eye Center, The Ohio State University, Columbus, Ohio, U.S.A.

Jocelyne S. Lapointe   Department of Radiology, Vancouver General Hospital, University of British Columbia, Vancouver, British Columbia, Canada

Kate Lazier   Thyroid Research Laboratory, Dalhousie University, Halifax, Nova Scotia, Canada

Martin Lubow   William H. Havener Eye Center, The Ohio State University, Columbus, Ohio, U.S.A.

Roy Ma   Department of Radiation Oncology, British Columbia Cancer Agency, Vancouver, British Columbia, Canada

Claudio Marcocci   Dipartimento di Endocrinologia e Metabolismo, Universita′ di Pisa, Varese, Italy

Michele Marinò   Dipartimento di Endocrinologia e Metabolismo, Universita′ di Pisa, Varese, Italy

Joseph C. Maroon   Presbyterian University Hospital, Pittsburgh, Pennsylvania, U.S.A.

Thomas R. Marotta   Diagnostic and Therapeutic Neuroradiology, St. Michael's Hospital, University of Toronto, Toronto, Ontario, Canada

Barbara Mazzi   Dipartimento di Endocrinologia e Metabolismo, Università di Pisa, Varese, Italy

Bruce M. McManus   Department of Pathology and Laboratory Medicine, St. Paul's Hospital, Providence Health Care, University of British Columbia, Vancouver, British Columbia, Canada

Alan A. McNab   Orbit, Plastic and Lacrimal Clinic, Royal Victorian Eye and Ear Hospital, Victoria, Melbourne, Australia

Francesca Menconi   Dipartimento di Endocrinologia e Metabolismo, Università di Pisa, Varese, Italy

Eugenia Morabito   Dipartimento di Endocrinologia e Metabolismo, Università di Pisa, Varese, Italy

Wieslaw L. Nowinski   Biomedical Imaging Laboratory, Agency for Science, Technology and Research (ASTAR), Singapore

Sylvia Pasternak   Department of Pathology, Dalhousie University, Halifax, Nova Scotia, Canada

Aldo Pinchera   Dipartimento di Endocrinologia e Metabolismo, Università di Pisa, Varese, Italy

Roberto Rocchi Dipartimento di Endocrinologia e Metabolismo, Università di Pisa, Varese, Italy

Jack Rootman Department of Ophthalmology and Visual Sciences, and Department of Pathology, University of British Columbia, Vancouver General Hospital, Vancouver, British Columbia, Canada

Peerooz Saeed Department of Ophthalmology, University of Amsterdam, Amsterdam, The Netherlands

Mario Salvi Cattedra di Endocrinologia, Universita di Panna, Panna, Italy

Kam Shojania Department of Medicine, University of British Columbia, Vancouver, British Columbia, Canada

Donald Smallman Thyroid Research Laboratory, Dalhousie University, Halifax, Nova Scotia, Canada

Terry J. Smith Division of Molecular Medicine, Harbor-UCLA Medical Center, Torrance, and School of Medicine, University of California, Los Angeles, California, U.S.A.

Diego Strianese Department of Ophthalmology, University of Naples, Naples, Italy

Roger E. Turbin Department of Ophthalmology, Allegheny General Hospital, Pittsburgh, Pennsylvania, U.S.A.

Sumalee Vangveeravong Department of Ophthalmology, Siriraj Hospital, Bangkok, Thailand

Jack R. Wall Thyroid Research Laboratory, Dalhousie University, Halifax, Nova Scotia, Canada

Valerie A. White Department of Pathology, Vancouver General Hospital, University of British Columbia, Vancouver, British Columbia, Canada

Wilmar M. Wiersinga Department of Medicine, Academic Medical Center, University of Amsterdam, Amsterdam, The Netherlands

1

Orbital Inflammatory Disease: Classification and New Insights

JACK ROOTMAN

Department of Ophthalmology and Visual Sciences, and Department of Pathology, University of British Columbia, Vancouver General Hospital, Vancouver, British Columbia, Canada

Over the last 20 years, our experience at the University of British Columbia Orbital Clinic in managing over 6000 orbital cases has led to a paradigm shift in terms of understanding orbital inflammatory disease. This is characterized by broad clinical definitions of inflammations shifting to diagnoses that are based on pathologic, anatomic, and systemic associations of disease. In recent years, we have seen increasing diagnostic specificity brought about by immunopathologic and molecular techniques, which in turn will link to specific treatment based on disease pathogenesis (1).

DEFINITION, CLASSIFICATION, AND CHANGING PARADIGM IN ORBITAL INFLAMMATORY DISEASE

In understanding orbital inflammatory disease, it is important to separate lymphoproliferative processes from the discussion of inflammatory disorders, since they are distinct entities that can be clearly defined pathologically and should no longer be included with the inflammatory processes. The noninfectious orbital inflammations can be viewed as either nonspecific or specific. In our series of patients with inflammation reviewed between 1976 and 1988, we have noted that 70% of noninfectious lesions were nonspecific while 30% were specific. Data from 2001 of all patients show that the ratio is now 1:1, demonstrating a significant shift toward specificity in diagnosis. The nonspecific inflammations are clinically acute and subacute, and are probably best understood in terms of their anatomic localization. We have defined these as myositic, lacrimal, anterior, diffuse, or apical, each of which have a constellation of findings based on their location. On the other hand, specific inflammations are defined on the basis of identification of a specific pathogen, specific local and/or systemic constellation of findings, or a specific kind of pathology. Examples of specific inflammation include microbial infection, granulomatous inflammation, many different types of vasculitis, and sclerosing inflammation (2). In the instance of vasculitic and granulomatous disorders, there is often a constellation of systemic associations that can define the orbital inflammations specifically. For example, Wegener's granulomatosis is distinct from some of the hypersensitivity or leukocytoclastic angiitides (3). Tables 1 and 2 outline the features of nonspecific and specific inflammations.

ROLE OF BIOPSY

We have noted that biopsy has allowed definition of more specific constellations, such as Wegener's granulomatosis that occur within the orbit (3). It has also led to a redefinition of lesions, such as sclerosing inflammation and xanthogranulomatous disease that have a very specific histopathology and constellation of findings. Indeed, 70% of our own biopsied inflammations have been associated with the discovery of a specific disorder, many of which have systemic implications as reported by Hamedani in this symposium. This paradigm should be applied carefully in the diagnosis of patients with so-called "nonspecific orbital inflammatory disease," particularly if the patient has an atypical onset, a particular location involved, or associated systemic findings. Our tendency is to define inflammations as a specific disorder before accepting a diagnosis of nonspecific orbital inflammatory diseases, particularly in certain locations, such as the lacrimal gland or the orbital apex. In the lacrimal gland, a high percentage (50%) of biopsied inflammatory lesions was associated with systemic disease. The range of diagnoses that we have experienced with lacrimal inflammations includes Wegener's granulomatosis (including in children), sclerosing inflammation, Sjögren's syndrome, sarcoidal reactions, and autoimmune diseases. Apical disease tends to be associated with either sight-threatening or even life-threatening disorders, and should rarely be accepted as nonspecific without meticulous investigation and consideration of biopsy.

Because of the paradigm shift based on our own experience, we tend to analyze orbital disease by defining the anatomy, looking at the pathology in terms of types of reactions that are based on the cell type and the focus of the infiltrate, then look for associated systemic or local features, and specific pathologic patterns thereby arriving at more specific diagnoses (Fig. 1).

Myositis is a good example of this shifting paradigm. In our experience, this disorder presents in an isolated, recurrent, or atypical fashion. Isolated myositis is acute or subacute, and typically when involving a single muscle is likely to be characterized by a single episode without systemic associations. On the other hand, recurrent myositis by definition is characterized as having repeated acute episodes or progressive sequential involvement of muscles. It typically involves

Table 1 · Comparative Features of Acute and Subacute Nonspecific Idiopathic Inflammations of the Orbit[a]

	Myositic	Lacrimal	Anterior	Diffuse	Apical
Clinical					
Number	51	25	23	3	11
Pain	On movement Painful	With tenderness	Moderate	Moderate	Can be severe
Ocular and orbital features	Decreased extraocular movement Normal vision Localized injection and chemosis	Lateral swelling S-shaped lid deformity Tenderness Pouting of lacrimal ducts Chemosis and injection localized	Uveitis Retinal detachment Decreased extraocular movement Decreased vision Anterior inflammation Chemosis Diffuse injection and swelling of lid	Uveitis Retinal detachment Decreased extraocular movement Decreased vision Anterior inflammation Chemosis Diffuse injection and swelling of lid	Decreased vision Decreased extraocular movement Mild proptosis and chemosis
Visual outcome	Good	Good	Good	Usually positive, rarely negative	Usually positive, rarely negative

Imaging

CT and MR	Muscle irregularly enlarged Swelling of tendon Local scleral and Tenon's capsule swelling Fusiform enlargement of whole muscle	Irregular swelling of lacrimal gland and adjacent tissues	Anterior: enhancing with irregular margins intimate to scleral envelope Variable extension along optic nerve Decreased fat density	Diffuse: enhancing with decreased fat density	Apical irregular infiltration Extends along muscle and optic nerve
Ultrasonography	Increased extraocular muscle size	Local swelling with increased Tenon's space	Sclerotenonitis with T sign	T sign	Negative

[a]From Rootman J. Diseases of the orbit: A Multidisciplinary Approach, 2nd. Ed.; Lippincott Williams and Wilkins: Philadelphia, 2002; 457.

Table 2 Examples of Specific Inflammations of the Orbit

Infections and infestations
  Microbial
  Fungal
    Mucormycosis
    Aspergillosis
  Tuberculosis and syphilis
  Parasitic
    Echinococcosis
    Cysticercosis
Other specific inflammations
  Vasculitis
    Wegener's granulomatosis
    Other respiratory vasculitides
    Polyarteritis nodosa
    Hypersensitivity (leukocytoclastic vasculitis)
  Sclerosing inflammation of the orbit
  Granulomatous inflammation
    Foreign body granuloma
    Sarcoidal inflammation
    Xanthogranulomatous inflammation
Transitional lesions
  Kimura's disease
  Sjögren's syndrome
  Sinus histiocytosis with massive lymphadenopathy
  Castleman's disease

more than one muscle in the first episode, and there is a higher incidence of associated systemic disorders. Finally, patients with atypical myositis (e.g., painless, characterized by a prolonged course, or with compressive features) should undergo biopsy, since this category has included such disorders as sclerosing inflammation, giant cell myositis (possibly associated with pericarditis and risk to life) (4), reactive lymphoid lesions, and more recently inflammation dominated either by T-cells or CD20-positive cells, which may have specific therapeutic implications. This definition of myositic disorders allows for a management algorithm that considers biopsy for bilateral, recurrent, and atypical presentations (Fig. 2).

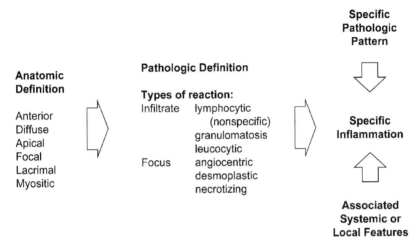

Figure 1 Algorithm for analysis of inflammation. (Borrowed with permission from Ref. 1, p. 499.)

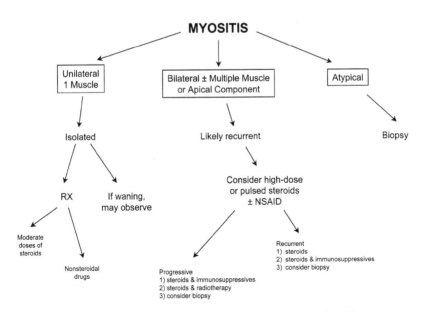

Figure 2 Suggested algorithm for the treatment of orbital myositis. (Borrowed with permission from Ref. 1, p. 462.)

THE ROLE OF IMMUNE MEDIATORS IN
SPECIFIC INFLAMMATIONS

Sclerosing inflammation was redefined by ourselves in a multicenter study done in the early 1990s (2,5). We define this inflammation as a de novo primary sclerosing process of the orbit with potential multisystem involvement (in particular, mediastinal and retroperitoneal fibrosis) that has a tendency to relentless progression. We found that the immunohistologic profile demonstrated a T-cell lymphocyte dominance with histiocytes and macrophages that was similar to retroperitoneal fibrosis. These new insights obtained from pathologic, pathophysiologic, and clinical inferences underline the necessity to understand the role or specific inflammatory and immune mediators. For example, T- and B-cells are found in different ratios depending on the nature of the disease process and may play an important role in inducing specific kinds of responses, such as fibroplasia. Indeed we found that in sclerosing inflammation and more recently in xanthogranulomatous disease that T-cells appear to play a significant role in the induction of either fibroplasia or a xanthogranulomatous reaction. In the case of thyroid orbitopathy, evidence suggests that in the early stages of the disease, T-cells play an important role with regard to activation of the fibroblast, leading to the production of glycosaminoglycans and fibrosis. With regard to adult xanthogranulomatous disease, as reported by Sivak in this symposium, there appear to be four syndromes with different local and constitutional features. The immunohistopathologic profile indicates a cytotoxic, T-cell mediated, local fibroblastic and lipophagic process in Erdheim–Chester disease and adult-onset asthma with peri-ocular xanthogranuloma (AAPOX). Systemic studies in this population also suggest a B-cell mediated component in AAPOX and necrobiotic xanthogranuloma. The T-cells implicated are of a cytotoxic CD8 cell type.

In thyroid orbitopathy, the orbital connective tissue, lipocytes, and possibly the extraocular muscles are thought to be targeted by T-lymphocytes as well. Activated lymphocytes infiltrate the tissues, particularly early in the disease, and induce the changes related to the disorder. This is brought about by cytokine release, oxygen-free radicals, and fibrogenic growth-factors leading to fibroblast stimulation and causing glycosaminoglycan deposition, cell growth, and preadipocyte transformation (6,7).

CHANGING PARADIGMS IN THE TREATMENT OF INFLAMMATION: THE RHEUMATOLOGIC APPROACH

Our experience in working with rheumatologists has made us aware of the changing approach to the management of rheumatologic disorders (as presented by Shojania in this symposium). Traditionally, diseases in this specialty have been treated in a pyramidal fashion, beginning with nonspecific anti-inflammatories, such as salicylates and nonsteroidal anti-inflammatory drugs (NSAIDs), moving up the ladder to disease-modifying treatments, such as antimalaria drugs, gold, methotrexate, and sulfadiazine, and more recently to drugs that target specific cytokines. The general shift, as noted in this symposium, has been to invert the pyramid and use more specific or aggressive therapy early in the course of the disease.

DIRECTED TREATMENTS OF DISTINCT ORBITAL INFLAMMATIONS

The recent trend in the management of rheumatologic disorders has prompted our unit to use their approach in managing certain orbital inflammations, thereby introducing more specific treatment for several disorders. This has led to improved results in the management of some complex inflammations. For instance since 1994, we have been treating newly diagnosed sclerosing inflammation with a combination of cytolytic doses of corticosteroids (intravenous methylprednisolone), T-cell inhibitors such as cyclosporine or methotrexate, and in some instances other immunosuppressive drugs.

This has led to significant improvement in some advanced cases and no recurrences or progression so far in eight patients treated following a biopsy-proven primary diagnosis of sclerosing inflammation of the orbit. Recently, in the instance of AAPOX, we have applied the same principle to attack the cytotoxic T-cells and have had several successes.

A recent case of a patient with AAPOX summarizes the role of immune mediation in establishing and promoting the disorder. This 46-year-old man presented with bilateral orbital involvement of AAPOX, which was associated with significant infiltration of the subcutaneous tissues of his cheek. He had an antecedent lymphoproliferative disorder and adult-onset asthma, signifying an immunoregulatory problem as the basis for his manifestations. The AAPOX heretofore had been unresponsive to corticosteroids alone. He was placed on cyclosporine, pulsed steroids, and immunosuppressives, which led to significant improvement of his periorbital and subcutaneous facial disease. Recently, he developed Burkitt's lymphoma that was treated with aggressive chemotherapy and autologous bone marrow transplantation, leading to further improvement of his orbital disease almost to the point of disappearance. Approximately 10 weeks after his bone marrow transplant, he developed an acute orbital infiltrate as his body repopulated with its own lymphocytes, which underlines the role of these cells and their cytokines in this specific inflammatory disease.

We have also encountered two different instances of myositis that were treated on the basis of the cellular infiltrate. One patient, previously unresponsive to corticosteroids, was found on biopsy to have a dominance of T-cells and responded well to methotrexate and cyclosporine. The second patient had a dominance of CD20 cells and responded to Rituximab, a specific chimeric drug directed against CD20 cells.

In review of the literature and from our own experience, T-cells and their mediators are now implicated in fibrotic responses in asthma, systemic sclerosis, sarcoidosis, murine viral myocarditis, thyroid orbitopathy, wound healing, lung

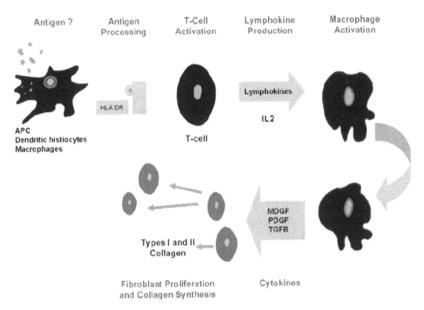

Figure 3 This diagram illustrates the inflammatory pathway and intermediaries that lead to fibroblast proliferation in collagen synthesis, emphasizing the multiple sites at which the process could be altered.

fibrosis, liver fibrosis, sclerosing inflammation, and retroperitoneal fibrosis, as well as AAPOX and Erdheim–Chester disease, which is reported in this symposium (8–21). In addition, fibroblasts isolated from conditions of pathologic fibrosis often display a persistently abnormal phenotype, which is apparently independent of exposure to initiating pathologic stimulus (22). This leads to the possibility of treating desmoplastic inflammatory diseases at many different points in their pathogenetic pathway (Fig. 3). This paradigm will define the future of management of inflammatory disease. In fact, the shift in our knowledge of inflammatory disease from nonspecific to specific is now allowing us to identify cytologic and molecular targets that will alter the fundamental approach to inflammatory disorders. Moreover, it emphasizes a need to define inflammatory disorders with greater specificity and accuracy.

REFERENCES

1. Rootman J. Diseases of the Orbit: A Multidisciplinary Approach. Lippincott, Philadelphia: Williams & Wilkins, 2003.

2. Rootman J, McCarthy J, White V, Harris G, Kennerdell J. Idiopathic sclerosing inflammation of the orbit: a distinct clinicopathologic entity. Ophthalmology 1994; 101(3):570–584.

3. Perry SR, Rootman J, White VA. The clinical and pathologic constellation of Wegener's granulomatosis of the orbit. Ophthalmology 1997; 104(4):683–694.

4. Selva D, Dolman PJ, Rootman J. Orbital granulomatous giant cell myositis: case report and review. Clin Exp Ophthalmol 2000; 28(1):65–68.

5. McCarthy JM, White VA, Harris G, Simons KB, Kennerdell J, Rootman J. Idiopathic sclerosing inflammation of the orbit: immunohistologic analysis and comparison with retroperitoneal fibrosis. Mod Pathol 1993; 6(5):581–587.

6. Kazim M, Goldberg RA, Smith TJ. Insights into the pathogenesis of thyroid-associated ophthalmopathy: evolving rationale for therapy. Arch Ophthalmol 2002; 120(3):380–386.

7. Pappa A, Lawson JMM, Calder V, Fells P, Lightman S. T cells and fibroblasts in affected extraocular muscles in early and late thyroid associated ophthalmopathy. Br J Ophthalmol 2000; 84(5):517–522.

8. Postlethwaite AE. Role of T cells and cytokines in effecting fibrosis. Int Rev Immunol 1995; 12(2–4):247–258.

9. Jimenez SA, Saitta B. Alterations in the regulation of expression of the alpha-1(I) collagen gene (COL1A1) in systemic sclerosis (scleroderma). Springer Semin Immunopathol 2000; 21(4):397–414.

10. Le Bousse-Kerdiles MC, Martyre MC. Myelofibrosis: pathogenesis of myelofibrosis with myeloid metaplasia. French INSERM Research Network on Myelofibrosis with Myeloid Metaplasia. Springer Semin Immunopathol 2000; 21(4):491–508.

11. Pinzani M. Liver fibrosis. Springer Semin Immunopathol 2000; 21(4):475–490.

12. Eckes B, Kessler D, Aumailley M, Krieg T. Interactions of fibroblasts with the extracellular matrix: implications for the understanding of fibrosis. Springer Semin Immunopathol 2000; 21(4):415–429.

13. Fonseca C, Abraham D, Black CM. Lung fibrosis. Springer Semin Immunopathol 2000; 21(4):453–474.

14. Chizzolini C. T lymphocyte and fibroblast interactions: the case of skin involvement in systemic sclerosis and other examples. Springer Semin Immunopathol 2000; 21(4):431–450.

15. Chizzolini C. Introductory note to: fibrosis year 2000. Springer Semin Immunopathol 2000; 21(4):377–382.

16. Wahl SM, Allen JB. T lymphocyte-dependent mechanisms of fibrosis. Prog Clin Biol Res 1988; 266:147–160.

17. Bellinghausen I, Brand U, Steinbrink K, Enk AH, Knop J, Saloga J. Inhibition of human allergic T-cell responses by IL-10-treated dendritic cells: differences from hydrocortisone-treated dendritic cells. J Allergy Clin Immunol 2001; 108(2):242–249.

18. Holgate ST, Djukanovic R, Howarth PH, Montefort S, Roche W. The T cell and the airway's fibrotic response in asthma. Chest 1993; 103(3):125S–128S.

19. Parkin J, Cohen B. An overview of the immune system. Lancet 2001; 357(9270):1777–1789.

20. Banchereau J, Steinman RM. Dendritic cells and the control of immunity. Nature 1998; 392(6673):245–252.

21. Cordeiro MF, Schultz GS, Ali RR, Bhattacharya SS, Khaw PT. Molecular therapy in ocular wound healing. Br J Ophthalmol 1999; 83(11):1219–1224.

22. Jelaska A, Strehlow D, Korn JH. Fibroblast hererogeniety in physiological conditions and fibrotic disease. Springer Semin Immunopathol 2000; 21(4):385–395.

2

Changing Paradigms in the Treatment of Inflammatory Disorders

KAM SHOJANIA

Department of Medicine,
University of British Columbia,
Vancouver, British Columbia, Canada

ABSTRACT

Inflammatory disorders are a heterogeneous group of idio-pathic diseases that typically involved several organ systems. Rheumatoid arthritis (RA) is a common inflammatory disorder of unknown etiology affecting 1% of the population. Rheuma-toid arthritis has been shown to be a systemic disease with a high morbidity and mortality rate. The treatment of RA has changed from a gradual "step up" or "pyramid" approach to a more aggressive paradigm using a combination of disease-mod-ifying anti-rheumatic drugs (DMARDs) and more recently, the anti-tumor necrosis factors (anti-TNF) and other biologic agents. These agents have been instrumental in improving the treatment of RA. The success of anti-TNF biologics in RA has spurred the use of these agents in other inflammatory disorders such as ankylosing spondylitis, psoriatic arthritis, and Wegener's granulomatosis.

Inflammatory diseases encompass a group of well-known and lesser-known diseases. The exact mechanisms underlying these disorders are unclear. For this reason, they are diagnosed primarily by a number of generally agreed-upon criteria, rather than a specific test. Rheumatoid arthritis (RA) is a good example of one of these conditions and is a common systemic autoimmune disease that affects all racial groups. It is a chronic, fluctuating disease of the joints with a symmetric, erosive, and eventually deforming polyarthritis. Nonarticular manifestations of RA are frequent and include subcutaneous nodules, serositis, vasculitis, and pulmonary, ocular and neurological involvement. The American Rheumatism Association revised the criteria for RA in 1987 for the purpose of classification in research studies (Table 1).

Rheumatoid arthritis presents usually with an insidious onset of fatigue and joint pain over weeks to months which may be transient early in the course of the disease. Eventually, joint inflammation becomes more persistent with warmth, effusion, tenderness, and loss of function. Some patients with RA have an acute onset within days. More often, patients have an intermediate onset over days to weeks (1,2).

Joint stiffness occurs in most patients, improves with physical activity and its duration after arising reflects the degree of synovial inflammation. The symmetrical polyarthritis classically involves the wrists, metacarpophalangeal (MCP) joints, metatarsophalangeal (MTP), and proximal interphalangeal joints (PIP) joints of the hands and feet. Joint damage usually becomes evident after one to two due to cartilage destruction and bony erosions as well as ligamentous laxity and tenosynovitis. Common structural deformities include loss of joint range of movement, subluxation, and angulation (Fig.1).

Table 1 The American Rheumatism Association 1987 Revised Criteria for the Classification of RA

Criterion	Definition
1. Morning stiffness	In joints, lasting at least 1 hr before maximal improvement
2. Arthritis of three or more areas	Soft-tissue swelling or fluid observed by a physician. Possible areas are PIP, MCP, wrist, elbow, knee ankle, and MTP joint
3. Arthritis of hand joints	At least one area in a wrist, MCP or PIP joint
4. Symmetric arthritis	Simultaneous involvement of the same joint areas on both sides of the body
5. Rheumatoid nodules	Subcutaneous nodules over bony prominences, extensor surfaces, or in juxta-articular regions observed by a physician
6. Serum rheumatoid factor	Any method in which results are positive in < 5% of normal population
7. Radiographic changes	Posterio-anterior hand and wrist radiographs which include erosions or periarticular osteopenia

For classification purposes, a patient shall be said to have rheumatoid arthritis if he/ she has satified at least 4 of these 7 criteria. Criteria 1 through 4 must have been present for at least 6 weeks. Patients with 2 clinical diagnoses are not excluded.

Systemic manifestations such as fatigue and generalized malaise are common with RA. Risk factors for extra-articular involvement are positive rheumatoid factor (RF) and rheumatoid nodules (2). The mortality of patients with severe RA (over 30 inflamed joints, positive RF) has been shown to be equivalent to three-vessel coronary artery disease and stage four Hodgkins disease (3).

Respiratory manifestations of RA are varied. Involvement of the cricoarytenoid joint may occur resulting in dysphonia. Interstitial lung disease with a predilection for basal involvement and less commonly, bronchiolitis obliterans, occurs. Rheumatoid nodules may affect the lung parenchyma and can cavitate. Pleural effusions occur but symptomatic pleuritis is uncommon. Pericardial effusions are common but

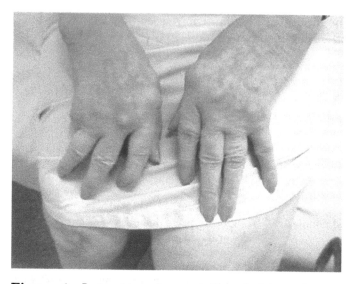

Figure 1 Late stage rheumatoid arthritis with ulnar deviation and subluxation at MCP joints.

generally asymptomatic. Neurologic manifestations are due to entrapment neuropathies, myelopathies from cervical spine instability, mononeuritis multiplex due to vasculitis or a mild peripheral sensory neuropathy. Felty's syndrome consists of RA, splenomegally, neutropenia, and, classically, leg ulcers. It may result in significant bacterial sepsis. It is also associated with thrombocytopenia and severe nodular RA. Dermal manifestations are rheumatoid nodules, pyoderma gangrenosum, and dermal drug side effects. Ocular manifestations include episcleritis, scleritis, and keratoconjunctivitis sicca.

The etiology of RA is unknown but there are data that point to both genetic and environmental etiologies. There are unique populations with a predilection to develop RA such as the Pima Indians in the United States (4). There are geographic clusters of erosive arthritis in archeological studies that indicate a possible environmental etiology (5). The pathogenesis of RA likely starts with an antigen-mediated activation of T-cells in an immunogenetically susceptible host, which leads to a cascade of multiple events such as proliferation of endothelial cells, synovial lining cells, recruitment of additional inflammatory cells from the bone marrow with secretion of cytokines and proteases and auto-antibody production. Once the immune response is triggered, additional antigens may be created and recognized by the T-cell to create an ongoing immune reaction.

Rheumatoid factors are immunoglobulins that react against the Fc portion of the immunoglobulin G (IgG) molecule. The RF is positive in 70–80% of patients with RA but only in 50–60% of patients with RA at onset (6). It is seen with many conditions besides RA such as chronic infections, viral diseases, and chronic inflammatory diseases. About 5% of the general population is RF positive with no evidence of disease. The prevalence of RF positive individuals increases with age (6).

The treatment of RA has changed over the past decade. Up to 1993, the step-up or "pyramid approach" was popular such that the pyramid even became the symbol for the American College of Rheumatology. This approach began with simple nonsteroidal anti-inflammatory medications (NSAIDs) and if needed, a slow progression was initiated through the milder disease-modifying anti-rheumatic drugs (DMARDs) such as the anti-malarials. If unsuccessful, "stronger" DMARDs such as gold salts and sulfasalazine were tried and eventually methotrexate was used if there was persistent disease. Unfortunately, it was found that many patients with RA developed severe joint damage and disability while moving up the steps of the therapeutic pyramid. The current approach to RA is that every patient with active, established RA should be on a DMARD as soon as possible, preferably within 3 months of disease onset. Patients with more severe disease and poor prognostic signs (RF positive, rheumatoid nodules) should be treated more aggressively than those with milder disease. Established DMARDs such as methotrexate, sulfasalazine, and the anti-malarials still play an important role in the management of RA.

Understanding the cytokine cascade in RA has helped produce novel new therapies. Cytokines are chemical messengers produced by activated immune cells that stimulate or inhibit various aspects of the immune response. Tumor necrosis factor alpha (TNFα) and Interleukin 1 (IL-1) are key proinflammatory cytokines in RA. These cytokines stimulate the production of each other and of other cytokines that cause synoviocyte proliferation, cartilage destruction, and bone erosions in RA. In clinical studies, inhibition of TNF and IL-1 has demonstrated a significant reduction in the manifestations of RA, improvement in function and retardation of X-ray progression (7–9).

Etanercept (Enbrel®) is a human soluble p75 TNFα receptor fusion protein that binds TNFα and is administered subcutaneously twice weekly. It has been demonstrated in several clinical trials that etanercept has remarkable efficacy in treating RA. In one of the earlier studies, a 3-month, double-blind study of etanercept vs. placebo in RA (7), etanercept at $16 \, mg/m^2$ given subcutaneously twice weekly showed an improvement in the American College of Rheumatology 20% (ACR 20) score of 75% compared to 14% for placebo. The onset of benefit in the treatment group was rapid and sustained with minimal side effects. There are minimal adverse events in patients on etanercept. Immunosuppression with resultant risk of infection is increased and there have been reports of demyelinating diseases.

Infliximab (Remicade®) is a chimeric (human/murine) IgG1 monoclonal antibody to TNFα given intravenously. In the ATTRACT study (8), patients with RA that was inadequately controlled with methotrexate were randomized to five groups: infliximab at 3 mg/kg every 8 weeks; infliximab at 3 mg/kg every 4 weeks; infliximab 10 mg/kg every 8 weeks; infliximab 10 mg/kg every 4 weeks; placebo. At 54 weeks in the lowest dose group (3 mg/kg every 8 weeks) the ACR 20, 50 and 70 were 42%, 21%, and 11%, respectively. The recommended initial dose is therefore 3 mg/kg by infusion at week 0, 2 and 6, then every 8 weeks. Given the modest dose–response at the higher doses in the ATTRACT study, the infliximab dose can be increased or the frequency interval can be decreased, based on the clinical response. Infliximab is generally well tolerated, but it has been shown to exacerbate congestive heart failure and predispose some patients to reactivation of *Microbacterium Tuberculosis* and other infections, including organisms that often infect immunocompromised hosts.

Anakinra (Kineret®) is a recombinant human interleukin 1 receptor antagonist (IL-1ra) given daily as a subcutaneous injection. In a 24 week, double-blind study, there was a significant improvement in the ACR 20 score at the 150 mg/day dose (9). Injection site reactions with anakinra are frequent, but mild and self-limiting. There is a small increase in incidence of pneumonia and urinary tract infections.

The success of the new biologic agents (etanercept, infliximab, and anakinra) in the treatment of RA has prompted further research into the treatment of other connective tissue diseases and vasculitides. Wegener's granulomatosis (WG) is a systemic vasculitis of the small and medium arteries (10). Classic WG primarily involves the upper and lower respiratory tracts and the kidneys, but can also involve the skin, eye, orbit (11) central and peripheral nervous system, cardiac and gastrointestinal tracts. These other manifestations may be organ or life-threatening. Without treatment, over 90% of patients with WG will die within 2 years. With current treatments, survival is over 80% at 5 years. Standard therapy includes high dose glucocorticoids and immunosuppressive therapy (often cyclophosphamide). Anti-TNF agents (infliximab and etanercept) have been used in the treatment of WG in limited studies. One open-label safety study of etanercept added to standard therapy in patients with WG was found to be safe and well tolerated with a resultant decrease in glucocorticoid use (10). There are two ongoing, large randomized studies of etanercept in WG in the United States.

Ankylosing spondylitis (AS) is a chronic inflammatory disease of the axial skeleton manifested by back pain and progressive spinal stiffness. It usually begins in young adults and can affect peripheral joints, eyes, heart, lungs, and skin. There are no therapies that can reliably prevent spinal fusion or deformity. In a randomized, double-blind study, 40 patients with AS were given etanercept 25 mg twice weekly or placebo (11). At 4 months, 80% of the patients in the treatment group had a treatment response, compared to 30% with placebo.

Improvements in many measurements of disease activity were seen, including morning stiffness, spinal pain, quality of life, enthesitis, chest expansion, and inflammatory laboratory tests.

Given the remarkable therapeutic benefit in RA, the biologic agents are being studied in the treatment of other rheumatic diseases such as psoriatic arthritis, adult Still's disease, scleroderma, and inflammatory myopathies. These agents have already changed the approach to the therapy of RA, and are poised to change the treatment strategy of other rheumatic diseases. The main limiting factor in the use of these new agents is the cost, which can be between 10,000 and 20,000 USD per year. Future therapies, including small molecules that can also target specific cytokines, may be less expensive alternatives to the current biologic therapies.

REFERENCES

1. Kelley WN, Harris ED Jr, Ruddy S, Sledge CB, eds. Textbook of Rheumatology. Philadelphia: WB Saunders Co., 1993: 822–873.

2. Utsinger PD, Zvaifler NJ, Ehrlich GE, eds. Rheumatoid Arthritis, Etiology, Diagnosis and Treatment. Philadelphia: JB Lippincott, 1985:1–934.

3. Wolfe F, Mitchell DM, Sibley JT, Fries JF, Bloch DA, Williams CA, Spitz PW, Haga M, Kleinheksel SM, Cathey MA. The mortality of rheumatoid arthritis. Arthritis Rheum 1994; 37(4):481–494.

4. Hirsch R, Lin JP, Scott WW Jr, Ma LD, Pillemer SR, Kastner DL, Jacobsson LT, Bloch DA, Knowler WC, Bennett PH, Bale SJ. Rheumatoid arthritis in the Pima Indians: the intersection of epidemiologic, demographic, and genealogic data. Arthritis Rheum 1998; 41(8):1464–1469.

5. Rothschild BM, Turner KR, DeLuca MA. Symmetrical erosive peripheral polyarthritis in the Late Archaic Period of Alabama. Science 1988; 241(4872):1498–1501.

6. Shojania K. Rheumatology: 2. What laboratory tests are needed? CMAJ 2000; 162(8):1157–1163.

7. Moreland LW, Baumgartner SW, Schiff MH, Tindall EA, Fleischmann RM, Weaver AL, Ettlinger RE, Cohen S, Koopman WJ, Mohler K, Widmer MB, Blosch CM. Treatment of rheumatoid arthritis with a recombinant human tumor necrosis factor receptor (p75)-Fc fusion protein. N Engl J Med 1997; 337(3):141–147.

8. Maini R, St Clair EW, Breedveld F, Furst D, Kalden J, Weisman M, Smolen J, Emery P, Harriman G, Feldmann M, Lipsky P. Infliximab (chimeric anti-tumour necrosis factor alpha monoclonal antibody) versus placebo in rheumatoid arthritis patients receiving concomitant methotrexate: a randomised phase III trial. ATTRACT Study Group. Lancet 1999; 354(9194):1932–1939.

9. Bresnihan B, Alvaro-Gracia JM, Cobby M, Doherty M, Domljan Z, Emery P, Nuki G, Pavelka K, Rau R, Rozman B, Watt I, Williams B, Aitchison R, McCabe D, Musikic P. Treatment of rheumatoid arthritis with recombinant human interleukin-1 receptor antagonist. Arthritis Rheum 1998; 41(12):2196–2204.

10. Stone JH, Uhlfelder ML, Hellmann DB, Crook S, Bedocs NM, Hoffman GS. Etanercept combined with conventional treatment in Wegener's granulomatosis: a six-month openabel trial to evaluate safety. Arthritis Rheum 2001; 44(5): 1149–1154.

11. Gorman JD, Sack KE, Davis JC Jr. Treatment of ankylosing spondylitis by inhibition of tumor necrosis factor alpha. N Engl J Med 2002; 346(18):1349–1356.

3

Bacterial Infections of the Orbit: Current Status and Future Challenges

GERALD J. HARRIS

Section of Orbital and
Oculoplastic Surgery,
Department of Ophthalmology,
Medical College of Wisconsin,
Milwaukee, Wisconsin, U.S.A.

In an age of antibiotic abundance, at least in the developed world, the treatment of bacterial infection would seem to be fairly straightforward: simply administer a broad-spectrum drug and observe the patient's recovery. If the patient does not respond, simply change drugs.

Unfortunately, bacterial infections can progress rapidly with sometimes devastating consequences, despite the use of appropriate drugs. Therefore, a simplistic approach may not be universally applicable.

We tend to think of all infections as assaults by organisms of extreme virulence—anthrax, for example—and that for each bug, there is an appropriate drug that can vanquish the invader. The theme of this essay is that the *primary* event in most orbital infections is not invasion by a lethal alien life form, but derangement of the host's normal physiology. Although antibiotics are powerful weapons, they may not be adequate, and our general objective should be restoration of homeostasis.

There are no bacteria within the orbit proper but there is a robust and diverse population lurking just beyond its borders: on the skin, eyelashes, and conjunctiva; in the nose and sinuses. We live in a state of peaceful coexistence—détente if you will—with these microbes, which is maintained by a wide range of host defenses, some anatomic and some immunologic. If those defenses are weakened, the balance is tipped in favor of the bacteria, converting them from inconsequential, normal flora to potentially life-threatening pathogens. That is when we are forced to mobilize our antibiotic arsenal. However, to restore the balance of power in the long term, our physiology must be normalized.

Dacryocystitis is an uncommon source of deep orbital infection, but it is a familiar example of how altered physiology can lead to clinical infection. In the normal state, the bacterial flora of the conjunctiva and eyelid margins never reach pathogenic proportions, because a stream of tears from the lacrimal gland continually washes them across the eye and into the nose. However, if the stream is "dammed up," the fluid stagnates, and the organisms multiply. Dacryocystitis results, and sometimes extends beyond the lacrimal sac. Antibiotics temporarily suppress the pathogens, but the problem is in the "plumbing," and different bugs will emerge until the plumbing is repaired.

With a penetrating injury, surface flora or foreign bacteria may be introduced into the orbit. Breach of the anatomic barriers now allows these organisms to proliferate in a more favorable environment. Our natural cellular and humoral immune responses may wall off the microbes but may not totally eradicate them. We enlist powerful antibiotics to further suppress bacterial growth. However, if there is foreign material retained in the orbit, it can mitigate—through numerous mechanisms—both natural and pharmacologic defenses. Again, surgery may be needed to restore homeostasis.

Among the varied sources of orbital infection, bacterial sinusitis is by far the most common, and clearly demonstrates how a better understanding of disease *mechanism* has refined treatment and improved outcomes.

The bacteria ultimately responsible for sinusitis are the varied normal flora of the upper respiratory tract. Continuing our theme, their growth from inconspicuous numbers to pathogenic levels depends on changes in their local environment (our sinuses). The first event is usually viral rhinitis, which obstructs the sinus ostia. Air is absorbed by the sinus mucosa, decreasing pO_2 and pH, and increasing pCO_2—conditions that favor aerobic and facultative flora.

Accumulation of inflammatory products further decreases the oxygen tension. Proliferating bacteria consume the remaining oxygen, and the anaerobic normal flora can then gain a foothold. This transition from simple aerobes to complex aerobes plus anaerobes may reflect the extent to which the sinuses are obstructed and the local physiology is altered, which will become relevant shortly.

Once the bacteria have reached pathogenic numbers, they can access the orbit fairly easily through shared venous channels and thin bony partitions. Orbital extension may be manifest as preseptal or true orbital cellulitis. Intraorbital abscess and cavernous sinus thrombosis are both extremely rare in this context. However, the accumulation of purulent material beneath the periorbita, a subperiosteal abscess (SPA), is quite common.

This condition results from simple direct extension from the sinuses. In cases secondary to ethmoiditis, the partition between sinus and orbit has merely shifted laterally. Because an SPA is a common, accessible collection of pathogens, it can inform us about all stages of orbital infection caused by bacterial sinusitis. In a series of studies at our institution during the past 15–20 years, we have demonstrated a strong relationship between the bacteriology and clinical responsiveness of this condition on one hand, and the age of the patient on the other (1–7). Briefly, children in the first decade tend to recover completely with antibiotic treatment, without orbital or sinus surgery. Among those who have had surgical drainage, cultures have either already become negative or have grown single aerobes. Older children and adults tend to have more refractory infections, with recovery of multiple, mixed aerobes and anaerobes, despite several days of treatment with appropriate antibiotics. These age-related differences lead us back to the degree of alteration of the normal physiology. With increasing age, the sinus cavities enlarge markedly, but the ostia remain the same size. Relative to the cavities drained, the ostia of young children are wide, and those of older children and adults are narrow. Younger children may rarely achieve strictly anaerobic conditions, while older children and adults are prone to more complete sequestration.

The orbital complications of sinusitis represent a local conflict between many host, bacterial, and drug factors. Although a correct choice of antibiotics favors the host, many other features support the pathogens, most notably in the complex infections of older children and adults. Consider one example: mixed infections permit synergy. Aerobes consume oxygen that would otherwise be toxic to most anaerobes; anaerobes can produce beta-lactamase, deactivating the antibiotics that are effective against aerobes in pure laboratory culture. Consider what happens to the culture material that is sent off to the microbiology lab. If there is mixed growth on culture media, individual colonies must be isolated and subcultured on plates with antibiotic disks to test for sensitivity of each organism. Those in vitro sensitivities of pure cultures do not reflect the interactions in a complex, in vivo ecosystem. This may explain, at least in part, why clinical infections in older children and adults can be refractory to antibiotics that are based on surgical drainage cultures.

So, we choose the best available antibiotic. Currently, ampicillin/sulbactam is effective against most of the aerobic and anaerobic organisms recovered in these cases; but again, our goal is restoration of the normal physiology. In this context, the requirement is ventilation of the subperiosteal space and sinuses. Can this be accomplished medically, or is surgical drainage needed? We might ask why every patient should not be surgically drained. The surgery is relatively simple. Why risk vision loss or progressive infection? There are case reports of brain abscesses caused by attempts at surgical drainage. In some series, the length of hospitalization without surgery was actually shorter. If the risk of general anesthesia can be avoided, so much the better. Finally, as we will see, surgery is not necessary in a large proportion of carefully chosen cases. We consider many factors in our therapeutic approach.

We perform *emergency drainage* (as soon as possible) of SPAs and sinuses for patients of any age whose optic nerve or retinal function is compromised by the simple mass effect of the abscess.

We perform *urgent drainage* (as soon as practical, but within 24 hr of presentation) for large SPAs in which the interval to vision compromise may be shorter than the time needed for pharmacologic control of the infection; for extensive superior or inferior abscesses that may not quickly resolve, even if the sinusitis clears medically; for intracranial complications at the time of presentation in which identification of the specific pathogens is critical; in frontal sinusitis, with a higher risk of intracranial extension, and in cases in which complex infections, including anaerobes, might be anticipated. Oxygen is the best weapon against anaerobes, and ventilation of the space can be curative. This group includes patients with infections of known dental origin, those with chronic sinusitis, and patients 9 years or older. The last comes from our early series, in which the youngest patient with anaerobic isolates was 9 years old.

We take an *expectant approach* to patients under 9 years of age, in whom simple infections might be predicted. This approach puts an added burden on the managing physicians and requires frequent monitoring.

In the course of close observation, patients still default to surgery if clinical improvement does not occur in a timely manner. However, decisions should not be made solely on the basis of serial computed tomographic (CT) scans. Enlargement of an SPA may occur in the first 12–24 hours of treatment, before local antibiotic levels reach therapeutic range. Thereafter, it may require several days to weeks for the space to contract, despite eradication of the organisms.

We prospectively applied this regimen during a 10-year interval to 40 patients under 9 years of age, among a much larger total group of SPAs of all ages (6). Eight of the 40 met criteria for early drainage and were so treated. Thirty-two met criteria for expectant observation. Among the 32, 3 patients did go to surgery for reasons beyond our control. Twenty-seven of the remaining 29 patients recovered with antibiotic treatment alone. Two failed to respond promptly, according to our guidelines, and defaulted to surgery. All 40 patients recovered without complications.

Orbital cellulitis secondary to sinusitis represents a spectrum of disease. Variations are age-related and, in turn, are associated with how much the normal physiology has been disturbed. This mechanistic approach has given us a fairly good handle on sinus-based orbital infections.

When we consider future challenges in the area of bacterial infection, we must look at the same interplay between microbe and host, and those factors that weaken the former or strengthen the latter. A good example is necrotizing fasciitis, most commonly caused by *Streptococcus pyogenes*, which may be increasing its virulence by altering its exotoxins (8–10). This infection can occur with diabetes, peripheral vascular disease, trauma, and relatively mild immunosuppression.

Necrotizing fasciitis involves vascular thrombosis in the subcutaneous planes, causing fascial necrosis and microabscesses. The disease has a 30% mortality rate, generally due to septic shock, respiratory distress syndrome, or renal failure.

The clinical features and management of necrotizing fasciitis can best be illustrated by a case we have encountered. A 66-year-old woman with rheumatoid arthritis, on a small dose of methotrexate and only 5 mg per day of prednisone, had a 2-day history of fulminant eyelid and orbital infection. On admission, she had fever and a white count of 28,000. Because of the fascial necrosis, the infection had spread rapidly within subcutaneous planes through her face and down her neck. There also had been extension into the retrobulbar orbit.

Treatment of this disease includes high-dose intravenous antibiotics. In this case, we used clindamycin and cefotaxime. Our objective, however, was to restore the normal physiology as soon as possible. The patient's immunosuppression could not be immediately reversed and, given the fulminant course, was a longer-term goal. At that moment, the intravascular thrombosis was causing ischemic necrosis, which provided additional substrate for the bacteria. To break that cycle, this patient was treated with hyperbaric oxygen (nine sessions of 90 min at 2.4 atm).

In addition, she was treated with serial debridement of necrotic tissue. A temporary tarsorrhaphy was placed because of the anticipated cicatricial changes.

With this treatment, the area of facial involvement contracted, and after about 2 weeks, a bed of sterile granulation tissue could be grafted. Six months later, eyelid function was normal and vision remained 20/20.

In summary, our successes and our challenges in the area of orbital infection relate to the ongoing dynamic between microbe and host. Bacterial infections will never be eliminated because they are caused by our normal flora, which simply gain the upper hand when our defenses are down. However, we can minimize the inflicted damage by promptly recognizing how, and to what degree, the normal physiology has been altered, and by taking measures that discourage bacterial growth and strengthen host defenses.

And don't forget the antibiotics.

ACKNOWLEDGEMENTS

Supported in part by core grant EY01931 from the National Eye Institute, Bethesda, Maryland, and by an unrestricted grant from Research to Prevent Blindness, Inc., New York U.S.A.

REFERENCES

1. Harris GJ. Subperiosteal abscess of the orbit. Arch Ophthalmol 1983; 101:751–757.

2. Harris GJ. Subperiosteal inflammation of the orbit: a bacteriological analysis of 17 cases. Arch Ophthalmol 1988; 106: 947–952.

3. Harris GJ. Subperiosteal abscess of the orbit: age as a factor in the bacteriology and response to treatment. Ophthalmology 1994; 101:585–595.

4. Harris GJ, Bair RL. Anaerobic isolates from a subperiosteal abscess in a 4-year-old patient. Arch Ophthalmol 1996; 114:98.

5. Harris GJ. Subperiosteal abscess of the orbit: computed tomography and the clinical course. Ophthal Plast Reconstr Surg 1996; 12:1–8.

6. Garcia GH, Harris GJ. Criteria for nonsurgical management of subperiosteal abscess of the orbit: analysis of outcomes 1988–1998. Ophthalmology 2000; 107:1454–1458.

7. Harris GJ. Subperiosteal abscess of the orbit: older children and adults require aggressive treatment Editorial. Ophthal Plast Reconstr Surg 2001; 173:395–397.

8. Bisno AL, Stevens DL. Streptococcal infections of the skin and soft tissues. N Engl J Med 1996; 334:240–255.

9. Feingold DS. Group A streptococcal infections: an old adversary reemerging with new tricks? Arch Dermatol 1996; 132:67–70.

10. Kronish JW, McLeish WM. Eyelid necrosis and periorbital necrotizing fasciitis: report of a case and review of the literature. Ophthalmology 1991; 98:92–98.

4

Inflammation: Definitions, Regulatory Mechanisms, and Contributions to Disease

BRUCE M. McMANUS and
JONATHAN C. CHOY

Department of Pathology and
Laboratory Medicine, St. Paul's Hospital,
Providence Health Care, University of British
Columbia, Vancouver, British Columbia, Canada

Inflammation is an old concept, originally recognized as a contributor to disease by the Romans. During that time inflammation was defined as "rubor, dolor, tumor, calor, functiolasae," or redness, pain, swelling, heat, and loss of function. Subsequent to these early observations, it was not until the 1800s that cellular processes were observed to contribute to inflammation, typically seen in microscopic analyses of human and experimental conditions. In the last 40 years, studies began to dissect the mechanisms of inflammation including identification of protein regulators of that control the cellular responses.

Inflammation is a multifactoral response to an injury and is comprised of innate and adaptive responses. The innate response to a pathogen/toxin is an antigen nonspecific process that is mediated largely by macrophages, neutrophils, natural killer (NK) cells, and complement. Adaptive responses to a pathogen/toxin are antigen specific responses. Activation of T- and B-cells by antigen presenting cells is required for acquired immunity, so the time course of this response is delayed in comparison to the innate response. The acquired immune response can be further divided into the humoral and cellular responses. Humoral responses are antibody driven and the down-stream effectors include complement activation and antibody-driven phagocytosis. Cellular responses are mediated largely by T-cells and include both T helper cell (Th) 1 and Th2 responses. The majority of this discussion will focus on the cellular responses in inflammation.

The contribution of inflammation to disease can be both beneficial and detrimental. Inflammation is a process that normally protects the host from injury and, as such, attenuation of this response can lead to increased susceptibility to infection. On the other hand, certain diseases are a result of dysregulated inflammation and in these instances inflammation may be viewed as detrimental. In these circumstances, down-regulation of specific aspects of the inflammatory response may be beneficial. Indeed, animal studies have shown that inhibition of certain immune functions can attenuate the development of atherosclerosis (1). Also, depletion of negative regulators of the immune response can increase the severity of atherosclerosis (2). Thus, determination of the specific mechanisms through which inflammation contributes to a disease process is necessary, and understanding the general mechanisms of the inflammatory response may aid in understanding specific events. Further, since one of the main mechanisms in the pathogenesis of many inflammatory disorders involves the effects of inflammation on the vasculature, specific focus will be given in this discussion to those components that affect vascular structure and function.

Once an inflammatory response is triggered, activated leukocytes must localize to the injured area in order to carry out their effector functions. This process requires leukocyte extravasation from the blood into the tissue, migration to the site of injury, and subsequent further activation. Leukocyte extravasation is generally believed to occur by distinct steps that consist of loose rolling, tight adhesion, and diapedesis. Each step is mediated by the interactions of particular molecules on the cell surface of leukocytes and endothelial cells (EC) . Although the exact mediators of these interactions differ slightly between types of leukocytes, the adhesive and migratory events are generally believed to be mediated in the following way. The initial interaction between leukocytes and endothelial cell (EC) is mediated by selectins on leukocytes and carbohydrate moieties (Sialyl-Lewis^X) on the surface of the endothelium. This loose binding slows the leukocyte to allow the stronger integrin–selectin interactions to proceed. Subsequent strong binding of leukocytes with cell adhesion molecules on the endothelial surface results in flattening and stopping of the rolling leukocytes, which then diapedeses through the endothelium (3). New reports have suggested that the molecular binding interactions between leukocytes and EC may also initiate signal transduction pathways that serve to provide outside-in signals to EC (4). Future work in determining the targets and cellular effects of these signal transduction pathways on endothelial biology will be helpful in further understanding the intricate leukocyte–endothelial interactions that occur during this process.

One of the main cellular mediators of the inflammatory response is the macrophage, which under steady-state conditions accumulates in tissues and serves two main functions. They phagocytose pathogens and toxins, and are also very important "professional" antigen presenting cells necessary for the activation of the adaptive immune response. After initiation of an inflammatory response, macrophages can aid in the clearance of pathogens/toxins by both antibody-dependent and independent mechanisms. Further, several recent reports have suggested that macrophages can contribute to the cytotoxic immune response by inducing apoptosis of target cells through a FasL-dependent mechanism (5,6).

Adaptive immunity is mediated by T-cell responses to pathogens or allogeneic tissue. The T-cell response can be loosely divided into those mediated by T helper cells (Th) and cytotoxic T-cells (CTL) . The Th response can be further divided into the Th1 and Th2 response, the balance of which is governed by the relative amounts of interleukin (IL)-4 and interferon-lambda (IFNγ) available. Recognition of foreign antigens by the T-cell receptor results in different cytokine profiles secreted by Th2 and Th1 cells. Th2 cells secrete many cytokines including IL-4, 5, and 6. These cytokines can activate B-cells and mobilize the humoral response. Th1 cells secrete IFN? and IL-2, leading to the activation of the cytotoxic immune response that is mediated largely by CTL (7). Recognition of foreign antigens by CTL results in the secretion of interferons (IFN) and activation of death inducing pathways. The IFN response protects target cells from viral infection by reducing proliferation and gene expression in these cells. Interferons can also induce apoptosis of some cell types. Activated T-cells also induce apoptosis of virus infected or foreign cells through FasL and granzyme/perforin-mediated pathways. FasL is a death inducing ligand that can activate caspases through the formation of death signaling complexes at the plasma membrane (8). Granzymes are a family of serine proteases that activate apoptosis through several mechanisms that include direct caspase activation, release of mitochondrial factors, and direct cleavage of cellular components (9).

Negative regulators of the inflammatory response, including IL-10 and transforming growth factor-beta (TGF-β), are important in ensuring the inflammatory response does not become pathologically dysregulated. IL-10 is secreted by macrophages and Th2 cells in a temporally delayed fashion as compared to proinflammatory cytokines. The majority of

IL-10 actions in vivo may depend on its ability to block nuclear factor kappaB (NF-κB) and mitogen-activated protein kinase (MAPK) activation, which in turn results in decreased proinflammatory cytokine secretion, EC–leukocyte interactions, antigen presentation, and Th1 activation (10,11). The importance of these regulatory actions can be observed in IL-10 knockout mice, which, although possessing an increased resistance to pathogenic infection, have an overall detrimental pathological enhancement of their inflammatory response to these infections (12–14). Transforming growth factor-β is a pleiotropic growth factor that is expressed as a latency-associated peptide (LAP) . Cleavage of LAP is required for the biological activity of TGF-β. This growth factor can inhibit several aspects of inflammation, including proinflammatory cytokine secretion, cell adhesion molecule expression, and inducible nitric oxide synthase (iNOS) and activation. Further, TGF-β can also affect vascular structure and function by inhibiting smooth muscle proliferation and normalizing vasodilation (15). Insight into the importance of TGF-β in regulating the inflammatory response is supplied by knockout models of TGF-β in which the mice die in utero due to excessive inflammation (16). Further, inhibition of TGF-β activity utilizing neutralizing antibodies promotes plaque destabilization in mouse models of atherosclerosis, implicating TGF-β in the pathogenesis of some inflammatory disorders (17).

Many biochemical mediators regulate the cellular components of the inflammatory response. Because of the impact of nitric oxide (NO) and eicosanoids on vascular structure, we will focus on the contribution of these factors to inflammation. Nitric oxide is a potent vasodilator that is synthesized by a constitutively expressed endothelial NO synthase (eNOS) and an inducible form of NO synthase (iNOS) . Low levels of NO, like those formed by eNOS, are normally secreted by the endothelium and negatively regulate inflammatory responses by inhibiting leukocyte adhesion, migration, and activation. However, in response to several stimuli and under many pathological conditions, increased expression and activation of iNOS results in the release of large amounts of

NO. These high levels of NO can increase cytokine secretion by surrounding cells, leukocyte activation, and apoptosis of some cell types (18). Eicosanoids are a family of lipid mediators that include prostanoids and leukotrienes. They have been shown to be both positive and negative regulators of inflammation. Since the same eicosanoid can at times either be pro- and anti-inflammatory, it has been suggested that the specific effect of these lipid mediators on inflammation may be dependent on the type of receptor expressed by target cells, one receptor signaling to activate or enhance inflammation and another to inhibit it. The proinflammatory effects of eicosanoids include leukocyte activation, control of T-cell development and maturation, and increased vasodilation and vascular permeability. The anti-inflammatory effects include inhibition of leukocyte activation and effector functions (19,20) (Fig. 1).

As noted, the endothelium is a selective barrier between circulating leukocytes and tissue. Many inflammatory responses can alter the endothelial structure in order to allow most effective access of leukocytes to clear pathogens/toxins

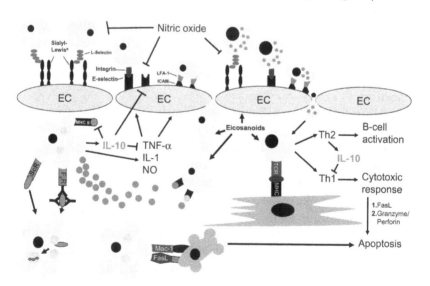

Figure 1 (*Caption on facing page*)

from the tissue. The increased release of inflammatory factors such as tumor necrosis factor-alpha (TNF-α), IL-1, vascular endothelial growth factor (VEGF), iNOS, and eicosanoids can either directly or indirectly enhance vascular permeability by altering endothelial cell structure or expression of adhesion molecules. For instance, the systemic release of large

---

Figure 1 (*Facing page*) Regulatory mechanisms in inflammation. Release of cytokines such as tumor necrosis factor-alpha (TNF-α) and interleukin (IL)-1β, and large amounts of nitric oxide (NO) by tissue macrophages activates the endothelium. Expression of carbohydrate moieties, selectins, and cell adhesion molecules (CAM) by this monolayer recruits leukocytes to the site of injury by facilitating leukocyte transmigration. This process of loose-rolling, tight adhesion, and diapedesis is followed by leukocyte chemotaxis toward the site of injury. Once activated, macrophages can elicit effector functions that include antibody-dependent and -independent phagocytosis, and induction of receptor-mediated apoptosis of some cells. Recognition of foreign antigen in areas of inflammation by T-cells can initiate either a T helper cell (Th)1 or Th2 response. The Th2 response activates B-cells, resulting in mobilization of the humoral response. The Th1 response can initiate a cytotoxic T-cell response towards cells expressing foreign antigen, leading to T-cell mediated apoptosis of target cells that is regulated primarily through FasL and granzyme/perforin pathways. Nitric oxide and eicosanoids can regulate inflammatory responses as well as affect vascular structure and function. When synthesized at low levels, NO can inhibit leukocyte transmigration and activation. However, when NO is synthesized at high levels, it can activate leukocytes, and induce vasodilation. Depending on the type of receptor expressed on effector cells, eicosanoids can either activate or inhibit leukocyte activation and transmigration. These lipid signal transduction mediators can also increase vasodilation. Negative regulators, such as IL-10 and transforming growth factor-beta (TGF-β), are important in reducing the inflammatory response once an infection has been cleared. IL-10 and TGF-β can both inhibit cytokine expression and secretion, cell adhesion molecule expression, antigen presentation, and activation of the Th1 response. Additionally, TGF-β can inhibit inducible nitric oxide synthase (iNOS) expression and activation, and can normalize vasodilation.

amounts of TNF-α during septic shock dramatically increases endothelial permeability, leading to damage of the surrounding tissue and eventual organ failure (21,22). The overall effect of this increased permeability may be observed as the fundamental characteristics of inflammation originally observed by the Romans.

Because one of the key requirements for a sustained and effective response to wound healing is the delivery of nutrients and cellular components to the site of injury, increased angiogenesis is an important event in many inflammatory responses. There are likely several angiogenic mediators that control the process at different stages of the inflammatory response. During the initial stage of a response to an injury, secretion of basic fibroblast growth factor (bFGF) has been suggested to induce the growth of new blood vessels. However, since bFGF is mainly expressed during the early stages of the healing process, other factors are likely involved in angiogenesis. During the later stages of wound healing, VEGF is expressed in high concentrations and may promote angiogenesis. VEGF is a very potent angiogenic factor that is secreted by macrophages and EC (23). Further, recent reports have suggested that CD40L, a T-cell activator and important regulator of immune responses, may also increase angiogenesis, potentially by up-regulating the secretion of VEGF from the endothelium (24).

Since several ocular and orbital conditions are a result of a dysregulated inflammatory response, appreciation of the processes is increasingly important to understanding the pathogenesis of these conditions. An example is the impact of inflammation on vascular structure and growth, since the neovascularization of several components of the eye is responsible for decreasing vision in conditions, such as age-related macular degeneration and diabetic retinopathy. Effective treatments, such as photodynamic therapy, are currently available to treat ocular neovascularization (25). However, understanding the inflammatory processes that contribute to ocular neovascularization may be important in the development of therapeutic regimens that are less injurious and more permanent in their effects.

REFERENCES

1. Laurat E, Poirier B, Tupin E, Caligiuri G, Hansson GK, Bariety J, Nicoletti A. In vivo downregulation of T helper cell 1 immune responses reduces atherogenesis in apolipoprotein E-knockout mice. Circulation 2001; 104:197–202.

2. Mallat Z, Besnard S, Duriez M, Deleuze V, Emmanuel F, Bureau MF, Soubrier F, Esposito B, Duez H, Fievet C, Staels B, Duverger N, Scherman D, Tedgui A. Protective role of interleukin-10 in atherosclerosis. Circ Res 1999; 85:e17–e24.

3. Delves PJ, Roitt IM. The immune system. First of two parts. N Engl J Med 2000; 343:37–49.

4. Hu Y, Szente B, Kiely JM, Gimbrone MA Jr. Molecular events in transmembrane signaling via E-selectin. SHP2 association, adaptor protein complex formation and ERK1/2 activation. J Biol Chem 2001; 276:48549–48553.

5. Boyle JJ, Bowyer DE, Weissberg PL, Bennett MR. Human blood-derived macrophages induce apoptosis in human plaque-derived vascular smooth muscle cells by Fas-ligand/Fas interactions. Arterioscler Thromb Vasc Biol 2001; 21: 1402–1407.

6. Seshiah PN, Kereiakes DJ, Vasudevan SS, Lopes N, Su BY, Flavahan NA, Goldschmidt-Clermont PJ. Activated monocytes induce smooth muscle cell death: role of macrophage colony-stimulating factor and cell contact. Circulation 2002; 105: 174–180.

7. Delves PJ, Roitt IM. The immune system. Second of two parts. N Engl J Med 2000; 343:108–117.

8. Granville DJ, Carthy CM, Hunt DW, McManus BM. Apoptosis: molecular aspects of cell death and disease. Lab Invest 1998; 78:893–913.

9. Bleackley RC, Heibein JA. Enzymatic control of apoptosis. Nat Prod Rep 2001; 18:431–440.

10. Schottelius AJ, Mayo MW, Saartor RB, Baldwin AS. Interleukin-10 signaling blocks inhibitor of kappaB kinase activity and nuclear factor kappaB DNA binding. J Biol Chem 1999; 274: 31868–31874.

11. Suttles J, Milhom DM, Miller RW, Poe JC, Wahl JC, Stout RD. CD40 signaling of monocyte inflammatory cytokine synthesis through an ERK1/2-dependent pathway. A target of interleukin (il)-4 and il-10 anti-inflammatory action. J Biol Chem 1999; 274:5835–5842.

12. Kane MM, Mosser DM. The role of IL-10 in promoting disease progression in leishmaniasis. J Immunol 2001; 166: 1141–1147.

13. Murray PJ, Young RA. Increased antimycobacterial immunity in interleukin-10-deficient mice. Infect Immun 1999; 67: 3087–3095.

14. Deckert M, Soltek G, Geginat S, Lutjen M, Montesinos-Rongen H, Hof H, Schluter D. Endogenous interleukin-10 is required for prevention of a hyperinflammatory intracerebral immune response in Listeria monocytogenes meningoencephalitis. Infect Immun 2001; 69:4561–4571.

15. Tedui A, Mallat Z. Anti-inflammatory mechanisms in the vascular wall. Circ Res 2001; 88:877–887.

16. Shull MM, Ormsby I, Kier AB, Pawlowski S, Diebold RJ, Yin M, Allen R, Sidman C, Proetzel G, Calvin D, Annunziata N, Doetschman T. Targeted disruption of the mouse transforming growth factor-beta 1 gene results in multifocal inflammatory disease. Nature 1992; 359:693–699.

17. Mallat Z, Gojova A, Marchiol-Fournigault C, Esposito B, Kamate C, Merval R, Fradelizi D, Tedgui A. Inhibition of transforming growth factor-beta signaling accelerates atherosclerosis and induces an unstable plaque phenotype in mice. Circ Res 2001; 89:930–934.

18. Abramson SB, Amin AR, Clancy RM, Attur M. The role of nitric oxide in tissue destruction. Best Pract Res Clin Rheumatol 2001; 15:831–845.

19. Funk CD. Prostaglandins and leukotrienes: advances in eicosanoid biology. Science 2001; 294:1871–1875.

20. Tilley SL, Coffinan TM, Koller BH. Mixed messages: modulation of inflammation and immune responses by prostaglandins and thromboxanes. J Clin Invest 2001; 108:15–23.

21. Penn MS, Saidel GM, Chisolm GM. Vascular injury by endo-toxin: changes in macromolecular transport parameters in rat aortas in vivo. Am J Physiol 1992; 262:H1563–H1571.

22. Dormehl IC, Hugo N, Pretorius JP, Redelinghuys IF. In vivo assessment of regional microvascular albumin leakage during coli septic shock in the baboon model. Circ Shock 1992; 38: 9–13.

23. Lingen MW. Role of leukocytes and endothelial cells in the development of angiogenesis in inflammation and wound healing. Arch Pathol Lab Med 2001; 125:67–71.

24. Melter M, Reinders ME, Sho M, Pal S, Geehan C, Denton MD, Mukhopadhyay D, Briscoe DM. Ligation of CD40 induces the expression of vascular endothelial growth factor by endothelial cells and monocytes and promotes angiogenesis in vivo. Blood 2000; 96:3801–3808.

25. Granville DJ, McManus BM, Hunt DW. Photodynamic ther-apy: shedding light on the biochemical pathways regulating porphyrin-mediated cell death. Histol Histopathol 2001; 16:309–317.

5

Future and Emerging Treatments for Microbial Infections*

ANTHONY W. CHOW

Division of Infectious Diseases, Department of
Medicine, University of British Columbia and
Vancouver Hospital Health Sciences Centre,
Vancouver, British Columbia, Canada

CHALLENGES IN THE TREATMENT OF INTRAOCULAR INFECTIONS

Despite significant advances in the past decade, major challenges still remain in our management of intraocular infections. I will address the current status and possible solutions in three specific areas related to the treatment of postoperative or posttraumatic endophthalmitis:

---

*Presented in part at the Vancouver Orbital Symposium, March 15–17, 2002, Vancouver, British Columbia, Canada

- *Microbiologic diagnosis*, particularly the use of molecular techniques.
- *New antimicrobials*, and pharmacokinetic–pharmaco dynamic principles to achieve greater therapeutic efficacy.
- *Emerging antibiotic resistance*, and what can be done to minimize the impact.

MICROBIOLOGIC DIAGNOSIS

The microbiologic diagnosis of postoperative or posttraumatic endophthalmitis remains problematic. Cultures from aqueous aspirates may be negative in up to 70% of cases, while vitreous cultures may be sterile in 30–40% of cases (1–3). In 1995, the Endophthalmitis Vitrectomy Study Group (EVS) examined the microbiology of postoperative endophthalmitis in one of the largest multicenter prospective studies of its kind (1). The overall culture positive rate was 69% among 420 patients with endophthalmitis within 6 weeks of cataract extraction or secondary intraocular lens implantation. Thus, the microbiologic diagnosis could not be established in fully one-third of these patients. Among those with positive cultures, gram-positive organisms were isolated from 94% of the patients, while gram-negative bacteria were isolated from 6% (Table 1). The most common isolates were coagulase-negative staphylococci (70%), followed by *Staphylococcus aureus* (10%), *Streptococcus* species (9%), *Enterococcus* species (2%), and miscellaneous gram-positive bacilli such as *Propionibacterium acnes* and *Bacillus* species (3%). In this study, a positive Gram stain from the aqueous or vitreous fluid was highly predictive of a positive culture from the eye, but a negative Gram stain had little predictive value for culture results (4). A more recent single-centre prospective study involving 206 vitreous samples from 206 patients yielded largely similar results (5). In this study, 46% of the specimens were sterile (Table 1). Among those with positive cultures, gram-positive bacteria (64%) were again more common than gram-negative bacteria (29%), which were recovered at a

Table 1 Microbiology of Postoperative or Posttraumatic Endophthalmitis[*]

Study population	Postoperative	Postoperative	Post-traumatic
Authors (reference)	EVS (1)	Kunimoto et al. (5)	Kunimoto et al. (6)
No. of patients	420	206	182
No. with positive cultures	291 (69%)	112 (54%)	113 (62%)
Total isolates recovered	123	126	138
Gram-positive	274 (94%)	72 (64%)	87 (77%)
Coagulase-negative staphylococci	226 (70%)	45 (36%)	25 (18%)
Staphylococcus aureus	32 (10%)	1 (1%)	5 (4%)
Streptococcus species	29 (9%)	13 (10%)	39 (22%)
Enterococcus species	7 (2%)	—	1 (1%)
Actinomycetes-related	—	5 (4%)	7 (5%)
Miscellaneous (*P. acnes, Bacillus* species, etc.)	10 (3%)	8 (6%)	24 (17%)
Gram-negative	19 (6%)	33 (29%)	25 (22%)
Filamentous fungi	—	21 (19%)	20 (18%)

[*]Postoperative cases included those following cataract extraction and lens implantation.
Note that the total is greater than 100% in each column because of polymicrobial infections.

higher rate than in previous reports. This study also identified Actinomycetes-related organisms (4%) and filamentous fungi (19%), mainly *Aspergillus* species. These results are contrasted to posttraumatic endophthalmitis in which a higher rate of *Streptococcus* species and gram-positive bacilli and a lower rate of coagulase-negative staphylococci were recovered (6) (Table 1).

Multiple studies have demonstrated that the usual source of organisms in postoperative endophthalmitis is endogenous from the lid or conjunctiva (7). Less common exogenous sources include airborne contaminants or contaminated intraocular solutions, lenses, or surgical instruments. The reasons for the low yield of positive cultures in postoperative endophthalmitis remain poorly explained. Cultures may be negative because of a small inoculum, sequestration of bacteria in a biofilm environment on solid surfaces, the fastidious nature of some microorganisms, and the use of antibiotics prior to sampling (8). Nevertheless, the presence of microorganisms in many culture-negative cases has been documented by transmission or scanning microscopy and by other means (9,10). Thus, improving the method for detection of microorganisms in postoperative endophthalmitis is an important task, and molecular techniques such as polymerase chain reaction (PCR) appear to hold considerable promise.

One of the earliest reports of the successful application of PCR for the detection of microorganisms in delayed postoperative endophthalmitis, particularly *Propionebacterium acnes*, was by Hykin et al. (11). These authors used nested PCR with universal eubacterial primers complimentary to regions of 16S rDNA-conserved sequences to detect bacterial DNA in vitreous samples obtained from vitrectomy. Twenty-three samples from patients with delayed postoperative endophthalmitis and 29 samples from patients who underwent vitrectomy for reasons unrelated to infection were studied. Seventeen (74%) specimens from patients with endophthalmitis and four (14%) from uninfected individuals gave positive results. Positive results with the *P. acnes* primers were obtained from 8 (35%) of 23 "endophthalmitis" specimens and none of 29 "normal" samples. Subsequent to this, three separate studies have confirmed the promising results with PCR (12–14) (Table 2). There is excellent correlation between positive PCR and positive cultures. The addition of PCR to culture improved the diagnostic yield of culture alone by 29–76%. False positive rates have been low ($\sim 5\%$). In addition, by using primers specific to gram-positive vs. gram-negative bacteria, the PCR method demonstrated an excellent capacity in discriminating gram-positive from gram-negative organisms (15).

All the PCR studies reported above utilized universal eubacterial primers directed at conserved sequences of the 16S rDNA gene. Research in my own laboratory has investigated the use of broad-range degenerate primers that amplify the 60-kDa heat shock protein (hsp60) gene, which is highly conserved and universally present in all microorganisms (16,17). The universal hsp60 primers amplify a 600-bp

Table 2 Molecular Detection of Intraocular Microorganisms by PCR

	Author		
	Therese et al. (12)	Lohmann et al. (13)	Okhravi et al. (14)
Suspected endophthalmitis	$n = 58$	$n = 25$	$n = 37$
Culture positive (%)	27 (47%)	6 (24%)	20 (54%)
PCR positive (%)	37 (64%)	23 (92%)	37 (100%)
Culture or PCR positive (%)	44 (76%)	25 (100%)	37 (100%)
"Uninfected" controls	$n = 20$	$n = 10$	$n = 53$
Culture positive (%)	0	0	0
PCR positive (%)	1 (5%)	0	2 (4%)

product that contains a hypervariable region in which the DNA sequence is unique for a given bacterial genus or species (16,17) (Fig. 1). Furthermore, PCR amplification followed by direct sequencing, dot blot hybridization, or restriction enzyme digestion has provided a convenient method for species-specific identification of both gram-positive and gram-negative microorganisms. Furthermore, the hsp60 method was found to be more discriminative than 16SrDNA sequences for species identification (17–19). An important advantage of this methodology is that multiple pathogens can be detected with a single set of universal hsp60 primers in a single clinical specimen. We have demonstrated proof of concept of this approach in the detection and identification of putative respiratory pathogens in the respiratory tract of patients with community-acquired pneumonia, and the etiologic diagnosis of enteric pathogens in infectious diarrhea (18). Its utility in the diagnosis of ocular infections remains to be determined by prospective study.

There are a number of advantages to molecular detection of intraocular organisms by PCR. The technique is extremely sensitive and can detect DNA from a single infectious agent. Results can be obtained within hours rather than days or weeks by conventional culture methods. It is particularly

*Hsp*60 gene

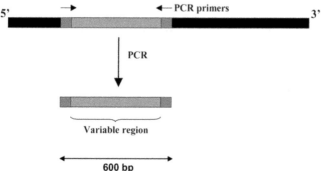

Figure 1 A schematic diagram depicting the 600-bp DNA product of the hsp60 gene amplified with our proprietary universal hsp60 degenerate primers. The primers are complimentary to highly conserved DNA sequences and amplify a hypervariable region, which contains sequences that are unique to each bacterial species or genus. The amplified product can be used as a DNA probe for diagnosis by hybridization, and can be analyzed by direct sequencing or restriction fragment length polymorphism.

suited for the detection of fastidious or non-cultivable microorganisms, and in cases where culture results may have been affected by the prior administration of antibiotics (8). Despite these advantages, PCR also has potential drawbacks. Because of the exquisite sensitivity of the test, scrupulous techniques are required to avoid contamination of the samples during collection and processing. Ocular specimens also contain substances that may inhibit the PCR reaction. This technical problem can be minimized by diluting the clinical samples or by the extraction of DNA prior to PCR (8). It should be noted that PCR does not directly test the ability of the microorganism to actively replicate, nor will it differentiate between an infection from contamination by extraneous or commensal organisms. Thus, clinical assessment of the patient remains critical for the evaluation of infection or inflammation, and PCR is unlikely to completely replace diagnostic cultures, which also provide information on antibiotic susceptibility or resistance. Finally, a significant number of newly determined microbial DNA sequences cannot be accurately identified due to the inadequacy of available GenBank databases.

NEW ANTIMICROBIALS AND PHARMACOLOGIC PRINCIPLES OF ANTIMICROBIAL THERAPY

The EVS study conducted, in 1995 was the first randomized clinical trial that evaluated the role of pars plana vitrectomy and systemic antibiotics in the management of postoperative endophthalmitis (20). The study concluded that vitrectomy was necessary only for patients who presented with the worst vision (light perception only), and that systemic antibiotics were not helpful when used in addition to intravitreal antibiotics. However, both the choice of systemic antibiotics used in the study (amikacin plus ceftazidime) and the conclusion about their lack of efficacy have been questioned (21). Since amikacin plus ceftazidime have little activity against coagulase-negative staphylococci, the most common organisms associated with postoperative endophthalmitis, it is not surprising that the addition of these antibiotics made no difference in outcome. Even if vancomycin was chosen instead of amikacin and ceftazidime against coagulase-negative staphylococci, its poor penetration into the vitreous would still likely produce similar results. In a study reported by Ferencz et al. (22), 14 patients with acute postoperative endophthalmitis were treated with 1 g intravenous vancomycin prior to vitrectomy and collection of vitreous samples. Intravitreal vancomycin and ceftazidime were then administered intraoperatively. Vitreous samples were cultured and their vancomycin concentrations were assayed. The intravitreal vancomycin levels following intravenous administration were below the minimal inhibitory concentrations (MIC) of the causative organisms in 44% of patients with positive cultures. Vitreous cidal activity against the causative organism was achieved in only 10% of these cases. Following a 1 mg intravitreal injection,

vancomycin levels and vitreous cidal activity were all therapeutic in a smaller subset of the patients. Thus, newer agents
with improved antimicrobial spectrum and pharmacologic
properties are needed for the optimal management of these
serious infections.

Some of the newer antimicrobials with potential for treating intraocular infections are listed in Table 3. These agents
either have improved antimicrobial spectrum or bioavailabil-
ity for organisms common in postoperative or posttraumatic
endophthalmitis. Many are still under investigation and their
efficacy in the treatment of endophthalmitis remains to be
determined by prospective, randomized clinical trials. Among
the newer antibacterial agents, the second or third generation
fluoroquinolones (e.g., levofloxacin, moxifloxacin, and gatiflox-
acin) deserve special mention, as these agents exhibit
improved activity against gram-positive and anaerobic pathogens, including penicillin-resistant pneumococci in contrast to
ciprofloxacin (2,23,24). Furthermore, they can penetrate the
eye even with oral administration (25,26). As a group, the

Table 3 New Antimicrobials with Potential Application in
Endophthalmitis

(A) Antibacterial	(a) Second and third generation fluoroquinolones
	Levofloxacin
	Moxifloxacin
	Gatifloxacin
	(b) Ketolides
	Telithromycin
	(c) Oxazolidinones
	Linezolid
	(d) Glycopeptides
	Teicoplanin
	(e) Streptogramins
	Quinupristin/dalfopristin (synercid)
	(f) Lipopeptides
	Daptomycin
(B) Antifungals	(a) Azoles
	Voriconazole
	(b) Echinocandins and pneumocandins
	Caspofungin

fluoroquinolones have excellent activity against gram-negative bacteria and thus may replace aminoglycosides or third generation cephalosporins in the treatment of bacterial endophthalmitis. However, intravenous or intravitreal administration may still be required since the concentrations achieved following oral administration may not be adequate (27). Whereas ofloxacin at intravitreal concentrations of 500 µg or higher may be toxic to the retina (28), ciprofloxacin and levofloxacin appear to be better tolerated (29,30).

The other newer antibacterials, listed in Table 2, all have improved activity against gram-positive bacteria. These include the ketolides (e.g., telithromycin) (31), which have improved activity against erythromycin resistant gram-positive cocci, and four other classes of antimicrobials with improved activity against methicillin-resistant staphylococci, coagulase-negative staphylococci, and vancomycin-resistant enterococci. These include the oxazolidinones (e.g., linezolid) (32), streptogramins (e.g., quinupristin/dalfoprisin or synercid) (33), lipopeptides (e.g., daptomycin) (34) and glycopeptides (e.g., teicoplanin) (35,36).

New antifungals include the azoles (e.g., voriconazole) (37) and echinocandins (e.g., caspofungin) (38), both with enhanced activity including *Aspergillus* and *Candida* species, including the fluconazole-resistant *Candida* species. A detailed discussion of these agents is beyond the scope of this review.

Perhaps more important is an understanding of some emerging pharmacologic principles that may improve therapeutic efficacy of antimicrobial therapy by optimizing the appropriate dosing regimens. Appropriate dosing requires knowledge of both the pharmacokinetic and pharmacodynamic (PK/PD) properties of different antimicrobial agents (39). Pharmacokinetic parameters determine what drug concentrations can be achieved in serum and tissue; pharmacodynamic parameters determine what antimicrobial effect can be achieved (Fig. 2). It is the time course of antimicrobial activity that determines which pharmacokinetic properties of a drug are the most important determinants of clinical efficacy (40). The critical question to ask is what kind

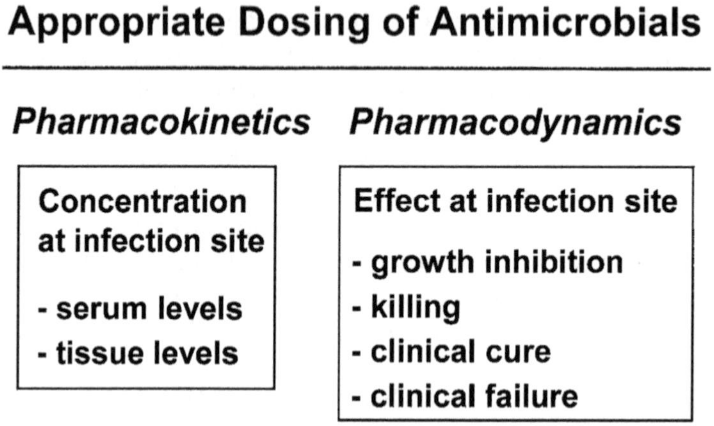

Appropriate Dosing of Antimicrobials

Pharmacokinetics   *Pharmacodynamics*

Concentration at infection site - serum levels - tissue levels	**Effect at infection site** - growth inhibition - killing - clinical cure - clinical failure

Figure 2 Overview of pharmacokinetics and pharmacodynamics in antimicrobial chemotherapy.

of killing pattern the drug has and whether the effect is short-lived or prolonged. Does it have concentration-dependent killing where higher levels will result in better killing? Or is it more time-dependent where higher concentrations will not necessarily kill the organism better but maintaining the concentration above the MIC of the organism for a longer period will? The specific PK/PD parameters that have been found to correlate best with outcome include the ratio of peak-to-minimum inhibitory concentration (peak/MIC ratio), the ratio of trough-to-minimum inhibitory concentration (trough/MIC ratio), the ratio of the 24-hr area under the curve to MIC (AUC_{24}/MIC ratio), and the duration of time when serum levels exceed the MIC, expressed as the percentage of the dosing interval (time above MIC) (41). The value of each of these PK/PD parameters in predicting a favorable outcome depends on the class of antibiotics.

Most antimicrobials fall into one of three categories based on their pattern of antimicrobial activity (Fig. 3). Agents such as aminoglycosides, fluoroquinolones, metronidazole, ketolides, and amphotericin B demonstrate concentration-dependent killing and persistent antimicrobial effects (Fig. 3A) (40). The goal of therapy with these agents is to maximize dosing in order to improve the killing and shorten the total duration of treatment and to minimize toxicity. The most important PK/PD parameters that correlate with clinical efficacy are the peak/MIC ratio and the AUC_{24}/MIC ratio. Agents such as betalactams and flucytosine exhibit time-dependent killing with minimal persistent effects (Fig. 3B), and the goal of therapy with these agents is to optimize the period of drug exposure during each dosing interval. With these agents, the frequency of administration and the dose are both important, and time above MIC is the most useful PK/PD parameter for predicting efficacy. Finally, agents such as glycopeptides, macrolides, azithromycin, clindamycin, tetracyclines, oxazolidinones, and fluconazole also exhibit time-dependent killing but with prolonged and persistent effects (Fig. 3C). The goal of therapy with these agents is to optimize the amount of drug delivered, but the dosing frequency is usually as important. The AUC_{24}/MIC and trough/MIC ratios are the most important PK/PD parameters that correlate with outcome. Thus, knowledge of the PK/PD characteristics of different antibiotics represents a major turning point in our approach to antimicrobial therapy, and a prerequisite for optimizing therapeutic efficacy and reducing the emergence of antibiotic resistance.

EMERGING ANTIBIOTIC RESISTANCE

Antibiotic resistance is a serious and world-wide concern. Resistance rates of ocular isolates to the fluoroquinolones, aminoglycosides, and third generation cephalosporins are increasing in almost all areas of the world (1,5,6). Methicillin-resistant *S. aureus* (MRSA) has become increasingly prevalent not only in the hospital setting but also in the community (42). Vancomycin intermediate susceptible (hetero-resistant) *S. aureus* and coagulase-negative staphylococci are increasingly recognized (43,44). At the Vancouver Hospital and Health Sciences Centre, fully 13% of bacteremic isolates of coagulase-negative staphylococci isolated during 1994 already exhibited vancomycin hetero-resistance (i.e.,

(A)

Concentration Dependent Killing

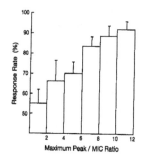

**Aminoglycosides
Fluoroquinolones
Ketolides
Metronidazole
Amphotericin B**

- **Maximize drug
  concentration**

  - Peak / MIC
  - AUC$_{24}$ / MIC

(B)

Time Dependent Killing
Minimal Persistent Effects

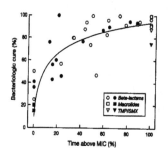

**Beta-lactams
Flucytosine**

- **Optimize
  exposure time**

  - Time above MIC

(C)

Time Dependent Killing
Prolonged Persistent Effects

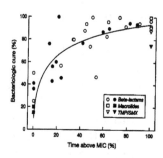

**Macrolides
Azithromycin
Clindamycin
Glycopeptides
Tetracyclines
Oxazolidinones
Fluconazole**

- **Optimize
  amount of drug**

  - AUC$_{24}$ /MIC
  - Trough / MIC

Figure 3 (*Caption on facing page*)

$MIC \geq 4\,mg/L$). The picture for the emergence of MRSA is even more alarming, with rates rapidly rising to 18% since 1997 (Fig. 4). Similar or even higher rates are reported elsewhere in Canada and abroad (45),(46). There are many factors that influence the emergence of antibiotic resistance (Fig. 5). Among these is the increasing susceptibility of hospitalized patients to nosocomial pathogens that are commonly antibiotic-resistant, inappropriate usage of antibiotics by physicians and patients, and budgetary restraints that adversely influence the optimal provision of health care and indirectly promote nosocomial transmission of antimicrobial resistant pathogens (47).

What can be done to control the emergence of antibiotic resistance? This will clearly require a multifaceted approach and a global effort. In this regard, Health Canada established some national goals following a consensus conference entitled "Controlling Antimicrobial Resistance: An Integrated Action Plan for Canada" in 1997 (48) (Table 4). Since the rate of antibiotic resistance can be clearly correlated with the total as well as inappropriate usage of antibiotics, reducing the overall and inappropriate prescribing is clearly a high priority (45). In the field of ophthalmology, although the total usage of antimicrobial agents is likely relatively small compared to other disciplines such as critical care, oncology, or transplantation, the potential for inappropriate or over-usage clearly exists. This includes the indiscriminant use of topical ophthalmic antibiotics, inappropriate surgical perioperative prophylaxis, and the wide practice of intracameral antibiotics in irrigating solutions (7). The combination of vancomycin and gentamicin is particularly popular, although the benefit of such practices remains poorly documented (49). The Centre for Disease Control in the United States strongly advocates

---

Figure 3 *(Facing page)* Three patterns of antimicrobial activity based on different pharmacokinetic and pharmacodynamic parameters: (A) concentration-dependent killing with persistent antimicrobial effects, (B) time-dependent killing with minimal persistent effects, and (C) time-dependent killing with prolonged and persistent effects.

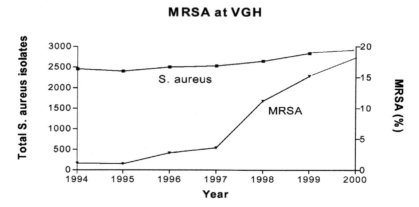

Data from E. Bryce et al.

Figure 4   Rate of isolation of MRSA at the Vancouver Hospital &
Health Sciences Centre during 1994–2000. Data provided by
Dr. Elizabeth Bryce, Clinical Microbiology Laboratory, Vancouver
Hospital and Health Sciences Centre, Vancouver, BC, Canada.

that vancomycin should be reserved for specific therapy and
should not be used routinely for surgical prophylaxis or for
topical irrigations (50). The American Academy of Ophthalmology also endorses these recommendations (51). In the final

**Clinical Challenges in the Management of
Antibiotic Resistance in the New Millennium**

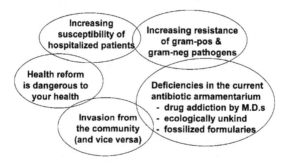

Figure 5   Factors that influence the emergence of antibiotic
resistance in the new millennium. (Adapted from Dr. Thomas Louie,
Division of Infectious Diseases, University of Calgary, Calgary, Alta.)

Table 4 Controlling Antimicrobial Resistance, the Canadian Action Plan

---

Reduce total and inappropriate usage of antimicrobials
  Change physician prescribing behavior
  Change patient expectations
  Curtail the use of prophylactic antibiotics
  Curtail the use of antibiotics in animal feeds
  Promote the use of vaccines
Control the nosocomial spread of resistance
  Strengthen infection prevention and control programs
  Improve the treatment of resistant infections
Enhance active surveillance of antimicrobial use and resistance trends
  Establish population-based surveillance programs in health care settings
    and the community
  Identify ecological niches including health care settings, dairy animals
    and the agriculture industry
  Improve methods for the detection of resistance, particularly laboratory
    tests that can be more predictive of in vivo events
Strengthen strategic partnerships
  Emphasize the need of a societal commitment that includes health care
    agencies, veterinary medicine, government, pharmaceutical industry,
    diary farming, agri-foods and aqua-culture sectors, as well as the public
  Encourage infrastructure costs as well as resources for surveillance
    networks, laboratory facilities as well as research and development of
    new vaccines

Adapted from Ref. 48.

analysis, the selection and administration of all antimicrobials must be carefully weighed based on several factors, including spectrum of activity, local susceptibility patterns, evolving resistance trends, cost, and most importantly, evidence of need and efficacy.

REFERENCES

1. Han DP, Wisniewski SR, Wilson LA, Barza M, Vine AK, Doft BH, Kelsey SF. Spectrum and susceptibilities of microbiologic isolates in the Endophthalmitis Vitrectomy Study. Am J Ophthalmol 1996; 122(1):1–17.

2. Montan P. Endophthalmitis. Curr Opin Ophthalmol 2001; 12(1):75–81.

3. Endophthalmitis Vitrectomy Study Group. Results of the Endophthalmitis Vitrectomy Study. A randomized trial of immediate vitrectomy and of intravenous antibiotics for the treatment of postoperative bacterial endophthalmitis. Endophthalmitis Vitrectomy Study Group. Arch Ophthalmol 1995; 113(12):1479–1496.

4. Barza M, Pavan PR, Doft BH, Wisniewski SR, Wilson LA, Han DP, Kelsey SF. Evaluation of microbiological diagnostic techniques in postoperative endophthalmitis in the Endophthalmitis Vitrectomy Study. Arch Ophthalmol 1997; 115(9):1142–1150.

5. Kunimoto DY, Das T, Sharma S, Jalali S, Majji AB, Gopinathan U, Athmanathan S, Rao TN. Microbiologic spectrum and susceptibility of isolates: Part I. Postoperative endophthalmitis. Am J Ophthalmol 1999; 128(2):240–242.

6. Kunimoto DY, Das T, Sharma S, Jalali S, Majji AB, Gopinathan U, Athmanathan S, Nagaraja Rao T. Micro biologic spectrum and susceptibility of isolates: Part II. Post-traumatic endophthalmitis. Am J Ophthal 1999; 128(2): 242–244.

7. Liesegang TJ. Use of antimicrobials to prevent postoperative infection in patients with cataracts. Curr Opin Ophthalmol 2001; 12(1):68–74.

8. Okhravi N, Adamson P, Lightman S. Use of PCR in endophthalmitis. Ocul Immunol Inflamm 2000; 8(3):189–200.

9. Kalicharan D, Jongebloed WL, Los LI, Worst JG. (An)aerobic bacteria found in secondary-cataract material. A SEM/TEM study. Doc Ophthalmol 1992; 82(1–2):125–133.

10. Busin M, Cusumano A, Spitznas M. Intraocular lens removal from eyes with chronic low-grade endophthalmitis. J Cataract Refract Surg 1995; 21(6):679–684.

11. Hykin PG, Tobal K, McIntyre G, Matheson MM, Towler HM, Lightman SL. The diagnosis of delayed post-operative endophthalmitis by polymerase chain reaction of bacterial

DNA in vitreous samples. J Med Microbiol 1994; 40(6): 408–415.

12. Therese KL, Anand AR, Madhavan HN. Polymerase chain reaction in the diagnosis of bacterial endophthalmitis. Br J Ophthalmol 1998; 82(9):1078–1082.

13. Lohmann CP, Linde HJ, Reischl U. Improved detection of microorganisms by polymerase chain reaction in delayed endophthalmitis after cataract surgery. Ophthalmology 2000; 107(6):1047–1051.

14. Okhravi N, Adamson P, Carroll N, Dunlop A, Matheson MM, Towler HM, Lightman S. PCR-based evidence of bacterial involvement in eyes with suspected intraocular infection. Invest Ophthalmol Vis Sci 2000; 41(11):3474–3479.

15. Carroll NM, Jaeger EEM, Choudhury S, Dunlop AAS, Matheson MM, Adamson P, Okhravi N, Lightman S. Detection of and discrimination between gram-positive and gram-negative bacteria in intraocular samples by using nested PCR. J Clin Microbiol 2000; 38(5):1753–1757.

16. Goh SH, Potter S, Wood JO, Hemmingsen SM, Reynolds RP, Chow AW. HSP60 gene sequences as universal targets for microbial species identification: studies with coagulase-negative staphylococci. J Clin Microbiol 1996; 34(4): 818–823.

17. Kwok AY, Chow AW. Phylogenetic study of Staphylococcus and Macrococcus species based on partial hsp60 gene sequences. Int J Syst Evol Microbiol 2003; 53(Pt 1):87–92.

18. Wong RS, Chow AW. Identification of enteric pathogens by heat shock protein 60 kDa (HSP60) gene sequences. FEMS Microbiol Lett 2002; 206(1):107–113.

19. Kwok AY, Wilson JT, Coulthart M, Ng LK, Mutharia L, Chow AW. Phylogenetic study and identification of human pathogenic Vibrio species based on partial hsp60 gene sequences. Can J Microbiol 2002; 48(10):903–910.

20. Doft BH, Barza M. Optimal management of postoperative endophthalmitis and results of the Endophthalmitis Vitrectomy Study. Curr Opin Ophthalmol 1996; 7(3):84–94.

21. Baker AS, Durand M. The endophthalmitis vitrectomy study [letter]. Arch Ophthalmol 1996; 114:1025.

22. Ferencz JR, Assia EI, Diamantstein L, Rubinstein E. Vancomycin concentration in the vitreous after intravenous and intravitreal administration for postoperative endophthalmitis. Arch Ophthalmol 1999; 117(8):1023–1027.

23. Ball P. Future of the quinolones. Semin Respir Infect 2001; 16(3):215–224.

24. Talan DA. Clinical perspectives on new antimicrobials: focus on fluoroquinolones. Clin Infect Dis 2001; 32(suppl 1): S64–S71.

25. Smith A, Pennefather PM, Kaye SB, Hart CA. Fluoroquinolones: place in ocular therapy. Drugs 2001; 61(6):747–761.

26. Fiscella RG, Nguyen TK, Cwik MJ, Phillpotts BA, Friedlander SM, Alter DC, Shapiro MJ, Blair NP, Gieser JP. Aqueous and vitreous penetration of levofloxacin after oral administration. Ophthalmology 1999; 106(12):2286–2290.

27. Morlet N, Graham GG, Gatus B, McLachlan AJ, Salonikas C, Naidoo D, Goldberg I, Lam CM. Pharmacokinetics of ciprofloxacin in the human eye: a clinical study and population pharmacokinetic analysis. Antimicrob Agents Chemother 2000; 44(6):1674–1679.

28. Wiechens B, Neumann D, Grammer JB, Pleyer U, Hedderich J, Duncker GI. Retinal toxicity of liposome-incorporated and free ofloxacin after intravitreal injection in rabbit eyes. Int Ophthalmol 1998; 22(3):133–143.

29. Wiechens B, Grammer JB, Johannsen U, Pleyer U, Hedderich J, Duncker GI. Experimental intravitreal application of ciprofloxacin in rabbits. Ophthalmologica 1999; 213(2):120–128.

30. Gurler B, Ozkul Y, Bitiren M, Karadede S, Gurkan T. A study on the toxicity of intravitreal levofloxacin in rabbits. Curr Eye Res 2002; 24(4):253–262.

31. Ackermann G, Rodloff AC. Drugs of the 21st century: telithromycin (HMR 3647)—the first ketolide. J Antimicrob Chemother 2003; 51(3):497–511.

32. Perry CM, Jarvis B. Linezolid: a review of its use in the management of serious gram-positive infections. Drugs 2001; 61(4):525–551.

33. Eliopoulos GM. Quinupristin-dalfopristin and linezolid: evidence and opinion. Clin Infect Dis 2003; 36(4):473–481.

34. Tally FP, DeBruin MF. Development of daptomycin for gram-positive infections. J Antimicrob Chemother 2000; 46(4): 523–526.

35. Abbanat D, Macielag M, Bush K. Novel antibacterial agents for the treatment of serious Gram-positive infections. Expert Opin Investig Drugs 2003; 12(3):379–399.

36. Schaison G, Graninger W, Bouza E. Teicoplanin in the treatment of serious infection. J Chemother 2000; 12(suppl 5): 26–33.

37. Johnson LB, Kauffman CA. Voriconazole: a new triazole antifungal agent. Clin Infect Dis 2003; 36(5):630–637.

38. Arathoon EG. Clinical efficacy of echinocandin antifungals. Curr Opin Infect Dis 2001; 14(6):685–691.

39. Craig WA. Does the dose matter? Clin Infect Dis. 2001 33 Suppl 3:S233–7. S233–S237.

40. Andes D, Craig WA. Animal model pharmacokinetics and pharmacodynamics: a critical review. Int J Antimicrob Agents 2002; 19(4):261–268.

41. Craig WA. Pharmacokinetic/pharmacodynamic parameters: rationale for antibacterial dosing of mice and men. Clin Infect Dis 1998; 26(1):1–10.

42. Naimi TS, LeDell KH, Boxrud DJ, Groom AV, Steward CD, Johnson SK, Besser JM, O'Boyle C, Danila RN, Cheek JE, Osterholm MT, Moore KA, Smith KE. Epidemiology and clonality of community-acquired methicillin-resistant *Staphylococcus aureus* in Minnesota, 1996–1998. Clin Infect Dis 2001; 33(7):990–996.

43. Hiramatsu K, Okuma K, Ma XX, Yamamoto M, Hori S, Kapi M. New trends in *Staphylococcus aureus* infections: glycopeptide resistance in hospital and methicillin resistance in the community. Curr Opin Infect Dis 2002; 15(4):407–413.

44. Srinivasan A, Dick JD, Perl TM. Vancomycin resistance in staphylococci. Clin Microbiol Rev 2002; 15(3):430–438.

45. Conly J. Antimicrobial resistance in Canada. Can Med Assoc J 2002; 167(8):885–891.

46. Haddadin AS, Fappiano SA, Lipsett PA. Methicillin resistant *Staphylococcus aureus* (MRSA) in the intensive care unit 1509. Postgrad Med J 2002; 78(921):385–392.

47. Taylor GD, McKenzie M, Kirkland T, Buchanan-Chell M, Wiens R. The impact of health care restructuring on nosocomially acquired blood stream infections. Can J Infect Dis 2000; 11(1):29–32.

48. Health Canada and the Canadian Infectious Disease Society. Controlling antimicrobial resistance: an integrated action plan for Canadians. Can Commun Dis Rep 1997; 23(suppl 7):1–32.

49. Alfonso EC, Flynn HW Jr. Controversies in endophthalmitis prevention. The risk for emerging resistance to vancomycin. Arch Ophthalmol 1995; 113(11):1369–1370.

50. Center for Disease Control. Recommendations for preventing the spread vancomycin resistance recommendations of the Hospital Infection Control Practices Advisory Committee (HICPAC). Morb Mort Wkly Rep 1995; 44:1–13.

51. AAO-CDC Task Force. The prophylactic use of vancomycin for intraocular surgery. A joint statement of the American Academy of Ophthalmology and the Centers for Disease Control and Prevention. Quality of care Publications, No. 515, American Academy of Ophthalmology, San Francisco, CA. October 1999.

6

The Science and Value of Lymphoma Classification

RANDY D. GASCOYNE

Department of Pathology,
British Columbia Cancer Agency
Vancouver, British Columbia, Canada

HISTORICAL PERSPECTIVE

The classification of lymphoid neoplasms has undergone significant change in the last several years. Previous systems were based primarily on morphologic criteria, as exemplified by the Rappaport classification, which served as the standard for almost 25 years. This approach to classification utilized both architectural features and cellular morphology to stratify cases into different categories (Table 1). Although it was both clinically useful and reproducible, it suffered from inappropriate terminology and failed to recognize specific disease entities. Large cell lymphomas of both B-cell and T-cell type

Table 1 Rappaport Classification

Nodular Diffuse
Lymphocytic, well differentiated
Lymphocytic, poorly differentiated
Mixed cell (lymphocytic and histiocytic)
Histiocytic
Undifferentiated

were included together in the category of diffuse histiocytic tumors. This was later recognized to be a problem, as virtually all of these neoplasms proved to be of lymphoid lineage and had no developmental relationship to tumors of histiocytes or so-called tissue-based macrophages. Therefore, the late 1960s saw the Rappaport classification fall into disfavor as it was replaced by a number of other classifications based upon new knowledge of the immune system. The two best known were the Lukes and Collins and the Kiel classifications. The former scheme was used heavily in North America, while the latter derives from Kiel, Germany and is still used frequently today in some parts of Europe. These two "competing" classifications incorporated new immunological data together with morphological assessment as the primary basis of classification. For the first time, lymphomas were separated into B- and T-cell types and clearly recognized in the context of normal lymphoid cell ontogeny. However, these two schemes were part of an explosion of different classification proposals that flooded the literature in the 1970s and led to mass confusion. No well-defined nomenclature existed to translate from one classification to another, rendering many clinicopathologic analyses virtually uninterruptible.

Our clinical colleagues recognized the problems with the various pathological classifications in use throughout the world, and sought to bring some order to the chaos. Thus, in the late 1970s and early 1980s, a large multicenter study was organized to develop a working nomenclature for translating from one classification to another. This effort brought together almost 1200 cases from North America and Europe as well as most of the recognized lymphoma classification experts in the world. The result was the Working Formulation for Clinical Usage (Working Formulation, WF).

As this effort was largely clinically driven, the resultant scheme separated the lymphoid tumors based primarily on their survival characteristics. Although never intended as a specific classification scheme, the WF became the predominant tool used throughout the world for the classification of malignant non-Hodgkin's lymphomas. The details of the WF are provided in Table 2. As is evident from the proposal, the diseases are separated into clinical grades and the scheme clearly lumps together lymphomas of various types and lineages. No effort was made to separate B-cell from T-cell diseases, and the effectiveness of therapy during the era in which these cases were accrued left some wondering whether this was really an analysis of the natural history of many of the proposed disorders. Nonetheless, this scheme remained

Table 2   Working Formulation for Clinical Usage

Low grade
  Small lymphocytic lymphoma (chronic lymphocytic
    leukemia) ± plasmacytoid differentiation
  Follicular lymphoma, small cleaved
  Follicular lymphoma, mixed small and large cell
Intermediate grade
  Follicular lymphoma, large cell type
  Diffuse small-cleaved cell lymphoma
  Diffuse mixed, small and large cell lymphoma
  Diffuse large cell lymphoma, cleaved and noncleaved types
High grade
  Diffuse large cell lymphoma, immunoblastic type
  Lymphoblastic lymphoma
  Small noncleaved lymphoma, Burkitt's
Miscellaneous
  Composite
  Mycosis fungoides
  True histiocytic
  Extramedullary plasmacytoma
  Unclassifiable
  Other

---

popular throughout the world until the hematopathologists got themselves properly organized and developed the REAL classification (Revised European–American Classification of Lymphoid Neoplasms) in 1994. The REAL classification was put forward by the International Lymphoma Study Group (ILSG), a small group comprised of North American and European hematopathologists. The REAL classification was essentially a consensus list of lymphoid neoplasms that pathologists could recognize using currently available techniques and that appear to be distinct disease entities. The most recent classification scheme for non-Hodgkin's lymphomas was put together by the World Health Organization classification (WHO). The various committees of the WHO proposal were for the most part under the leadership of different ILSG members; thus, the WHO classification as shown in Table 3 is essentially a recapitulation of the REAL scheme with minor modifications.

The approach to classification of non-Hodgkin's lymphomas uses all available information including morphology, immunophenotype, genetic and cytogenetic data, and clinical features to define a disease entity. Monoclonal antibody technology and refinements in molecular genetic techniques have been paramount to our ability to recognize these entities and specifically define diseases using routinely archived paraffin material. Several caveats are important to understand the new approach to classification. Firstly, the relative importance of any of these features varies among disease entities, and there is no one "gold standard." Some diseases continue to be defined primarily by morphology, with immunophenotype only required in difficult cases. Other disorders have a unique or "signature" immunophenotype, such that one would hesitate to make the diagnosis in the absence of the immunophenotype. Still other lymphoma subtypes have a specific molecular genetic alteration that essentially defines the disease. As our level of understanding has improved, we are now recognizing that many of these diseases have unique genetic alterations that translate into the production of highly specific proteins. These then serve as unique immunophenotypic markers of disease and have greatly facilitated the routine application

Table 3   World Health Organization Classification

B-cell neoplasms
Precursor B-cell neoplasms
   Precursor B-cell lymphoblastic leukemia/lymphoma
Mature B-cell neoplasms
   Small lymphocytic lymphoma/chronic lymphocytic leukemia
   B-cell prolymphocytic leukemia
   Lymphoplasmacytic lymphoma
   Splenic marginal zone lymphoma
   Hairy cell leukemia
   Plasma cell myeloma
   Monoclonal gammopathy of undetermined significance
   Solitary plasmacytoma of bone
   Extraosseus plasmacytoma
   Primary amyloidosis
   Heavy chain disease
   Extranodal marginal zone B-cell lymphoma of mucosa-associated
      lymphoid tissue (MALT)
   Nodal marginal zone lymphoma
   Follicular lymphoma
   Mantle cell lymphoma
   Diffuse large cell lymphoma
   Mediastinal (thymic) large B-cell lymphoma
   Intravascular large B-cell lymphoma
   Primary effusion lymphoma
   Burkitt's lymphoma/leukemia
T-cell neoplasms (including natural killer (NK) cell neoplasms)
Precursor T-cell neoplasms
   Precursor T-cell lymphoblastic lymphoma/leukemia
Mature T-cell neoplasms
   T-cell prolymphocytic leukemia
   T-cell large granular lymphocytic leukemia
   Aggressive NK cell leukemia
   Adult T-cell leukemia/lymphoma (HTLV 1)
   Mycosis fungoides
   Sézary syndrome
   Primary cutaneous anaplastic large cell lymphoma
   Lymphomatoid papulosis
   Extranodal T/NK cell lymphoma, nasal type
   Enteropathy-type T-cell lymphoma
   Hepatosplenic T-cell lymphoma
   Subcutaneous panniculitis-like T-cell lymphoma
   Angioimmunoblastic T-cell lymphoma

(Continued)

Table 3 (*Continued*)

Peripheral T-cell lymphoma, unspecified
Anaplastic large cell lymphoma
Blastic NK cell lymphoma

NPM-ALK: nucleophosmin-anaplastic lymphoma kinase.

of accurate lymphoma subtyping. Examples of a signature immunophenotype or characteristic genetic alterations are shown in Table 4. This list is not meant to be comprehensive. Secondly, within any specific lymphoma entity there may be a spectrum of morphologies, which may have a basis in genetic alterations. Thirdly, any lymphoma subtype may have a spectrum of clinical behavior and therefore cannot be defined simply by survival characteristics as recognized in the WF. Frequently, cytogenetic clonal evolution and genetic alterations that accompany progression reflect the variable clinical behavior. These may or may not have a morphological correlate. For example, patients with MCL tend to do very poorly, with estimated 5-year overall survival rates of only 30%. However, within MCL there is a subgroup of patients who do very poorly, often characterized by blastoid or pleomorphic morphology, peripheral blood involvement at diagnosis, mutations

Table 4   Unique Lymphoma Features

Disease entity	Cytogenetics	Gene	Protein expressed signature phenotype
Small lymphocytic leukemia	None	None	B-cell, CD5$^+$, CD23$^+$, dim CD20
Mantle cell lymphoma	t(11;14)(q13;q32)	Cyclin D1	B-cell, CD5$^+$, CD23$^-$
Hairy cell leukemia	None	None	CD19$^+$, CD20$^+$, CD11c$^+$, CD25$^+$, CD103$^+$
Anaplastic large cell lymphoma	t(2;5)(p23;q35)	NPM-ALK	ALK1$^+$
Follicular lymphoma	t(14;18)(q32;q21)	Bcl-2	B-cell, CD10$^+$, Bcl-6$^+$

NPM-ALK: nucleophosmin-anaplastic lymphoma kinase.

in tumor suppressor genes such as *p16* or *p53*, and often have a complex karyotype including tetraploidy (92 chromosomes). Thus, although all such cases can now be recognized within the spectrum of MCL because of characteristic staining for cyclin D1, the diverse clinical behavior is beginning to be explained by specific genetic alterations evident within the neoplastic cells.

CURRENT APPROACH

The current approach to the classification of non-Hodgkin's lymphomas takes advantage of all of the diagnostic tools available to reach an accurate diagnosis. As detailed above, some lymphoma entities can be reliably diagnosed using morphology alone. Examples would include most follicular lymphomas and small lymphocytic lymphoma (SLL). A diffuse infiltrate of large lymphoid cells now requires that one first establish lineage (B-cell vs. T-cell) followed by more targeted immunophenotypic studies that help with specific classification. For example, mediastinal large B-cell lymphoma requires clinical input to know that the patient's main site of tumor is the mediastinum. Primary effusion lymphoma typically occurs in the setting of HIV infection, characterized by an effusion without mass-like lesions. The immunophenotype is often ambiguous (lack of B-cell-associated markers, CD19 and CD20), but molecular genetic evidence of commitment to a B-cell lineage with clonal immunoglobulin gene rearrangements is virtually always present. The neoplastic cells usually show coinfection with both Epstein–Barr virus (EBV) and human herpes virus-8 (HHV-8). Nasal T-/natural killer (T/NK) cell lymphoma most frequently occurs in the nasopharynx and is virtually always associated with latent EBV infection in the neoplastic cells. The tumor cells express CD56, but often lack T-cell gene rearrangements reflecting their true natural killer (NK) cell lineage. Anaplastic large cell lymphomas can occur as systemic lymphomas or as isolated cutaneous lesions. Biopsies of either disorder reveal a pleomorphic lymphoid infiltrate with large, CD30-positive malignant cells and evidence of T-cell clonality. However, the primary cutaneous lesions do not express anaplastic lymphoma kinase (ALK)

Table 5   Approach to Diagnosis of Lymphoma

---

1. Clinical correlation
2. Morphologic assessment
3. Immunophenotypic studies
4. Molecular genetic data
5. Cytogenetics
6. Gene expression analysis (not routine)

---

protein, whereas virtually all of the systemic cases do, providing a unique immunophenotypic signature to distinguish these tumors. Both SLL and MCL are examples of CD5-positive B-cell lymphomas. However, they are clinically quite distinct. MCL is an aggressive lymphoma whereas SLL tends to be quite indolent. A combination of immunophenotypic data and molecular cytogenetic results can be used to clearly distinguish these two neoplasms. SLL is usually dim CD20-positive, expresses CD23, and may express CD11c. MCL on the other hand, brightly expresses CD20, and does not express CD23 or CD11c. MCL is characterized by a recurrent cytogenetic abnormality, the t(11;14), which is not seen in SLL. Importantly, as a result of the t(11;14), MCL expresses cyclin D1, which is not expressed by the neoplastic cells of SLL. Moreover, MCL cases with pleomorphic morphology were not considered part of the spectrum of MCL; however, the routine use of immunostains to cyclin D1 is now used to make the diagnosis in such cases, establishing them as extreme examples of the morphologic diversity of MCL. In summary, the current approach to lymphoma classification may take advantage of all of these approaches in any given case to more precisely render an accurate diagnosis (Table 5). The ultimate goal of these efforts is to provide our clinical colleagues with precise diagnoses that may have both prognostic and therapeutic consequences.

LYMPHOMAS OF THE OCULAR ADNEXA AND EYE

While lymphomas of the eye itself are very rare, extranodal lymphomas of the ocular adnexal, including the conjunctiva, eyelids, lacrimal gland, and orbit, constitute as many as 5–8% of all extranodal non-Hodgkin's lymphomas. The vast majority of the ocular adnexa lymphomas are extranodal marginal zone B-cell lymphomas of MALT type, while intraocular lymphomas are virtually all diffuse large B-cell lymphomas (DLBCL). Most of the progress in distinguishing low-grade non-Hodgkin's lymphomas involving the orbit from atypical lymphoid hyperplasia (so-called pseudolymphoma) has been the result of improvements in diagnostic techniques for the demonstration of B-cell monoclonality using either immunohistochemical techniques for light chain restriction or gene rearrangement studies showing monoclonal immunoglobulin (IgH) rearrangements. Although clonality is not synonymous with malignancy, it certainly favors a lymphoma. Importantly, the presence of clonality does not necessarily translate into clinically aggressive disease.

MALT lymphomas at this site are thought to arise following acquired reactive MALT tissue that follows chronic antigenic stimulation. Hence, a proliferation of polyclonal B-cells occurs followed in some cases by the emergence of a dominant B-cell clone. The histopathology is characteristic of MALT lymphomas at other sites, with reactive lymphoid follicles, plasma cells, a proliferation of centrocytes-like cells, and lympho-epithelial lesions. Scattered, large transformed cells may be present. The diagnosis can typically be established by immunostains demonstrating an excess of B-lymphocytes with light chain restriction evident in some cases. B-cells are seen lying within the epithelium (lympho-epithelial lesions) and can be highlighted with stains for cytokeratin. Gene rearrangement studies typically reveal a clonal IgH rearrangement. If cytogenetic studies are performed, presence of a t(11;18)(q21;q21) may be found. This novel translocation has been documented in MALT lymphomas from a variety of different anatomical sites. Others lymphomas at this site are uncommon, but include primary follicular lymphoma, lymphoplasmacytic lymphoma, and mantle cell lymphoma. Immunostains together with molecular genetic studies can usually provide the necessary data to allow a distinction between these lymphoma subtypes.

FUTURE DIRECTIONS

Current research efforts in non-Hodgkin's lymphoma are taking several directions. Most are designed to improve our understanding of the biology, but may also have the added advantage of providing insights into determining prognosis and providing rationale targets for future therapies. One of the new technologies that is critical in this effort is gene expression profiling using microarrays. These techniques utilize tumor tissue mRNA to survey genome-wide expression profiles from individual cases. Consequently, in contrast to the past where typically a single marker was studied in a cohort of patients, this technique allows 15,000–30,000 data points to be generated for each patient. The overwhelming amount of data now requires bio-informatic assistance for proper interpretation, but has already led to significant insights into the heterogeneous biology of some lymphoid tumors, the most recent example being DLBCL. The WHO currently groups the majority of such cases under the rubric "unspecified DLBCL." Gene expression profiling has now revealed at least two or three major subtypes of disease based on cell of origin. Not only have these data provided an improved understanding of the biology, but also have been shown to be powerful predictors of clinical behavior. In the near future, similar techniques using customized "mini-chips" may become part of the routine diagnostic armamentarium.

REFERENCES

1. Anonymous. National Cancer Institute sponsored study of classifications of non-Hodgkin's lymphomas: summary and description of a working formulation for clinical usage. The Non-Hodgkin's Lymphoma Pathologic Classification Project. Cancer 1982; 49(10):2112–2135.

2. Anonymous. A clinical evaluation of the international lymphoma study group classification of non-Hodgkin's lymphoma. Blood 1997; 89(11):3903–3918.

3. Harris NL, Jaffe ES, Diebold J, Flandrin G, Muller-Hermelink HK, Vardiman J, Lister TA, Bloomfield CD. World Health Organization classification of neoplastic diseases of the hemato-poietic and lymphoid tissues: report of the Clinical Advisory Committee Meeting, House, Virginia, November 1997. J Clin Oncol 1999; 17(12):3835–3849.

4. Harris NL, Jaffe ES, Stein H, Banks PM, Chan JK, Cleary ML, Delsol G, De Wolf-Peeters C, Falini B, Gatter KC. A revised European–American classification of lymphoid neoplasms: a proposal from the International Lymphoma Study Group. Blood 1994; 84(5):1361–1392.

5. Jaffe ES, Harris NL, Stein H, Vardiman JW. World Health Organization Classification of Tumours: Tumours of Haemato-poietic and Lymphoid Tissues. Lyon: IARC Press, 2001.

6. Rosenwald A, Wright G, Chan WC, Connors JM, Campo E, Fisher RI, Gascoyne RD, Muller-Hermelink HK, Smeland EB, Giltnane JM, Hurt EM, Zhao H, Averett L, Yang L, Wilson WH, Jaffe ES, Simon R, Klausner RD, Powell J, Duffey PL, Longo DL, Greiner TC, Weisenburger DD, Sanger WG, Dave BJ, Lynch JC, Vose J, Armitage JO, Montserrat E, Lopez-Guillermo A, Grogan TM, Miller TP, LeBlanc M, Ott G, Kvaloy S, Delabie J, Holte H, Krajci P, Stokke T, Staudt LM. The use of molecular profiling to predict survival after chemotherapy for diffuse large-B-cell lymphoma. N Engl J Med 2002; 346(25): 1937–1947.

7

Non-Hodgkin's Lymphoma

JOSEPH M. CONNORS

Division of Medical Oncology,
University of British Columbia and
British Columbia Cancer Agency,
Vancouver, British Columbia, Canada

INCIDENCE AND EPIDEMIOLOGY

The incidence of non-Hodgkin's lymphoma (NHL) in North America has been rising for the past 50 years at a rate of approximately 2–3% per year. It has become the fourth most common type of cancer for adult men (after lung, prostate, and colorectal) and women (after lung, breast, and colorectal) reaching an incidence of approximately 15 cases per 100,000 per year in women and 25 cases per 100,000 per year in men and causing approximately 60,000 new cases annually. The reason for this rise is unknown, though three observations may be relevant. Firstly, although a modest contribution to this rise has come from the cases seen in patients with

AIDS, most of the increase has occurred in the elderly. Secondly, workers in occupations such as farming, processing of forestry products, paper processing, and others that involve long-term exposure to bioactive solvents and reagents have an increased risk of developing NHL, which is 1.5–4.0 times normal. Thirdly, the increase in lymphomas is exactly parallel to that seen in melanoma, the only other cancer with a rising incidence unrelated to smoking. It is possible that exposure to solar radiation plays a role in both increases.

There is a 50-fold increase in incidence of NHL between infancy and old age, and the average lifetime risk of developing NHL in North America is 1/50. The median age of patients with NHL is at least 60–65 years, and approximately one-third of patients are over 70 years at the time of diagnosis.

ETIOLOGY AND RISK FACTORS

The cause of NHL is unknown. Individuals with the following risk factors have an increased likelihood of developing NHL:

1. congenital immunodeficiency,
2. acquired immunodeficiency syndrome (AIDS),
3. organ transplant-related immune suppression, and
4. chronic immunoregulatory or autoimmune diseases such as rheumatoid arthritis, Hashimoto's thyroiditis, or celiac sprue and more recently, autoimmune thyroid disease [editor's comment].

The theme common to these conditions is dysregulation of the immune system. Although some authorities think this leads to the increased risk of lymphoma by causing diminished immune surveillance, it is more likely that these conditions are associated with overactivity (hyperstimulation) of a damaged system leading to genetically stable loss of growth control, perhaps through loss of usual apoptosis (programmed cell death).

Certain viruses are associated with NHL.

1. *Human immunodeficiency virus* (HIV) is the cause of acquired immunodeficiency syndrome (AIDS). It

appears to increase the risk of developing lymphoma primarily by profoundly depleting the pool of T-cells, which in turn leads to an immunodeficiency state that is permissive for the development of lymphomas, especially those associated with Epstein–Barr virus. Patients with AIDS have a markedly increased risk of developing lymphoma and the risk seems to be closely related to the degree of T-cell depletion. These lymphomas are often seen at unusual extranodal sites, such as the central nervous system (CNS) where 5% of the lymphomas seen in AIDS patients occur compared to only 1% of the lymphomas in the normal population.

2. *Human lymphotrophic virus type I (HTLV-I)* (1) is a retrovirus endemic to parts of Southern Japan and the Caribbean basin and sporadic elsewhere. It is transmitted in intact lymphocytes, therefore, by breast feeding, sexual contact, and blood product transfusion. Approximately, 1% of individuals infected in infancy, but none of those infected in adult life develop a T-cell lymphoma typically associated with leukemic peripheral blood involvement, skin and CNS infiltration, and hypercalcemia. Treatment is only transiently effective (2).

3. *Epstein-Barr virus* (EBV), the herpes virus that causes infectious mononucleosis, is present intracellularly in virtually all cases of Burkitt's lymphoma and many of the NHLs seen in association with AIDS or transplant related immunosuppression. Epstein–Barr virus also can immortalize lymphocytes in vitro. Thus, it is strongly suspected to contribute causally to the development of some types of NHL but its precise role is unknown.

4. *Hepatitis C virus* has been found much more frequently than expected in patients with lymphoplasmacytic lymphomas (formerly called small lymphocytic lymphoma with plasmacytoid differentiation or Waldenström's macroglobulinemia) in approximately 30% of

cases (3). The viral DNA is present in the malignant cells implying but not proving a possible etiologic role.

5. *Human Herpes Virus 8, HHV-8* (Kaposi's Sarcoma Herpes Virus, KSHV) is closely associated with AIDS-related and sporadic Kaposi's sarcoma and may have a role in their etiology. It is also closely associated with body cavity associated or primary effusion lymphoma, a large cell B-cell lymphoma presenting primarily with pleural or peritoneal malignant effusion (4). HHV-8 has been recovered from virtually all studied cases and it is probably a crucial etiologic agent for this rare lymphoma whether it is seen sporadically or with AIDS.

Certain specific cytogenetic abnormalities and dysregulated expression of associated oncogenes are associated with specific lymphomas. Typically a known or putative tumor promoter gene is moved to a new location where it is upregulated or a tumor suppressor gene is mutated or suppressed. Any translocation involving the immunoglobulin H chain gene on 14q32 can occasionally alternatively involve the κ light chain gene at 2p12 or the λ light chain gene at 22p11. Hence, instead of a t(8;14)(q24;q32), one might encounter a t(2;8)(p12;q24), which has an equivalent effect. Table 1 contains a partial list of the most common lymphoma-associated oncogenes.

DIAGNOSIS, CLASSIFICATION, AND STAGING

Table 2 identifies the diagnosis, classification, and staging of non-Hodgkin's lymphomas.

TREATMENT

The treatment plan for NHLs is listed in Table 3. This overall approach can be expected to produce results that reflect both the effectiveness of the treatment and the underlying natural history of the lymphoma (Table 4).

Table 1 Partial List of Common Lymphoma-Associated Oncogenes

Oncogene	Chromosome location	Gene product	Lymphoma	Frequency (%)	Typical t
Bcl-1	11q13	Cyclin D1	Mantle cell	95	11;14
Bcl-2	18q21.3	Antiapoptosis	Follicular	85	14;18
Bcl-6	3q27	Zinc fing tran factor	Diffuse large B-cell	40	3;14
PAX-5	9q13	B-cell specific activator protein	Lymphoplasmacytic	50	9;14
Myc	8q24	DNA spec transcript factor	Burkitt's	100	8;14
ALK	5q35	Nucleophosmin (NPM) ALK fusion protein	T-cell anaplastic large cell	30–50	2;5

Table 2 Diagnosis, Classification, and Staging of non-Hodgkin's Lymphomas

Type	B-cell	T-cell
Indolent	Small lymphocytic/CLL	Mycoses fungoides
	Lymphoplasmacytic [a]	Primary cutaneous
	Follicular,[b] any type	anaplastic large cell
	Marginal zone	Lymphoproliferative
	MALT	disease of large
	Nodal (monocytoid	granular lymphocytes
	B-cell)	
	Splenic	
Aggressive	Mantle cell	Peripheral T-cell, unspecified
	Diffuse large cell,[c] any	Peripheral T-cell, specified
	subtype	Angioimmunoblastic
	Burkitt-like (small	(AILD[d]-type)
	noncleaved cell)	Nasal T/NK cell-type
		Subcutaneous panniculitic
		Intestinal enteropathy
		associated
		Hepatosplenic
		Anaplastic large cell
		including null cell
Acute leukemia-like	Lymphoblastic	Lymphoblastic
	Burkitt	
Viral	Primary effusion (HHV-8[e]	HTLV-1 associated
	associated)	

[a] Formerly plasmacytoid small lymphocytic with or without IgM paraprotein (Waldenström's macroglobulinemia).
[b] Small cleaved, mixed or large cell subtypes.
[c] Mixed large and small cell, immunoblastic, primary mediastinal, T-cell rich B-cell, intravascular or B-cell anaplastic subtypes.
[d] Angioimmunoblastic lymphadenopathy with dysproteinemia.
[e] Human herpes virus type 8.

SPECIAL COMMENTS ON LYMPHOMA ASSOCIATED WITH THE EYE

Malignant lymphoma involves the structures of the eye and orbit in two quite distinct patterns (5–8). The most common presentation is in the periorbital soft tissues, particularly the conjunctival mucosal surfaces and around the lacrimal gland. Previously, the majority of these localized soft-tissue

Table 3 Treatment Regimens for non-Hodgkin's Lymphomas

Type	Stage	Frequency	Age (years)	Treatment
Indolent	Limited	10%	—	Irradiation
	Advanced	90%	—	Watchful waiting
				Single-agent chemotherapy
				Local irradiation
				Escalate to multiagent chemotherapy
Aggressive	Limited	30%	—	Brief chemotherapy[a] plus irradiation
	Advanced	70%	< 70	Prolonged chemotherapy[a] full dose, on time
				Tailored chemotherapy
Acute leukemia-like	All	100%	< 60–70	Intensive chemotherapy
				+CNS prophylaxis +Heme stem cell transplant
			> 60–70	Palliative chemotherapy

[a] The chemotherapy for aggressive type lymphoma should include doxorubicin, cyclophosphamide, vincristine, and prednisone in full standard doses. Acceptable regimens include CHOP, ACOP-12, and similar combinations.

lymphomas presenting in periorbital soft tissue were classified as small lymphocytic lymphomas or pseudolymphoma. With the ability to identify clonal B-cell disease on the basis of immunoglobulin gene rearrangement studies, it has become clear that these are definite clonal neoplasms of B-cells. Most fit best into the new category designated "MALT" for mucosa associated lymphoid tumor. Radiation is highly effective in eradicating this type of lymphoma and is potentially curative in the majority who present with localized disease (5–7). The dose of irradiation need not be high and should be kept in the range of 2500–3000 cGy to reduce the risk of cataract formation, xerophthalmia, and retinal damage. Shielding of the lens is also mandatory if cataract

Table 4 Prognosis of Treatment Regimens for non-Hodgkin's
Lymphomas

Type	Stage	Prognosis
Indolent	Limited	Fifty to seventy percent disease-free survival for 10 + years
		Late relapse not uncommon
	Advanced	Median survival for all: 8–9 years
		Median survival for age < 60: 10–12 years
		Most patients relapse but long survival with disease is common
Aggressive	Limited	Disease-free survival 80–90% for 10 + years
	Advanced	Disease-free survival for age < 70: 55–60%
		Disease-free survival for age > 70: 20–30%
Acute leukemia-like	All	Disease-free survival > 50% but only after intensive chemotherapy plus CNS prophylaxis ± heme stem cell transplantation

formation is to be avoided. Chemotherapy with agents
suitable for low grade lymphoma is also capable of inducing
prolonged remission and is the best choice if disease is widespread at diagnosis, recurs after irradiation, or if the
morbidity of the irradiation might be excessive. Interestingly,
bilateral eye involvement with MALT is not uncommon and
may be synchronous or metachronous and can occur without
other evidence of systemic disease, a pattern of spread implying a special interaction between these malignant B-cells and
the mucosal microenvironment of the eye.

The periorbital soft tissues and bones may be involved
with lymphoma of other indolent types than MALT or
occasionally with variants of large cell lymphoma. In such
cases, there is nothing unique about the natural history.
Treatment should be based on the overall clinical picture
and should take into consideration the histologic subtype,
stage, age, and frailty of the patient and expected toxicity of
the chosen regimen. When this is done, results identical to
those obtained for other sites of presentation can be secured.
When the periorbital disease also involves the paranasal

sinuses, special precautions to avoid spread to the central nervous system must be employed.

The rarest presentation of lymphoma involving the eye is also the most unusual. Intraocular lymphoma (6) constitutes less than 1% of lymphomas and can be quite difficult to diagnose. Although almost all are B-cell large cell lymphomas, they often pursue a more indolent course and are frequently mislabeled as chronic uveitis or unexplained vitritis for months or even years before diagnosis, a mistake abetted by this lymphoma's marked responsiveness to corticosteroids which may have been given empirically. The diagnosis is best established by vitrectomy performed when the patient has been off corticosteroids for at least several weeks. Although an experienced ophthalmologist can often recognize this distinct entity by appearance alone, the seriousness of the diagnosis still necessitates vitrectomy for certain diagnosis. Other important peculiarities of the natural history of intraocular lymphoma are its tendency to be bilateral, seen in at least 50% of cases, and its frequent association with brain or leptomeningeal involvement, also seen in at least 50% of cases. Slit lamp examination of the other eye, computerized tomographic scanning or magnetic resonance imaging of the brain and cytologic examination of the cerebrospinal fluid must be included in the staging evaluation. Current treatment results for intraocular lymphoma are unsatisfactory. Irradiation is the mainstay and should be extended to include the other eye or brain if necessary. Despite irradiation, however, most patients relapse within the eye or brain. Unfortunately, chemotherapeutic agents other than corticosteroids and antimetabolites penetrate the eye and brain poorly, limiting additional treatment. Presently most patients can be offered excellent palliation for months to years with irradiation and corticosteroids but recurrence is usual. Investigational approaches include the use of high dose antimetabolites (8). Recently, it has been shown that very high dose methotrexate (> 8000 ma/m^2) does penetrate the interior structures of the eye reaching therapeutic levels; subconjunctival antimetabolites have also been used [editor's comment]. If preliminary observations of useful responses are confirmed, this will constitute an alternative systemic treatment. Unfortunately, eventual progression in the eye or CNS usually leads to blindness or death indicating a clear need for more effective approaches.

REFERENCES

1. Hollsberg P, Hafler DA. Seminars in medicine of the Beth Israel Hospital, Boston. Pathogenesis of diseases induced by human lymphotrophic virus type I infection. N Engl J Med 1993; 328(16):1173–1182.

2. Gill PS, Harrington W Jr, Kaplan MH, et al. Treatment of adult T-cell leukemia-lymphoma with a combination of interferon alpha and zidovudine. N Engl J Med 1995; 332(26): 1744–1748.

3. Silvestri F, Pipan C, Barillari G, et al. Prevalence of hepatitis C virus infection in patients with lymphoproliferative disorders. Blood 1996; 87(10):4296–4301.

4. Nador RG, Cesarman E, Chadburn A, et al. Primary effusion lymphoma: a distinct clinicopathologic entity associated with the Kaposi's sarcoma-associated herpes virus. Blood 1996; 88(2):645–656.

5. Esik O, Ikeda H, Mukai K, Kaneko A. A retrospective analysis of different modalities for treatment of primary orbital non-Hodgkin's lymphomas. Radiother Oncol 1996; 38(l): 13–18.

6. Whitcup SM, de Smet MD, Rubin BI, et al. Intraocular lymphoma. Clinical and histopathologic diagnosis. Ophthalmology 1993; 100(9):1399–1406.

7. Smitt MC, Donaldson SS. Radiotherapy is successful treatment for orbital lymphoma. Int J Radiat Oncol Biol Phys 1993; 26(l):59–66.

8. Plowman PN, Montefiore DS, Lightman S. Multiagent chemotherapy in the salvage cure of ocular lymphoma relapsing after radiotherapy. Clin Oncol (R Coll Radiol) 1993; 5(5): 315–316.

8

Epithelial Lacrimal Gland Tumors: Pathologic Classification and Current Understanding

THOMAS J. JOLY and JACK ROOTMAN

Department of Ophthalmology, University of British Columbia, Vancouver General Hospital, Vancouver, British Columbia, Canada

HIND M. AL-KATAN

Department of Ophthalmology, Security Forces Hospital, Riyadh, Saudi Arabia

GUILIO BONAVOLONTA and DIEGO STRIANESE

Department of Ophthalmology, University of Naples, Naples, Italy

KENNETH A. FELDMAN

Department of Ophthalmology, Kaiser Permanente Medical Center, Harbor City, California, U.S.A.

JOCELYNE S. LAPOINTE

Department of Radiology, Vancouver General Hospital, University of British Columbia, Vancouver British Columbia, Canada

KENNETH W. BEREAN and VALERIE A. WHITE

Department of Pathology, University of British Columbia, Vancouver General Hospital, Vancouver British Columbia, Canada

SYLVIA PASTERNAK

Department of Pathology, Dalhousie University, Halifax Nova Scotia, Canada

PEEROOZ SAEED

Department of Ophthalmology, University of Amsterdam, Amsterdam, The Netherlands

SUMALEE VANGVEERAVONG

Department of Ophthalmology, Siriraj Hospital, Bangkok, Thailand

Prior to the advent of histopathology, there was no distinction between various types of epithelial tumors of the lacrimal gland, and thus no valid basis for clinical prognostication regarding specific types. Warthin, in his review of 132 cases in 1901, came to the conclusion that many previous diagnoses could be subsumed under the diagnosis of mixed tumor (1). As recently as 1939, this trend continued with the publication of a series by Sanders of 12 cases of mixed tumor with no distinction between benign and malignant lesions, even though the clinical outcome varied tremendously between cases (2). In 1948, a series by Godtfredsen was the first to distinguish benign from malignant lacrimal gland tumors according to histologic features, and to note that the clinical prognosis was different for the two classes (3). Since that time, classification schemes have evolved with a general trend toward more specific histopathologic diagnoses. Duke-Elder and MacFaul listed seven diagnoses in 1974 (4), and the most recent World Health Organization (WHO) classification of 1980 similarly lists seven diagnoses (5) (Table 1).

Because of the more frequent occurrence of salivary gland tumors and the biologic similarity between salivary and lacrimal gland tumors, classification schemes for lacrimal tumors have traditionally been adapted from those for salivary gland tumors. In 1953, Foote and Frazell reviewed 877 cases of salivary gland tumors to arrive at a classification scheme of 13 diagnoses that clearly distinguished benign from

Table 1   Epithelial Lacrimal Tumor Classification Listed in the World Health Organization International Histological Classification of Tumors

---

Pleomorphic adenoma
Other adenomas
Mucoepidermoid tumor
Carcinoma in pleomorphic adenoma
Adenoid cystic carcinoma
Adenocarcinomas
Other carcinomas

From Ref. 5.

malignant tumors (6). Based on this work, the first American Armed Forces Institute of Pathology (AFIP) classification, published in 1954, listed five benign and nine malignant diagnoses (7). Since that time, both the WHO and AFIP have published updated classification schemes, including the most recent WHO classification of 1991, which lists 14 adenomas and 17 carcinomas (8), and the most recent AFIP classification of 1996, which lists 13 benign and 23 malignant tumors (9).

A re-evaluation of lacrimal tumor classification is needed to reflect the recent advances in salivary tumor classifications. At the University of British Columbia, we reviewed a series of lacrimal gland epithelial tumors contributed from four orbital disease centers: the University of Naples, University of Amsterdam, and Kaiser Permanente Medical Center of Southern California combined with our own series. Our goal is to apply the most recent salivary classification schemes to lacrimal tumors, and to correlate clinical outcomes with histologic tumor type.

The combined series includes a total of 118 cases, with diagnoses as listed in Table 2. The most frequent diagnosis is pleomorphic adenoma, with 57 cases (48%) of the total series. Adenoid cystic carcinomas are next most numerous, with 38 cases (32%). There are nine cases of carcinoma ex pleomorphic adenoma, and 11 cases of various other rare diagnoses, including adenocarcinoma, mucoepidermoid carcinoma, ductal carcinoma, myoepithelial carcinoma, squamous cell carcinoma, myoepithelioma, and oncocytoma. Three tumors were found to be unclassifiable. Two of these were considered to have malignant features histopathologically, while the third was indeterminate.

We have confirmed that benign tumors by histologic criteria typically run a benign course clinically. All pleomorphic adenomas were treated with local excision only, without adjuvant therapy or more radical surgery. No patient with pleomorphic adenoma has died with disease, and no patient whose tumor was first diagnosed at one of our centers has had recurrence after surgical excision (median follow-up 3.0 years, range 0–25 years). This includes five cases of pleomorphic adenoma with various degrees of cellular atypia

Table 2 Histological Diagnoses of Epithelial Lacrimal Gland Tumors Determined upon Case Series Review, with Clinical Outcomes for Each Diagnosis

Diagnosis	Number of cases	Number of cases with over 1 year follow-up	Clinical outcome			
			Died with disease	Metastasis	Local recurrence	No recurrence or metastasis
Pleomorphic adenoma	51	41	0	0	3	38
Pleomorphic adenoma with cellular atypia	5	5	0	0	0	5
Pleomorphic adenoma variant with atypical features	1	0	0	0	0	0
Myoepithelioma	1	0	0	0	0	0
Oncocytoma	1	1	0	0	0	1
Spindle cell tumor	1	1	0	0	0	1
Adenoid cystic carcinoma	38	34	14	5[a]	6[a]	12
Carcinoma ex pleomorphic adenoma, circumscribed	3	2	0	0	0	2
Carcinoma ex pleomorphic adenoma, noncircumscribed	6	5	2	0	1	2
Adenocarcinoma	3	2	1	0	0	1
Mucoepidermoid carcinoma	2	2	1	0	0	1
Ductal carcinoma	2	2	0	0	0	2
Squamous cell carcinoma	1	0	0	0	0	0
Myoepithelial carcinoma	1	1	1	0	0	0
Unclassifiable carcinoma	2	2	1	0	0	1

[a]Three patients had both local recurrence and metastasis.

(median follow-up 4.1 years, range 2.4–8.8 years). Of three patients who initially presented with recurrent disease after initial diagnosis and treatment elsewhere, one had further recurrence after treatment at our centers; none has died with disease (follow-up 0.4, 3.0, and 3.1 years after initial treatment at our centers). There was no recurrence over 5 years in the single case of oncocytoma. Follow-up data were not available for a single, very recent case of myoepithelioma.

In contrast, malignant tumors by histologic criteria are associated with a much worse prognosis. Carcinomas were treated with combinations of local excision, exenteration, orbitectomy, and local irradiation. No statistically significant correlation was seen between type of treatment and clinical outcome. Of 43 patients with primary malignant tumors (adenocarcinoma, adenoid cystic, mucoepidermoid, lacrimal duct, myoepithelial, or unclassifiable carcinoma but excluding malignant mixed tumors) with over 1 year of follow-up, 18 died with disease within a median of 2 years of diagnosis (range <1–25 years). Another eight patients are living with recurrence or metastasis. The remaining 17 patients remain disease free with a median of 10.6 years follow-up (range 1.2–17.8 years). Ductal carcinoma of the lacrimal gland was the one diagnostic category with a suggestion of better prognosis, with two patients disease-free after 3 and 4 years of follow-up, although the small number of cases makes any conclusion tenuous.

There were nine cases of malignant mixed tumor in our series, all of which were cases of carcinoma arising in pleomorphic adenoma, or "carcinoma ex pleomorphic adenoma." (The diagnostic category "malignant mixed tumor" also includes carcinosarcoma and metastasizing pleomorphic adenoma, neither of which was seen in our series.) We were able to distinguish two subtypes of carcinoma ex pleomorphic adenoma based on histopathologic findings. One subtype had the carcinoma completely circumscribed within the pleomorphic adenoma or its pseudocapsule. We found three cases of this subtype, all with no recurrence within the follow-up period (range 0.4–3.0 years) with no adjuvant therapy or additional surgery beyond initial excision. The other subtype, comprising six cases, had extension of the carcinoma beyond the margins of the pleomorphic adenoma. Patients with this subtype did poorly: of five patients with follow-up, two patients died with disease within 3 years of diagnosis and one patient developed recurrence 1 year and again 2 years after initial treatment.

Malignant transformation of pleomorphic adenoma appears to manifest a continuum of changes from minor atypia to clearly invasive carcinoma with little residual evidence of the original pleomorphic adenoma. Typical pleomorphic adenoma, pleomorphic adenoma with atypia, and circumscribed carcinoma ex pleomorphic adenoma (not extending beyond the margins of the pleomorphic adenoma) all appear to behave in a benign manner clinically. In contrast, for noncircumscribed carcinoma ex pleomorphic adenoma (where the carcinoma extends beyond the margins of the pleomorphic adenoma), the prognosis is much worse, similar to that of primary carcinomas. We recommend clearly distinguishing between the two diagnostic entities, "circumscribed carcinoma ex pleomorphic adenoma" and "noncircumscribed carcinoma ex pleomorphic adenoma." Decisions regarding therapy should be made recognizing the prognostic differences among the various types of lacrimal gland tumors. Clinically, benign tumors can be treated with simple excision alone, sparing the added morbidity and mutilation of more aggressive surgery or adjuvant therapy. Clinically, malignant tumors may require additional treatment, such as exenteration, orbitectomy, and high-dose radiotherapy, and may well be fatal even with these measures.

Our proposed classification scheme for lacrimal gland tumors is listed in Table 3 and emphasizes the increasing range of potential epithelial tumor diagnoses arising from this site. It comprises the diagnoses included in our series, as well as a few diagnoses not seen in our series but described in the lacrimal or salivary tumor literature. The ambiguous term "malignant mixed tumor" has been deleted, and its three constituents, carcinoma ex pleomorphic adenoma, carcinosarcoma, and metastasizing pleomorphic adenoma are listed separately. The category "carcinoma

Table 3 Proposed Classification of Epithelial Lacrimal Gland Tumors

---

Benign epithelial neoplasms
Pleomorphic adenoma
  Without atypia
  With atypia
Myoepithelioma
Oncocytoma
Malignant epithelial neoplasms
Adenoid cystic carcinoma
Carcinoma ex pleomorphic adenoma
  Circumscribed
  Noncircumscribed
Mucoepidermoid carcinoma
Adenocarcinoma
Lacrimal duct carcinoma
Myoepithelial carcinoma
Squamous cell carcinoma
Carcinosarcoma[a]
Acinic cell carcinoma[a]
Sebaceous adenocarcinoma[a]
Basal cell adenocarcinoma[a]
Epithelial-myoepithelial carcinoma[a]
Polymorphous low-grade adenocarcinoma[a]
Metastasizing pleomorphic adenoma[a]

---

[a]Not seen in our series, but reported in the literature.

ex pleomorphic adenoma" is subdivided into circumscribed and noncircumscribed carcinomas to reflect their different clinical prognoses.

REFERENCES

1. Warthin A. Endothelioma of the lacrimal gland. Arch Ophthalmol 1901; 30:601–620.

2. Sanders TE. Mixed tumor of the lacrimal gland. Arch Ophthalmol 1939; 21:239–260.

3. Godtfredsen E. Pathology of mucous and salivary gland tumors in the lacrimal gland and the relation to extra orbital mucous and salivary gland tumors. Br J Ophthalmol 1948; 32:171–179.

4. Duke-Elder S, MacFaul PA. The ocular adnexa. Part II. Lacrimal, orbital and para-orbital diseases. In: Duke-Elder S, ed. System of Ophthalmology. London: Henry Kimpton, 1974: 596–1163.

5. Zimmerman L, Sobin L. Histological typing of tumors of the eye and its adnexa. International Histological Classification of Tumors. Geneva: World Health Organization,1980:24.

6. Foote FW Jr, Frazell EL. Tumors of the major salivary glands. Cancer 1953; 6:1065–1133.

7. Foote F, Frazell E. Tumors of the major salivary glands. Atlas of Tumor Pathology. Series 1, Fascicle 11. Washington, DC: Armed Forces Institute of Pathology, 1954.

8. Seifert G, Sobin L. Histological classification of salivary gland tumours. International Histological Classification of Tumors. Berlin: Springer-Verlag, 1991.

9. Ellis GL, Auclair PL. Tumors of the salivary gland. Atlas of Tumor Pathology. 3rd Series, Fascicle 17. Washington, DC: Armed Forces Institute of Pathology, 1996.

9

Chemotherapy of Epithelial Lesions: New Approaches and Directions

JAMES H. GOLDIE
University of British Columbia, Vancouver
British Columbia, Canada

ABSTRACT

The significant insights gained in recent years into the molecular processes underlying the malignant state are making possible the development of new, more specific classes of antineoplastic agents. Together with the availability of sophisticated diagnostic technology such as DNA array analysis, it is becoming feasible to fashion drug programs that will be tumor specific and less toxic for the patient. There are, however, major obstacles to be overcome. DNA array technology is still early in its development and there remain problems in reproducibility, cost, and clinical correlation. The whole field of drug discovery is hampered by a drug approval process that is out of date and not attuned to what is required at the clinical evaluation stage. Emphasis on unwieldy and time consuming clinical trials makes it very difficult to develop drug combination protocols in a timely manner. Finally, the biomedical community has been slow to consider the implications that many types of cancer may have as their necessary cause infectious agents, including both viruses and bacteria.

INTRODUCTION

Malignancies arising in epithelial tissues constitute by far the largest number of clinically occurring cancers. Although cancers arising in orbital structures are relatively uncommon compared to carcinomas of the aerodigestive tract and breast, collectively the epithelial cancers represent a formidable clinical and scientific challenge. While there has been some progress made in the management of certain of these tumors, the distressing fact remains that the great majority of these malignancies remain incurable once they have reached an advanced stage.

In the last few years there have been a number of conceptual advances made in our understanding of cancer at the molecular level and for the first time it has become possible to envisage rationally constructed treatment strategies. There remain many problems, however, not the least of which are (in this writer's opinion) overly conservative thinking by the biomedical research community and the entrenchment of a drug development and approval process that is excessively bureaucratic and poorly set up to expedite novel treatment approaches.

STEPS TOWARD TUMOR SPECIFIC THERAPY

For more than 50 years the principal drugs used in the treatment of metastatic cancer have been a variety of cytotoxic chemicals that have been found in the process of empirically screening many hundreds of thousands of both synthetic and naturally produced organic compounds. From this huge inventory, some 50–60 agents have been discovered, which have at least some clinical activity against some cancers and which have a satisfactory therapeutic index. In addition, a number of hormonal agents such as androgen and estrogen analogues and corticosteroids have been found to have a useful role in the management of certain types of malignancy.

Virtually all of the cytotoxic agents act by interfering in DNA function or synthesis or by damaging the mitotic spindle. This in turn triggers a cellular auto-destruct sequence (apoptosis) with resultant cell death (1). Hormonal agents likewise can initiate apoptosis in certain cell types. However, only a minority of cancer types are highly susceptible to cytotoxic drug inhibition and for the most part these do not include the common epithelial cancers of middle and older age. Hormonal agents are active in breast and prostate cancers but do not appear able to yield cures against advanced disease, even when used in combination with cytotoxic agents.

New cytotoxic agents are always being added to the inventory but all suffer from the same limitations as the older drugs and they have not significantly expanded the range of tumors that can be effectively treated. It appears self-evident that new strategies will be required to develop drugs that will have both different spectra of activities as well as superior therapeutic indices.

CANCER SPECIFIC MOLECULAR TARGETS

Recent studies have produced comprehensive molecular models of the transformation of a normal cell to the malignant state (2). Three broad categories of alterations are required to produce the full blown malignant phenotype. The first involves one or other of the signal pathways that provide growth signals to the cell nucleus. This usually is a consequence of overexpression or constitutive activity of one or more of the many growth factor receptors. Many of these growth factor receptors have regions that function as tyrosine kinases (3). That is, they are able to catalyze the transfer of a phosphate group to a specific tyrosine residue in an adjacent protein. This changes the shape of the protein and permits interaction with other proteins in turn altering their shape, activity, etc. A common biochemical mediator of these signals consists of a series of phosphorylation–dephosphorylation reactions, which ultimately initiate DNA synthesis by activating DNA transcription factors.

Another critical change involves activating the genes that block the various programmed cell death pathways. As a result, processes that would normally act to put a brake on continuous cell division and to cull cells that are expressing abnormal growth signals are suppressed, allowing the neoplastic cell unimpeded growth.

It appears that human cells require a third fundamental change to permit continuous cell proliferation. This involves activation of the enzyme telomerase, which acts to prevent the shortening of the telomeres at the ends of chromosomes. Progressive shortening of the telomeres normally provides a signal for the cell to stop dividing after a set number of divisions. This occurs in all normal somatic cells with the exception of stem cells and germ cells. However, normal stem cells still respond to appropriate physiological stimuli to regulate their growth and total numbers. Malignant cells that have largely lost their capacity to respond to these signals are thus not constrained in their relentless expansion.

The identification of these molecular alterations also suggests that inhibition of one or more of these steps might represent the basis for potent and specific antitumor drug treatments. Preclinical data as well as preliminary clinical trials indicate that this is indeed the case and that whole new classes of antitumor agents can be produced, which can be rationally used against specific categories of clinical malignancy.

Some of the most promising of these newer agents are specific inhibitors of the tyrosine kinase growth factor receptors. A particularly interesting drug is STI 151, a 2-phenylaminopyrimide compound that is undergoing large-scale clinical evaluation (4). This drug has been found to be particularly effective in inhibiting the abnormal fusion protein, bcr-abl, which is a hallmark of chronic myelogenous leukemia (CML). The bcr-abl protein functions as a continuously active tyrosine kinase growth factor receptor in CML and plays a major role in the continuous proliferation of myeloid cells in this disease. Treatment with STI 151 results in greater than 95% remission rate in CML with very little toxic side effects. Turning off bcr-abl results in massive apoptosis of leukemic cells without concomitant damage to the normal myeloid elements as they lack the *bcr-abl* gene, which arises due to a chromosomal translocation. Shutting down the growth stimulus provided by the abnormal protein removes the block to apoptosis that would otherwise occur to regulate cell numbers (5–7).

STI 151 also is a powerful inhibitor of the *c-kit* oncogene, which is structurally similar to bcr-abl. *c-kit* is overexpressed in the rare gastrointestinal malignancy, gastrointestinal stromal tumor, or GIST, which is a slow growing mesenchymal tumor of the gastrointestinal tract. More than 50% of these otherwise refractory malignancies show an excellent clinical response to treatment by STI 151 (8).

The responses seen with this drug are not permanent in most cases, with relapse by drug resistant tumors being the rule. This clearly argues for combination therapy with agents that act on the new pathways that are activated in the drug resistant state. As will be mentioned below, scientific validation and demonstrated clinical need of a drug is no assurance that the drug approval process will actively encourage it.

Another drug that has entered clinical trial is the quinazoline compound ZD 1839 (Iressa), which inhibits the epidermal growth factor receptor (EGFR) that is commonly dysregulated in many epithelial malignancies (9). Iressa has shown responses in nonsmall cell lung carcinoma (NSCLC), a tumor which is typically unresponsive to standard cytotoxic drug protocols. However, the responses tend not to be complete or highly durable, indicating that this agent will have to be employed as part of a sophisticated drug combination.

A large number of other compounds are being evaluated, which act at various points in the growth factor signaling pathways. Immediately downstream from the EGFR kinase are members of the ras family of transduction proteins. Activating mutations of ras occur in a high proportion of gastrointestinal tract carcinomas as well as in lung and breast carcinomas and in myeloid leukemia. To express their function, these proteins require the attachment of a specific cofactor, farnesyl alcohol, a reaction which requires the action of a special enzyme, farnesyl transferase. Inhibitors of farnesyl transferase are capable on their own of producing clinical responses in approximately 15% of patients with a variety of refractory malignancies (10). Early clinical trials indicate that these responses can be significantly increased by the addition of standard cytotoxic agents.

A feature of these drugs is that they are highly tumor class specific and they have relatively little toxicity as compared with the older cytotoxic agents. However, their specificity of action makes it essential that a molecular characterization of the patient's tumor be carried out with a degree of precision that until quite recently was not possible. This requires the application of a new technology known as DNA array analysis that makes it feasible to obtain a comprehensive picture of the pattern of gene expression in an individual patient's cancer (11).

DNA ARRAY ANALYSIS

The basic principle of DNA arrays involves the production of slides that contain hundreds (or thousands) of discrete spots each consisting of single stranded DNA molecules corresponding to a different gene. The investigator can choose the genes that he wishes to investigate, which could in principle include the entire list of defined human genes. In practice, one would initially select those genes that are known or suspected of being involved in a particular cancer. Messenger RNA is extracted from a clinical biopsy and cDNA is produced from the RNA. Fluorescent tags are added to the DNA and the tagged cDNA is reacted with the slide. The cDNA will bind to its complementary gene "spot" and the amount of binding will be reflected in the intensity of the fluorescent signal produced, which can then be read off by computer scanning. The result is a pattern of red and green spots that will be specific to an individual patient and more generally to a particular tumor type and subtype (12).

This type of analysis has already identified hitherto unsuspected tumor subtypes that display significant differences in prognosis and response to treatment. There is an obvious potential for greatly refining pathological diagnosis and for rational selection of agents "tailor made" for an individual patient (13).

The technology is still in its infancy and there are many practical problems that need to be solved before a high measure of confidence can be assigned to these determinations. However, even in its present state of development it is now possible to carry out an analysis in a couple of days that would have taken a dozen technologists the better part of a year to complete using older methods of molecular biology. For example, in a variation of the technique described above, one can "spot" a slide with oligonucleotides corresponding to every conceivable single nucleotide change in the gene that codes for ras. The cDNA from a biopsy can be applied to the slide and one can immediately determine if mutant ras is present and if so, where the mutation occurred. This can be accomplished in a few minutes as opposed to several weeks.

The implications of this technology has yet to be fully determined but it clearly has the potential for revolutionizing our ability to make precise diagnoses as well as aid in the development of newer and far more effective therapies.

WHICH MOLECULAR TARGETS?

Even in the preliminary reports that have appeared to date, DNA arrays have documented large numbers of gene expression differences between normal cells and their malignant counterparts. Up to several hundred differentially expressed genes have been identified and this almost certainly will represent the lower range of numbers we can expect (14). It is imperative that guidelines be developed for determining which of these many potential targets are likely to be the ones that will yield the most positive results in terms of turning off the neoplastic process.

Mention was made earlier that researchers have identified the minimum number of alterations required to transform normal cells. It seems reasonable to assume that these steps will also be the ones that are the most vulnerable to some kind of therapeutic intervention. The observation that inhibition of abnormal growth factor receptor function can be dramatically effective even on its own is consistent with this hypothesis. However, even within the three classes of transforming events, there are many different distinct processes involved. It would be very useful to have more specific rules as to which of these mechanisms will be the most important. Relying simply on trial and error approaches will have many of the problems associated with current empirical drug screening strategies. Clearly, a deeper understanding of what truly drives the neoplastic process is required.

WHAT IS THE FUNDAMENTAL "CAUSE" OF CANCER?

Up till now, we have discussed what are in effect the molecular mechanisms that produce cancer, and this has been the focus of much of cancer research over the past 20 years. Issues such as what truly constitutes the basic or *necessary* cause of cancer tends to be put aside or more specifically, it is assumed that cancers do not have a single underlying cause but rather arise from the interaction of a long list of "risk factors" that combine to produce the disease state (15,16). Despite the growing body of evidence that many human cancers have as their underlying cause the action of some type of infectious organism, the biomedical community tends to dismiss such evidence almost contemptuously. The example of the role of the bacterium *Helicobacter pylori* in human disease causation is particularly instructive.

H. pylori is a ubiquitous gram negative bacterium that colonizes many regions of the gastrointestinal tract in man and many other species. It has finally been accepted, many years after the case was proven, that *H. pylori* is the *cause* of peptic ulcers (17)—not stress, spicy foods, smoking, alcohol, or a "type A" personality. Moreover, if the bacteria are eradicated the patient is cured, usually permanently. Of potentially, even greater import is the observation that *H. pylori* is also the cause of virtually all types of gastric carcinoma (18) and if the bacteria are eradicated before the neoplastic transformation is initiated, gastric carcinoma can then be prevented in a high proportion of cases (perhaps even in all cases). The relative indifference to these stunning conclusions by the medical community (and the nonreportage in the lay press) strikes this writer as perplexing.

It is not as if there has not been abundant evidence of the causative role of oncogenic viruses in human cancer presented in the last few years. The significance of hepatitis B and C in hepatocellular carcinoma has been established (19) as well as human papilloma virus in cervical cancer (20) (and likely many other types of anogenital carcinoma) and the role of Epstein-Barr virus in many forms of malignant lymphoma (21). Several other examples could be cited, but the point is that establishing an infectious organism as the cause of a malignancy not only provides a clear strategy for prevention but in the case of oncogenic viruses, for identifying the critical molecular events that initiate and sustain the malignant state. The great majority of clinicians and researchers are still strongly wedded to their lists of risk factors, however, and it will take more time and more evidence to "shift the paradigm."

BUREAUCRATIC OBSTACLES IN DRUG DEVELOPMENT

From the considerations discussed in this paper, it is apparent that truly effective drug treatment for tumors will require the concurrent administration of at least several different types of compounds. The combinations will be tumor class specific and perhaps even individual patient specific. The problem is that the drug approval process is built around assessing individual drugs on their own and looking for levels of activity that are greater than existing "standards." If the level of activity is simply equivalent, even if the mechanism of action is different, then it is likely that the new agent will not be approved. The whole process is based on the discredited notion that there are magic bullets for cancer and that combination therapy is something that can be done after a single agent is approved. Unfortunately, if the new agents are not dramatically effective on their own, they will not be approved and we will continue on the fruitless search for a magic bullet. A process that was developed for sleeping pills has to be harmonized with what will likely be required for effective cancer therapies (22).

CONCLUSIONS

The management of most kinds of epithelial cancers has in a sense "hit the wall." It seems reasonable to expect, however, that common sense will prevail in the drug development and approval process. Scientific and technological advances have given us immensely powerful tools for expanding our understanding of cancer and for producing therapeutic agents of greatly enhanced specificity and effectiveness. Also, if it can be convincingly demonstrated that many of the major clinical malignancies have an infectious basis then truly efficacious prevention strategies can be initiated.

REFERENCES

1. Lowe SW, Ruley HE, Jacks T, Housman DE. p53-dependant apoptosis modulates the cytotoxicity of anticancer agents. Cell 1993; 74(6):957–967.

2. Martin SJ, Green DR. Apoptosis and cancer: the failure of controls on cell death and survival. Crit Rev Oncol Hematol 1995; 18(2):137–153.

3. Hahn WC, Counter CM, Lundberg AS, Beijersbergen RL, Brooks MW, Weinberg RA. Creation of human tumour cells

with defined genetic elements. Nature 1999; 400(6743): f464–468.

4. Levitzki A. Protein tyrosine kinase inhibitors as novel therapeutic agents. Pharmacol Ther 1999; 82(2–3):231–239.

5. Donato NJ, Talpaz M. Clinical use of tyrosine kinase inhibitors: therapy for chronic myelogenous leukemia and other cancers. Clin Cancer Res 2000; 6(8):2965–2966.

6. Counter CM, Hirte HW, Bacchetti S, Harley CB. Telomerase activity in human ovarian carcinoma. Proc Natl Acad Sci USA 1994; 91(8):2900–2904.

7. Druker BJ, Talpaz M, Resta DJ, Peng B, Buchdunger E, Ford JM, Lydon NB, Kantarjian H, Capdeville R, Ohno-Jones S, Sawyers CL. Clinical efficacy and safety of an Abl specific tyrosine kinase inhibitor as targeted therapy for chronic myelogenous leukemia. Blood 1999; 94:368a.

8. Strickland L, Letson GD, Muro-Cacho CA. Gastrointestinal stromal tumors. Cancer Control 2001; 8(3):252–261.

9. Arteaga CL, Johnson DH. Tyrosine kinase inhibitors-ZD1839 (Iressa). Curr Opin Oncol 2001; 13(6):491–498.

10. Karp JE, Kaufmann SH, Adjei AA, Lancet JE, Wright JJ, End DW. Current status of clinical trials of farnesyltransferase inhibitors. Curr Opin Oncol 2001; 13(6):470–476.

11. Friend SH, Stoughton RB. The magic of microarrays. Sci Am 2002; 286(2):44–49, 53.

12. Alizadeh AA, Eisen MB, Davis RE, Ma C, Lossos IS, Rosenwald A, Boldrick JC, Sabet H, Tran T, Yu X, Powell JI, Yang L, Marti GE, Moore T, Hudson J Jr, Lu L, Lewis DB, Tibshirani R, Sherlock G, Chan WC, Greiner TC, Weisenburger DD, Armitage JO, Warnke R, Levy R, Wilson W, Grever MR, Byrd JC, Botstein D, Brown PO, Staudt LM. Distinct types of diffuse large B-cell lymphoma identified by gene expression profiling. Nature 2000; 403(6769):503–511.

13. Perou CM, Sorlie T, Eisen MB, van de Rijn M, Jeffrey SS, Rees CA, Pollack JR, Ross DT, Johnsen H, Akslen LA, Fluge O, Pergamenschikov A, Williams C, Zhu SX, Lonning PE, Borresen-Dale AL, Brown PO, Botstein D. Molecular portraits of human breast tumours. Nature 2000; 406(6797):747–752.

14. Bittner M, Meltzer P, Chen Y, Jiang Y, Seftor E, Hendrix M, Radmacher M, Simon R, Yakhini Z, Ben-Dor A, Sampas N, Dougherty E, Wang E, Marincola F, Gooden C, Lueders J, Glatfelter A, Pollock P, Carpten J, Gillanders E, Leja D, Dietrich K, Beaudry C, Berens M, Alberts D, Sondak V. Molecular classification of cutaneous malignant melanoma by gene expression profiling. Nature 2000; 406(6795):536–540.

15. Goedret JJ, ed. Infectious Causes of Cancer: Targets for Intervention. Totawa, NJ: Humana Press, 2000.

16. Ewald P. Plague Time. New York: Anchor Books, 2002.

17. Marshall BJ, Warren JR. Unidentified curved bacilli in the stomach of patients with gastric and peptic ulceration. Lancet 1984; 1(8390):1273–1275.

18. Uemura N, Okamoto S, Yamamoto S, Matsumura N, Yamaguchi S, Yamakido M, Taniyama K, Sasaki N, Schlemper RJ. Helicobacter pylori infection and the development of gastric cancer. N Engl J Med 2001; 345(11):784–789.

19. Kew MC. Hepatocellular carcinoma. In: Goedert JJ, ed. Infectious Causes of Cancer: Targets for Intervention. Totawa, NJ: Humana Press, 2000:331–338.

20. Wolf JK, Ramirez PT. The molecular biology of cervical cancer. Cancer Invest 2001; 19(6):621–629.

21. de Thé G. Epstein-Barr virus and Burkitt's lymphoma. In: Goedert JJ, ed. Infectious Causes of Cancer: Targets for Intervention. Totawa, NJ: Humana Press, 2000:77–92.

22. Fernandes M. Cancer science vs. archaic bureaucracy [Letter to editor]. Wall Street J, March 4, 2002.

10

Malignant Lacrimal Gland Tumors

GEORGE B. BARTLEY

Mayo Clinic, Jacksonville, Florida, U.S.A.

With the possible exception of melanomas that arise within or around the eye, malignancies of the lacrimal gland arguably are the most deadly tumors that an ophthalmologist may encounter in clinical practice. As with most cancers, survival is improved with early detection, and early detection is more likely when the practitioner is prepared to recognize and follow-up signs and symptoms that may be relatively subtle. In this short review, I will pose a series of questions that the ophthalmologist should be considering when he or she is examining a patient with a possible lacrimal gland malignancy.

First, who are the "players" in the cast of malignant lacrimal gland tumors? Lymphoma and adenoid cystic carcinoma are the antagonists we will encounter most frequently. Malignant mixed tumors and primary adenocarcinomas play secondary roles, and an additional half dozen tumors make appearances only occasionally: mucoepidermoid carcinoma, primary squamous cell carcinoma, primary ductal adenocarcinoma, anaplastic adenocarcinoma with sebaceous differentiation, acinic cell carcinoma, and clear cell epithelial–myoepithelial carcinoma. Rarely, the lacrimal gland is the site of metastatic spread.

Table 1 summarizes the distribution of primary malignant lacrimal gland tumors seen at the Mayo Clinic in Rochester, Minnesota. These data were compiled by John W. Henderson, whose study of orbital tumors began in the 1940s and has been a life-long passion. Dr. Henderson's classic text, *Orbital Tumors*, has been published in three editions (14). The fourth edition, which comprises a half-century of clinical experience from one institution, is currently in preparation.

The frequency of pleomorphic adenomas is included in Table 1 for comparison, and it is interesting that the number of patients with this tumor has been almost identical to that of adenoid cystic carcinoma during the 50-year span of the survey. Additionally, we were surprised that no new benign mixed tumors were seen in our practice (Dr. James A. Garrity and myself) during the decade 1987–1997.

Because Table 1 includes only primary lacrimal gland tumors, metastatic or lymphomatous involvement was excluded. A fair question, therefore, is to ask how often lymphomas manifest in the lacrimal gland. The answer: "too often." Unpublished data from our institution, compiled by one of our fellows (Dr. Seyda Ugurlu), included 111 patients with orbital lymphoma examined between 1970 and 1997. Of these, 45 (40.5%) involved the lacrimal gland plus other tissues and 21 (19%) involved the lacrimal gland only. These results are similar to those reported by Coupland et al. (5). Their group studied a series of 112 patients with lymphoproliferative lesions of the ocular adnexa. Forty-four (39%) localized to the orbit. Of these 44 orbital lymphomas, 6 (14%) involved the lacrimal gland exclusively. Looking at the issue from another angle, how many patients with disseminated lymphoma have lacrimal lesions? Bairey et al. (2) reported

Table 1 Primary Malignant Lacrimal Gland Tumors: The Mayo Clinic series

	Edition 1, 1948–1966, 465 orbital tumors	Edition 2, 1948–1974, 764 orbital tumors	Edition 3, 1948–1987, 1376 orbital tumors	Edition 4, 1948–1997, 1790 orbital tumors
Adenoid cystic carcinoma	9	12	22	29
Percentage of orbital tumors	1.9	1.6	1.6	1.6
Malignant mixed tumor	7	10	10	11
Percentage of orbital tumors	1.5	1.3	0.7	0.6
Adenocarcinoma	4	4	5	8
Percentage of orbital tumors	0.9	0.5	0.4	0.4
Mucoepidermoid carcinoma	1	1	2	3
Percentage of orbital tumors	0.2	0.1	0.1	0.2
Primary squamous cell carcinoma	0	1	2	2
Percentage of orbital tumors		0.1	0.1	0.1
NB: benign mixed tumor	9	13	25	25

that 10 (5%) of 187 patients with systemic non-Hodgkin's lymphoma had orbital involvement. One of the 10 had a lacrimal gland tumor.

A parenthetical digression: when one encounters an isolated, circumscribed marginal zone B-cell lymphoma of the lacrimal gland, is excision of the involved gland without supplementary therapy (radiation therapy, chemotherapy, or both) a reasonable approach? Harris et al. (12) opined that "localized tumors may be cured with local treatment." I have treated a small number of patients in this manner with seemingly good results but admittedly have not "closed the loop" with appropriate long-term follow-up. What has been the experience of others? Coupland et al. (5), again in her excellent paper, described two patients with localized disease who were treated with excision only. One patient had no recurrence, but the length of follow-up was unspecified. A second patient was lost to follow-up. More recently, Ness et al. (20) similarly reported two patients with localized disease who were treated solely with surgical excision of the lacrimal gland tumor. Complete remission was achieved in both patients, with follow-up intervals of 42 and 150 months, respectively. Lymphoma specialists at the Mayo Clinic, when queried about this scenario, recommend supplementary radiation therapy or chemotherapy in virtually all cases, a stance echoed in print by Auw-Haedrich et al., "Primary EMZL [extranodal marginal zone lymphoma] would be treated best with an excisional biopsy, where possible, combined with radiotherapy." In the absence of a prospective randomized clinical trial to compare the long-term outcomes of various therapeutic options, most orbital surgeons feel comfortable treating presumed lacrimal gland lymphoma by performing an incisional biopsy followed by radiotherapy or chemotherapy after appropriate tumor staging.

Let us move back from treatment to diagnosis. When examining a patient in the clinic, can we predict preoperatively whether a lacrimal gland tumor is benign or malignant? With regard to lymphomas, I agree with Coupland et al. (5) who concluded that "benign and malignant lymphoid proliferations of the ocular adnexa cannot be diagnosed accurately on the basis of clinical or radiologic criteria." When dealing with primary lacrimal gland tumors, we have a better chance of heading down the correct diagnostic path if we follow the thoughtful algorithm created by Rose and Wright (12) from Moorfields Eye Hospital in London and published in 1992. In short, malignant tumors tend to present fairly rapidly, with pain, sensory loss, or other symptoms that may belie the lesion's size. The margins of the mass often are poorly defined, and the tumor may mold to the globe and contain calcium. Bony invasion obviously is a worrisome sign. This algorithm is summarized in Table 2 .

If a lacrimal gland tumor is confirmed to be malignant, what is the best treatment? Published reports have focused on adenoid cystic carcinoma because it is the most common primary malignant lacrimal gland tumor. Perhaps the fundamental question is whether radical resection (orbitectomy) yields superior survival to a more conservative surgical approach. In their study of 38 patients with adenoid cystic carcinoma published, Wright et al. (30) concluded that "disease free survival after treatment of adenoid cystic carcinoma appears unaltered by cranio-orbital resection, though these latter patients form a relatively greater proportion of those surviving for more than 10 years." More recently, Font et al. (9) reported 12 patients with lacrimal gland adenoid cystic carcinoma, all of whom had local recurrence, with an average interval of 39 months until tumor reappearance. Tumor-related death occurred in

Table 2 Algorithm for the Diagnosis of Primary Lacrimal Gland Tumors

Think malignancy	Think benignancy
Symptoms < 10 months	Symptoms > 10 months
Persistent pain	Minimal or no pain
Sensory loss	Sensation intact
Poorly defined mass	Well-defined mass
Molding to globe or bone	No molding
Calcification	No calcification
Bone invasion	No bone invasion
Size > symptoms	Symptoms > size

60% of the patients, with a mean survival of 4.5 years. The longest survivors (13 and 16 years, respectively) had undergone early exenteration, radiation therapy, and subsequent cranio-orbital resection, perhaps suggesting that an aggressive approach is preferable. The authors concluded, however, that "the problem with arriving at a consensus for treatment is that the number of long-term survivors with adenoid cystic carcinoma is so low that all studies advocating any particular treatment modality are anecdotal."

As regards nonsurgical therapy, either as primary or adjunctive treatment, the picture is equally cloudy. Conventional radiation therapy has not been demonstrated to eradicate all tumor cells in the treated field. Neutron radiotherapy has yielded impressive results in some patients with head and neck adenoid cystic carcinoma, but side effects from treatment of orbital tumors frequently are severe and significant. Anecdotal reports concerning proton beam irradiation are promising; published results are anticipated with great eagerness. The most encouraging intervention in recent years may be the use of adjunctive intraarterial chemotherapy, as described by Meldrum et al. (19). Harris (3) and I summarized the current state of treatment options in an editorial.

When are we "out of the woods" with a malignant lacrimal gland tumor? Unfortunately, the answer is "probably never." Although patients with lacrimal gland lymphoma typically respond well to a combination of incisional biopsy, chemotherapy, and radiation therapy, long-term surveillance nevertheless is required. Survival rates for primary lacrimal gland malignancies, in contrast, have improved only negligibly over the past several decades, with gains likely the result of improved imaging techniques rather than novel and robust therapeutic regimens. Even when diagnosed early and treated assertively, long-term "cures" of such tumors remain an elusive goal.

REFERENCES

1. Auw-Haedrich C, Coupland SE, Kapp, A, et al. Long term outcome of ocular adnexal lymphoma subtyped according to the REAL classification. Br J Ophthalmol 2001; 85:63–69.

2. Bairey O, Kremer I, Rakowsky E, et al. Orbital and adnexal involvement in systemic non-Hodgkin's lymphoma. Cancer 1994; 73:2395–2399.

3. Bartley GB, Harris GJ. Adenoid cystic carcinoma of the lacrimal gland: is there a cure . . . yet? Ophthal Plast Reconstr Surg 2002; 18:315–318.

4. Buchholz TA, Shimotakahara SG, Weymuller EA Jr, et al. Neutron radiotherapy for adenoid cystic carcinoma of the head and neck. Arch Otolaryngol Head Neck Surg 1993; 119: 747–752.

5. Coupland SE, Krause L, Delecluse HJ, et al. Lymphoproliferative lesions of the ocular adnexa. Analysis of 112 cases. Ophthalmology 1998; 105:1430–1441.

6. Douglas JG, Laramore GE, Austin-Seymour M, et al. Treatment of locally advanced adenoid cystic carcinoma of the head and neck with neutron radiotherapy. Int J Radiat Oncol Biol Phys 2000; 46:551–557.

7. Eviatar JA, Hornblass A. Mucoepidermoid carcinoma of the lacrimal gland: 25 cases and a review and update of the literature. Ophthal Plast Reconstr Surg 1993; 9:170–181.

8. Font RL, Gamel JW. Adenoid cystic carcinoma of the lacrimal gland. A clinicopathologic study of 79 cases. In: Nicholson DH, ed. Ocular Pathology Update. New York: Masson, 1980:277–283.

9. Font RL, Smith SL, Bryan RG. Malignant epithelial tumors of the lacrimal gland. A clinicopathologic study of 21 cases. Arch Ophthalmol 1998; 116:613–616.

10. Froula PD, Bartley GB, Garrity JA, Forbes G. The differential diagnosis of orbital calcification as detected on computed tomographic scans. Mayo Clin Proc 1993; 68:256–261.

11. Gamel JW, Font RL. Adenoid cystic carcinoma of the lacrimal gland: the clinical significance of a basaloid histologic pattern. Hum Pathol 1982; 13:219–225.

12. Harris NL, Jaffe ES, Stein H, et al. A revised European–American classification of lymphoid neoplasms: a proposal from the international lymphoma study group. Blood 1994; 84:1361–1392.

13. Heaps RS, Miller NR, Albert DM, et al. Primary adenocarcinoma of the lacrimal gland. A retrospective study. Ophthalmology 1993; 100:1856–1860.

14. Henderson JW. Orbital Tumors. 3rd ed. New York: Raven Press, 1994.

15. Henderson JW. Adenoid cystic carcinoma of the lacrimal gland, is there a cure? Trans Am Ophthalmol Soc 1987; 85:312–319.

16. Henderson JW, Farrow GM. Primary malignant mixed tumors of the lacrimal gland. Report of 10 cases. Ophthalmology 1980; 87:466–475.

17. Katz SE, Rootman J, Dolman PJ, et al. Primary ductal adenocarcinoma of the lacrimal gland. Ophthalmology 1996; 103:157–162.

18. Lee DA, Campbell RJ, Waller RR, Ilstrup DM. A clinicopathologic study of primary adenoid cystic carcinoma of the lacrimal gland. Ophthalmology 1985; 92:128–134.

19. Meldrum ML, Tse DT, Benedetto P. Neoadjuvant intracarotid chemotherapy for treatment of advanced adenocystic carcinoma of the lacrimal gland. Arch Ophthalmol 1998; 116:315–321.

20. Ness GO, Lybœk H, Arnes J, Rødahl E. Chromosomal imbalances in lymphoid tumors of the orbit. Invest Ophthal Vis Sci 2002; 43:9–14.

21. Ostrowski ML, Font RL, Halpern J, et al. Clear cell epithelial–myoepithelial carcinoma arising in pleomorphic adenoma of the lacrimal gland. Ophthalmology 1994; 101:925–930.

22. Perzin KH, Jakobiec FA, Livolsi VA, Desjardins L. Lacrimal gland malignant mixed tumors (carcinomas arising in benign mixed tumors): a clinico-pathologic study. Cancer 1980; 45:2593–2606.

23. Rodgers IR, Jakobiec FA, Gingold MP, et al. Anaplastic carcinoma of the lacrimal gland presenting with recurrent subconjunctival hemorrhages and displaying incipient sebaceous differentiation. Ophthal Plast Reconstr Surg 1991; 7:229–237.

24. Rose GE, Wright JE. Pleomorphic adenoma of the lacrimal gland. Br J Ophthalmol 1992; 76:395–400.

25. Rosenbaum PS, Mahadevia PS, Goodman LA, Kress Y. Acinic cell carcinoma of the lacrimal gland. Arch Ophthalmol 1995; 113:781–785.

26. Shields JA, Shields L. Malignant transformation of presumed pleomorphic adenoma of lacrimal gland after 60 years. Arch Ophthalmol 1987; 105:1403–1405.

27. Tellado MV, McLean IW, Specht CS, Varga J. Adenoid cystic carcinomas of the lacrimal gland in childhood and adolescence. Ophthalmology 1997; 104:1622–1625.

28. Tibolt RE, Meyer DR, Wobig JL. Small-cell carcinoma metastatic to the lacrimal gland. Arch Ophthalmol 1991; 109: 921–922.

29. Tse DT, Neff AG, Onofrey CB. Recent developments in the evaluation and treatment of lacrimal gland tumors. Ophthalmol Clin North Am 2000; 13:663–681.

30. Wright JE, Rose GE, Garner A. Primary malignant neoplasms of the lacrimal gland. Br J Ophthalmol 1992; 76:401–407.

11

The Management of Optic Nerve Sheath and Sphenoid Wing Meningiomas

JOHN S. KENNERDELL,
KIMBERLY P. COCKERHAM, and
ROGER E. TURBIN
Department of Ophthalmology,
Allegheny General Hospital, Pittsburgh,
Pennsylvania, U.S.A.

JOSEPH C. MAROON
Presbyterian University Hospital,
Pittsburgh, Pennsylvania, U.S.A.

Meningiomas, a term introduced by Cushing (1922), arise from the meninges and appear to originate from the arachnoid cap cells which line the outer surface of the arachnoid. There is disagreement as to their origin—neural crest or mesenchyme. They occur in the intracranial area, the spine or orbit. They represent 13–18% of all primary intracranial tumors in most large series. Up to 4% of primary intracranial meningiomas occur in children, and there is general agreement that they tend to be more aggressive in children than in adults. Meningiomas favor the elderly and are two to three times more prevalent in women, a gender bias that may be related to the estrogen or progesterone receptors in these tumors. It is not uncommon for meningiomas to be multiple, especially in patients with neurofibromatosis type 2 (NF2). The usual course is slow progression, but variable growth rates may occur resulting in acute onset of functional defects. Because meningiomas are characteristically indolent, discovery is often incidental at autopsy or when computed tomography (CT) or magnetic resonance imaging (MRI) is performed for unrelated reasons.

Although, there are five cytologic types, these subtypes do not significantly influence clinical activity, particularly with sphenoid wing and optic nerve sheath meningiomas. Although the presence of a syncytial pattern with whorls and psammoma bodies is helpful in histologic diagnosis of meningioma, malignancy is determined by rapidity of growth and recurrence rather than the presence of mitotic figures. The malignant form of meningioma is uncommon. Meningiomas can be associated with other intracranial tumors, particularly in patients with neurofibromatosis.

The diagnosis of meningioma has been revolutionized by CT and MRI, particularly with contrast enhancement. *This is one tumor in which both scans are helpful to identify the characteristics of the lesion.* The soft-tissue characteristics and the relationship to the optic nerve are best seen with gadolinium-enhanced MRI. The presence of calcium and involvement of bone are best evaluated with the CT.

Until the development of these diagnostic entities, many meningiomas were not identified until functional loss was profound. Magnetic resonance angiography and traditional angiography are of limited value in the evaluation of the meningioma; however, if the tumor appears highly vascular on neuro-imaging, angiography is utilized to identify the large feeder vessels, which may require embolization prior to removal of the tumor.

The optic nerve sheath meningioma arises from the intraorbital portion of the optic nerve secondarily by spread from an intracranial meningioma located in the sphenoid wing (particularly the inner third), tuberculum sella, or olfactory groove. The intraorbital meningioma may spread along the optic nerve within the dura (endophytic), actually surrounding and crushing it, even to the point of central retinal artery or vein occlusion. Rarely, optic nerve meningiomas exit the dura almost immediately and surround the optic nerve, acting like an intraconal orbital tumor compressing the optic nerve (exophytic). A combination of the intra- and extradural components can occur, having both characteristics. This variable growth pattern has made the optic nerve meningioma difficult to manage, particularly those tumors that remain within the dura. The primary optic nerve sheath meningioma follows the gender bias and age patterns of other meningiomas. Most are unilateral, but bilateral cases can occur, primarily in the younger age group or with NF2. They usually present initially with blurred vision and loss of color vision with a relative afferent pupillary defect. Occasionally, there is limitation of ocular motility, slight ptosis (usually upgaze), or slight proptosis. Upper or lower eyelid edema may be present. Transient visual obscurations can occasionally occur, and visual field loss is variable, but can consist of a central scotoma and/or arcuate field loss. Optic nerve meningiomas characteristically progress to an irregular depression of the central visual field and finally to total blindness.

The optic disc of the affected eye may be normal, pale, or edematous (often with a chronic appearance). In advanced cases, opticociliary shunt vessels may develop on the optic disc to bypass the induced constriction of venous drainage of the distal nerve. Optic nerve edema can occasionally be caused by an optic canal meningioma but more commonly is associated with a primary optic nerve sheath meningioma in the mid or anterior orbit. Primary optic nerve sheath meningiomas usually do not cause significant pain, but mild discomfort has been reported.

The visual acuity and visual field loss early in the course of the optic nerve sheath meningioma usually progresses slowly and can remain at relatively normal levels for a considerable period of time. However, nearly all patients with primary optic nerve sheath meningiomas gradually lose vision, often to total blindness of the involved eye. Therefore, treatment modalities have been sought to preserve function as long as possible. In 1977, we were able to remove a meningioma that was eccentric to the optic nerve and restored vision in a woman from 20/200 to 20/20. Her visual field recovered nearly completely as well. She has now been followed for more than 20 years and the meningioma has recurred in the medial orbit, but does not compress the optic nerve at this time. She will need removal of the tumor through an anterior medial orbitotomy if afferent dysfunction recurs.

In contrast, most of the primary optic nerve sheath meningiomas are located in the intradural space or as a combination of intra- and extradural components. On MRI, they have a characteristic appearance with the nerve surrounded by gadolinium-enhanced tumor (the tram track sign). On CT, the nerve appears thickened and may be calcified. These are more difficult to manage, and although biopsy of the extradural component is usually safe, biopsy or attempted removal of the intradural component leads to marked decrease in vision, probably due to the interruption of the blood supply to the optic nerve. We also have learned that a neurosurgical approach that allows successful removal of most of the intradural portion of the meningioma results in further postoperative orbital progression. The clinical course, in combination with neuro-imaging, allows us to diagnosis most intradural primary optic nerve sheath meningiomas with confidence, when agreement is reached between the ophthalmologist, neurosurgeon, and neuro-radiologist regarding the nature of the tumor. Therefore, we developed a strategy of treating these patients with progressive vision loss before the loss was profound: radiotherapy (5000–5500 rad) is directed from a lateral portal with global protection without a biopsy, or with biopsy of the extradural portion only.

THERAPEUTIC RECOMMENDATIONS

1. If visual acuity is between 20/20 and 20/30, OBSERVE.
2. If visual acuity is 20/30 or worse with progressive visual fields, RADIATION.

3. If vision is no light perception, SURGICAL EXCISION.

Based on 30 years of experience, we have found that patients with progressive vision loss due to presumed or biopsied primary optic nerve sheath meningiomas can maintain or improve their usual functional vision following radiotherapy.

In 1988, we reported a series of 39 optic nerve sheath meningiomas: 18 were observed, 6 radiated, 10 totally removed, and 5 had partial excision or biopsy followed by radiation therapy. Only the six who were radiated, retained or improved vision in the affected eye for 3–6 years (Fig. 1). Recently, we have completed a multicenter study that confirms that radiotherapy preserves long-term visual function in patients with primary optic nerve sheath meningiomas. In the study, we compared long-term visual outcome in patients with primary optic nerve sheath meningiomas managed by traditional treatments. The group evaluated consisted of 55 women and 9 men. We used a decimal visual acuity scale limiting the investigation to assessment of visual acuity. In addition, we used a nonparametric testing plan and statistical analysis to determine the effect of various management methods. The treatment methods analyzed were observation (13 patients), surgery only (12), radiation only after radiologic diagnosis (18 patients),

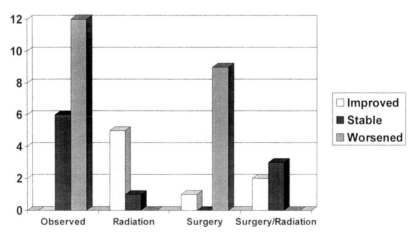

Figure 1   1988 Optic Nerve Sheath Meningioma Study.

and surgery consisting of a biopsy followed by radiation (16 patients). The patients treated with radiation only clearly had better long-term visual outcomes than patients who were simply observed. As suspected, patients with surgical removal of the optic nerve suffered profound visual loss and patients who underwent surgery followed by radiation did not have good visual preservation (Fig. 2). The radiation dosage was 4000–5500 rad with the majority receiving between 5000 and 5500 rad. The radiation often improved vision with long-term maintenance of the improvement.

Our conclusion is that patients with optic nerve sheath meningiomas receiving radiation treatment only, after convincing radiologic diagnosis, demonstrated the best visual outcome during the period of follow-up. We recommend radiation for patients who have optic nerve sheath meningiomas, characteristic in clinical course and neuroradiologic findings, for long-term preservation of visual function.

Radiation complications were seen in 33% of the patients and included vascular occlusion or retinopathy in four patients, persistent iritis in one, and temporal lobe atrophy in one. The patients with surgery only or radiation and surgery had significant complication rates of 66.0% and 62.5%, respectively. This also convinces us that the complications of other treatments

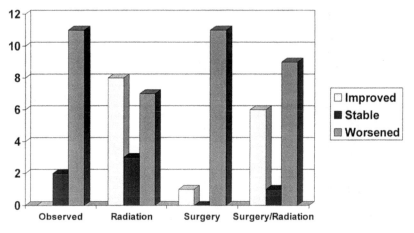

Figure 2   2001 Optic Nerve Sheath Meningioma Study.

justify the management of these patients with radiation without the necessity of biopsy in characteristic cases.

Of course, children with optic nerve meningiomas are treated more aggressively with complete surgical removal in unilateral cases and radiation of at least one nerve in aggressive bilateral optic nerve cases.

SPHENOID WING MENINGIOMAS

Sphenoid wing meningiomas arise from the arachnoid adjacent to the sphenoid wing. The sphenoid wing is about 5 cm long, but the tumors are usually divided into those arising from the outer, middle, or inner wing. We manage all sphenoid wing meningiomas in a similar fashion.

Sphenoid wing meningiomas can grow quite large intracranially. They have a propensity to invade the bone causing significant boney thickening, which results in proptosis and fullness of the temporalis fossa, often prior to functional loss of vision or extraocular movement. Of course, the more medial the tumor, the earlier effect on visual function and the less tendency for significant proptosis. Outer sphenoid wing meningiomas often have a significant boney component and are often confused with fibrous dysplasia, although they characteristically occur in an older age group. The soft-tissue components of these meningiomas tend to invade the superior orbital fissure, the cavernous sinus, and the lateral superior orbit. The outer wing meningiomas, if they grow large intracranially, can cause dementia or personality changes as an initial clinical sign. Occasionally, they are quite vascular and can hemorrhage into themselves with catastrophic neurologic sequelae. The orbital extension is typically extraconal and superolateral between the lateral and/or superior recti muscles and the adjacent orbital wall. Occasionally, they invade the intraconal space, making them more difficult to remove from the orbit.

These meningiomas are usually easily diagnosed with MRI or CT. Both techniques are recommended as MRI better shows the soft-tissue component, especially with gadolinium, and CT better shows better the extent of boney involvement.

The treatment of the sphenoid meningiomas continues to be surgical resection as complete as possible. Unfortunately, subtotal excision is common due to the proximity to and infiltration of the orbit and cavernous sinus. In the late 1970s, we realized that we were frequently operating on meningiomas which had recurred, so we sought a therapy to prevent recurrence following surgery. It was found that external beam radiation can effectively delay recurrence following subtotal removal. It is often impossible to totally remove the sphenoid wing meningioma, particularly when it invades the crevices of the superior orbital fissure, cavernous sinus, or the orbit. In addition, radiation therapy can preserve the remaining visual function, as it does with primary optic nerve sheath meningiomas. The dose is 5000–5500 rad of external beam radiation from a lateral port. In 1996, we previously reported the effectiveness of radiation therapy following subtotal excision of sphenoid wing meningiomas, thus preventing recurrences (Figs. 3 and 4). We have found that radiation therapy following subtotal removal of these tumors delays recurrences in both primary and recurrent tumors. Recently, after a review of our sphenoid wing meningiomas with a longer follow-up period, we again found that recurrence is prevented if radiation therapy is delivered approximately 2 months following

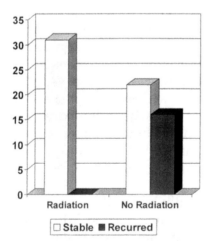

• 69 subtotally excised primary tumors

• 38 surgery alone
  – 16 recurred
  – Mean time to recurrence: 5 years

• 31 surgery and radiation
  – No recurrences
  – Mean follow-up: 4 years

Figure 3 Primary sphenoid wing meningiomas, 1996.

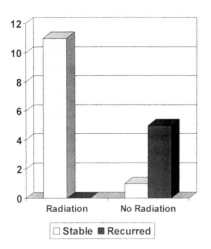

- 17 recurrent tumors

- 6 surgery alone

- 11 surgery and radiation

- No patient receiving radiation recurred during follow-up (mean: 3.5 years)

Figure 4 Recurrent sphenoid wing meningiomas, 1996.

the initial tumor excision, and appears to delay recurrence in already recurrent tumors (Figs. 5 and 6).

In our study, 65 primary sphenoid meningiomas were evaluated. No patients receiving radiation 2 months after their initial excision recurred. In contrast, 28 patients not

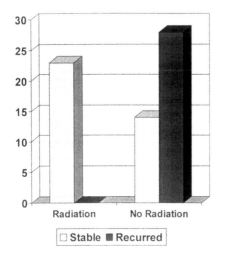

- 65 primary tumors

- 42 surgery alone
  - 28 recurred
  - Mean time to recurrence: 5 years

- 23 surgery and radiation
  - No recurrences
  - Mean follow-up: 7 years

Figure 5 Primary sphenoid wing meningiomas, 2002.

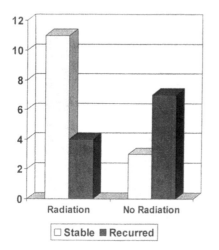

- 10 surgery alone
  - 7 recurred, all symptomatic
  - Mean time to recurrence: 2 years

- 15 surgery and radiation
  - 4 recurred, 2 symptomatic
  - Mean time to recurrence: 5 years

Figure 6 Recurrent sphenoid wing meningiomas, 2002.

receiving radiation recurred (14 were stable). For already recurrent tumors, 70% of patients who did not receive radiation recurred. This contrasts with 27% recurrence rate in the recurrent tumors who received postoperative radiotherapy.

Other therapies for large intracranial meningiomas have been tried. Hormonal therapy is of limited effectiveness. Hydroxyurea therapy is somewhat useful in inoperable or aggressive intracranial meningiomas, but not of value in sphenoid wing or optic nerve sheath meningiomas. Gene therapy is promising in meningiomas but because of their indolent course and other priorities for gene therapy, it will be some time before these may be of practical use.

Finally, studies on the social and functional aspect of patients treated surgically with or without radiotherapy show that the majority of patients undergoing treatment for intracranial meningioma remain functional, productive, and capable of independent living. Timely radiation in optic nerve sheath meningiomas and surgical debulking augmented with radiation in sphenoid wing meningiomas maximizes patients' long-term visual and neurologic functions.

REFERENCES
Optic Nerve Sheath Meningiomas

1. Alper MG. Management of primary optic nerve sheath meningiomas. J Clin Neuro Ophthalmol 1981; 1(2):101–117.

2. Dutton JJ. Optic nerve sheath meningiomas. Survey Ophthalmol 1992; 37(3):167–183.

3. Jakobiec FA, Depot MJ, Kennerdell JS, Shults WT, Anderson RL, Alper ME, Citrin CM, Housepian EM, Trokel SL. Combined clinical and computed tomographic diagnosis of orbital glioma and meningioma. Ophthalmology 1984; 91(2):137–155.

4. Kennerdell JS, Maroon JC, Garrity J, Warren F. The management of optic nerve sheath meningiomas. Am J Ophthalmol 1988; 106:450–457.

5. Smith JL, Vuksanovic MM, Yates BM, Bienfang DC. Radiation therapy for primary optic nerve meningiomas. J Clin Neuro Ophthalmol 1981; 1(2):85–99.

6. Sibony PA, Kennerdell JS, Slamovits TI, Lessell S, Krauss HR. Intrapapillary retractile bodies in optic nerve sheath meningioma. Arch Ophthalmol 1985; 103:383–385.

Sphenoid Wing Meningiomas

1. Al-Mefty O, Kersh JE, Routh A, Smith RR. The long-term side effects of radiation therapy for benign brain tumors in adults. J Neurosurg 1990; 73:502–512.

2. Cockerham KP, Kennerdell JS, Maroon JC. Tumors of the meninges and related tissues: meningiomas and sarcomas. In: Miller NR, Newman NJ, eds. Walsh and Hoyt Textbook of Neuro-Ophthalmology. Vol. 2. 5th ed. Baltimore: Williams & Wilkins, 1997:2017–2082.

3. Goldsmith BJ, Wara WM, Wilson CB, Larson DA. Postoperative irradiation for subtotally resected meningiomas. A retrospective analysis of 140 patients treated from 1967 to 1990. J Neurosurg 1994; 80:195–201.

4. Maroon JC, Kennerdell JS, Vidovich DV, Abla A, Sternau L. Recurrent spheno-orbital meningioma. J Neurosurg 1994; 80(2):202–208.

5. Newman SA. Meningiomas: a quest for the optimum therapy. J Neurosurg 1994; 80:191–194.

6. Peele KA, Kennerdell JS, Maroon JC, Kalnicki S, Kazim M, Gardner T, Malton M, Goodglick T, Rosen C. The role of post-operative radiation in the surgical management of sphenoid wing meningiomas. Ophthalmology 1996; 103(11):1761–1766.

12

Gliomas of the Anterior Visual Pathway

JONATHAN J. DUTTON

University of North Carolina,
Chapel Hill, North Carolina, U.S.A.

Intrinsic tumors of the optic nerve include optic gliomas and optic sheath meningiomas. Together, they account for less than 4% of all orbital tumors, with optic gliomas representing approximately 65% and meningioma 35% of this group (1). Despite the large literature that has accumulated concerning anterior visual pathway gliomas, there is still considerable controversy regarding their natural history and appropriate management (2).

In 1816, Antonio Scarpa gave the first clinical description of optic nerve tumors. His patients clearly had several different diseases, including extraocular extension of retinoblastoma and adult optic sheath meningioma. However, some were children who appear to have had gliomas of the optic nerve extending to the chiasm and even infiltrating the hypothalamus. Treatment was by enucleation and extirpation of the optic nerve within the orbit. Since that time, the disease has been characterized and defined more precisely as a distinct clinical entity.

CLINICAL CHARACTERISTICS

Demographics

The mean age at presentation for all optic gliomas is 8–9 years with a median age of 7 years (1). It has been reported in patients from birth to 79 years of age, but 70% are in the first decade of life. Although several studies suggest that age predilections are associated with specific tumor locations, this has not been confirmed with larger series. There is no sex predilection, with 50% of patients being male and 50% female.

Location

Gliomas may occur at any location along the visual pathway from the optic nerve to the occipital cortex. Reliable data are available only from more recent series where computer tomographic (CT) or magnetic resonance imaging (MRI) studies were obtained. Many older series relied upon clinical data to deduce tumor location. Among 600 cases where reliable data are available, 7% are confined to the chiasm alone, and 69% occur in the chiasm and adjacent optic nerve or brain (1). Only 24% of gliomas are confined to the optic nerve. Rarely, the tumor may extend to the optic disk. It has been stated that in patients with neurofibromatosis, there is a greater incidence of pure optic nerve gliomas, and this has been reiterated in several more recent studies.

Association with Neurofibromatosis

An association between neurofibromatosis and optic pathway gliomas was first noted as early as 1873, and has since been confirmed in all larger series. Among patients with neurofibromatosis, the incidence of optic gliomas determined on CT scan is about 15%, although only about 20% will show evidence of visual impairment. It is therefore important that all patients with neurofibromatosis type 1 have periodic neuroimaging studies.

The exact incidence of neurofibromatosis among patients with optic pathway gliomas has been a matter of some debate, with estimates varying from 10% to 70%. When all data are taken together, however, about 29% of children with optic gliomas show stigmata of neurofibromatosis type 1 (1). The true incidence may be higher since many studies fail to mention the presence or absence of such findings.

PRESENTING SIGNS AND SYMPTOMS

The signs and symptoms of optic pathway gliomas depend largely on tumor location. When confined to the orbital optic nerve, symptoms are those associated with an orbital tumor, including unilateral proptosis, diplopia, ptosis or eyelid retraction, and optic disk edema (Fig. 1A). With tumors of the chiasm and little or no orbital component, there may be minimal or no orbital signs.

Regardless of tumor location, most patients experience some degree of visual dysfunction. Overall, 88% show some visual loss with 25% having good vision of 20/40 or better, and 55% having significant visual loss of 20/300 or worse. More than 75% of patients show optic nerve disturbance with a relative afferent papillary defect, visual field defect, and decreased color vision. Optic atrophy is common, seen in 60% of patients, most with involvement of the orbital optic nerve.

With extension of tumor into the midbrain, hypothalamic signs may predominate. These include precocious puberty, obesity, diabetes insipidus, panhypopituitarism, and dwarfism. Hydrocephalus may follow third ventricle involvement. Seizures and diencephalic syndrome have also been reported.

RADIOGRAPHIC IMAGING

With the advent of CT imaging, diagnostic accuracy for this lesion has increased considerably. On CT, the orbital glioma

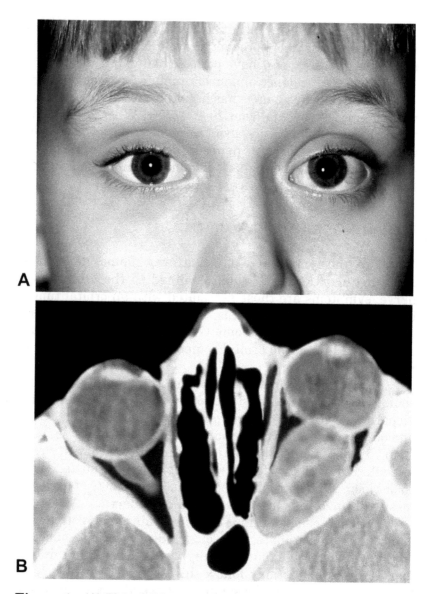

Figure 1   (A) This child presented with left proptosis, visual loss, elevation of the disk, and some lateral episcleral venous dilatation. (B) CT revealed a fusiform, heterogeneous, well-delineated expansion of the optic nerve by a tumor mass that is causing indentation of the globe and expansion of the orbital apex.

appears as a well-outlined enlargement of the optic nerve that is usually fusiform, but may be more rounded or even multi-lobulated (Fig. 1B). Increased tortuosity or kinking of the nerve is a common finding (3). The optic canal may be enlarged compared to the contralateral side when the canalicular portion of the nerve is involved. The tumor is isodense to brain but typically shows a heterogeneous structure. Less dense cystic spaces correspond to areas of mucinous accumulation. Small high-attenuation foci of calcification are rare. Following contrast administration, enhancement is heterogeneous and variable from imperceptible to moderate. For patients with neurofibromatosis, it should be kept in mind that a normal CT scan in younger children does not preclude the future development of an optic nerve glioma, and these studies should be repeated at intervals.

On the T1-weighted MRI study, gliomas are isointense or slightly hypointense with respect to cortical gray mater (Fig. 2) (4). A dilated subarachnoid space filled with cerebrospinal fluid may image as a hypointense zone surrounding the tumor. Low signal hypointense areas within the lesion represent cysts of mucinous degeneration and necrosis. On T2-weighted images, the signal may be more variable. Small fusiform tumors can be homogeneously hyperintense due to the proton-rich water component and prolonged relaxation time. Larger lesions are usually heterogeneous with a peripheral zone of hyperintense arachnoidal hyperplasia and cerebrospinal fluid, and a hypointense inner zone of optic nerve and glial cells. There is moderate to marked enhancement with gadolinium, but less than with meningioma.

ULTRASOUND

Standardized echography allows the evaluation of the orbital optic nerve that is complimentary to radiographic studies. B-scan typically shows widening of the optic nerve void (Fig. 3A). Large gliomas appear as a smooth, fusiform, or oval mass of low density replacing the normal wedge-shaped optic nerve shadow (5). The optic nerve may be kinked behind

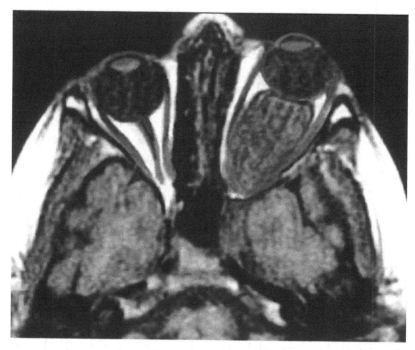

Figure 2 T1-weighted MR scan demonstrates a fusiform tumor mass of the optic nerve, which was found to be an optic nerve glioma.

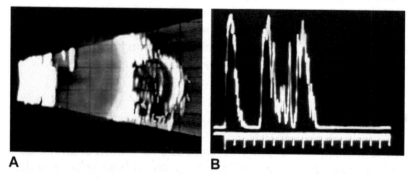

A   B

Figure 3 (A) B-scan ultrasound of an optic nerve tumor demonstrates a well-delineated margin. Irregular echoes are seen on A-scan, which also shows low internal reflectivity consistent with glioma (B).

the globe. The A-scan cross-section shows marked widening of the optic nerve defect within the orbital fat. The internal structure is regular and reflectivity is low (Fig. 3B).

HISTOPATHOLOGY

The histologic picture is that of a benign pilocytic ("hair like") astrocytoma (Fig. 4). Elongated spindle-shaped astrocytes with uniform oval nuclei form intersecting bundles that distend the fibrous pial septa of the optic nerve. The astrocytes are cytologically benign and mitotic figures are not apparent. In most tumors, there are some astrocytes with spherical or cylindrical, swollen cell processes that stain brightly eosinophilic ("Rosenthal fibers"). There are usually pale cystic areas scattered among the astrocytes; these contain mucin (glycosaminoglycans) that can be highlighted using histochemical

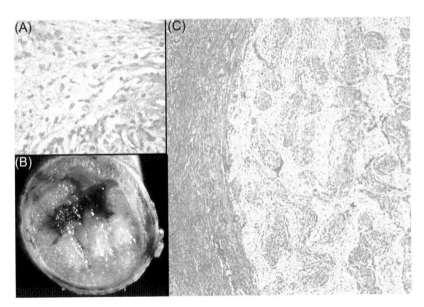

Figure 4   (A) Intraoperative photograph of an optic nerve glioma. (B) Gross and (C) Histologic features of an optic nerve glioma demonstrate expansion of the optic nerve by a loosely arranged pilocytic astrocytoma confined within the dural sheath.

stains. Mucin may be particularly prominent in longstanding tumors. If the tumor infiltrates the surrounding meninges, then the astrocytes are accompanied by fibroblasts and meningothelial cells. Though not usually necessary for diagnosis, the astrocytic nature of the neoplasm can be immunohistochemically confirmed in paraffin sections using antibodies against glial fibrillary acidic protein (GFAP).

TREATMENT AND PROGNOSIS

There remains some controversy over the appropriate management of optic gliomas (6). Much of the debate results from a general lack of understanding of the natural history of this disease, and from small series of patients and short follow-up intervals. Nevertheless, it is clear that gliomas are true neoplasms with the potential for growth and spread into adjacent tissues, and therefore must be treated with this risk in mind.[1]

For lesions confined to the orbit with good vision and minimal proptosis, observation with serial MR imaging is appropriate. Visual loss is common, but typically stabilizes with time. If severe proptosis and blindness result, surgical excision should be considered for palliation and cosmesis. However, if the tumor remains stable, no specific therapy is necessary.

With documented posterior extension that threatens the chiasm, surgical excision should be considered because of the associated increased morbidity and mortality (Fig. 5). For large tumors already involving the chiasm, surgical debulking followed by adjunctive therapy may delay other CNS complications, but contralateral visual loss is a significant risk of any surgery. Although the data are inconclusive, radiotherapy may be effective in advanced cases but may cause major CNS morbidity in young children. Multiple agent chemotherapy for chiasmatic or recurrent tumors may delay progression. Preliminary studies are encouraging, but longer follow-up intervals and larger series will be needed before any firm conclusions can be drawn.

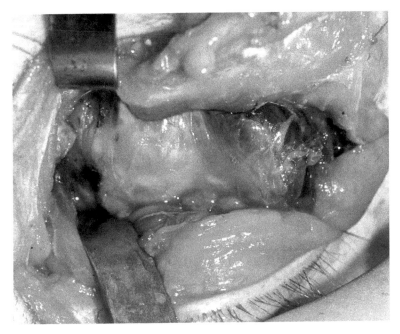

Figure 5 Surgical excision of optic gliomas.

The prognosis for vision is variable. After initial visual deterioration seen in 80% of patients, vision tends to stabilize. In 26% of cases, vision remains better than 20/40, and in 45% better than 20/200. The prognosis for life depends on tumor location and involvement of adjacent structures. For orbital lesions, the prognosis for life is excellent, with a mortality rate less than 5%. With chiasmal involvement, mortality rises to 20%, from ultimate midbrain invasion. Once the hypothalamus or third ventricles are involved, mortality rises to 55% over 10 years.

REFERENCES

1. Dutton JJ. Gliomas of the anterior visual pathway. Surv Ophthalmol 1994; 38(5):427–452.

2. Garvey M, Packer RJ. An integrated approach to the treatment of chiasmatic–hypothalamic gliomas. J Neurooncol 1996; 28(2–3):167–183.

3. Jakobiec FA, Depot MJ, Kennerdell JS, Shults WT, Anderson RL, Alper ME, Citrin CM, Housepian EM, Trokel SL. Combined clinical and computed tomographic diagnosis of orbital glioma and meningioma. Ophthalmology 1984; 91(2):137–155.

4. Haik BG, Saint-Louis L, Bierly J, Smith ME, Abramson DA, Ellsworth RM, Wall M. Magnetic resonance imaging in the evaluation of optic nerve gliomas. Ophthalmology 1987; 94(6): 709–717.

5. Ossoinig KC, Cennamo Byrne SF. Echographic differential diagnosis of optic nerve lesions. In: Thijssen JM, Verbeek AM, eds. Ultrasonography in Ophthalmology: Proceedings of the 8th SIDUO Congress. Dordrecht: Dr. W. Junk, 1981:327.

6. Listernick R, Louis DN, Packer RJ, Gutmann DH. Optic pathway gliomas in children with neurofibromatosis1: consensus statement from the NF1 Optic Pathway Glioma Task Force. Ann Neurol 1997; 41(2):143–149.

13

Stereotactic Radiotherapy for Optic Nerve and Meningeal Lesions

ROY MA

Department of Radiation Oncology,
British Columbia Cancer Agency,
Vancouver, British Columbia, Canada

BACKGROUND

Meningiomas and other tumors arising from the optic nerve often present with progressive visual deficits, which may be indolent in the case of meningioma. Treatment with radiotherapy is often indicated for tumor control and visual preservation. Since the tumor is usually small and is located in close proximity to many radiosensitive and critical structures, the technique of stereotactic irradiation is ideal for the delivery of a finely focused beam of radiation to the tumor with maximal sparing of adjacent normal tissue.

139

DEFINITIONS

Stereotactic irradiation is defined as the accurate delivery of high doses of radiation to a stereotactically defined target (the tumor) in such a way that the dose fall-off outside the target volume is very sharp. The radiation prescription can be given in one of two ways: (1) when the treatment is delivered in a single fraction, the term "stereotactic radiosurgery" (SRS) is used, and (2) when the treatment is delivered in a fractionated manner over a number of weeks, it is called "stereotactic radiation therapy" (SRT). For patients with salvageable vision, the latter is more appropriate because fractionation optimizes the effect of radiation on cycling tumor cells and minimizes the damage to late responding neural tissue such as the optic nerve.

METHODS OF STEREOTACTIC RADIATION THERAPY

The three essential components of SRT are precise immobilization, precise tumor localization, and conformal treatment planning and delivery. Each will be described briefly as follows.

Precise Immobilization

To allow for fractionation of stereotactic irradiation, several devices that provide a relocatable coordinate system have been developed. Generally, these are rigid thermoplastic mask and/or bite block systems with a repositioning accuracy of ±1.0 mm both axially and in the superior to inferior direction (Fig. 1).

Precise Tumor Localization

In SRT, the location of the tumor to be irradiated must be defined to within 1 mm accuracy in three-dimensional (3D) space. The task of tumor localization starts with acquisition of thin-slice, contrast-enhanced axial computed tomographic

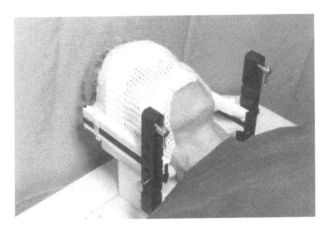

Figure 1 Thermoplastic mask and bite block for SRT.

(CT) and magnetic resonance images (MRI) done in the immo-bilization system. In order to achieve the required level of precision, an external fiducial system is commonly employed (Fig. 2). This allows for the accurate transfer of the tumor location, with respect to a known 3D coordinate system, from the planning image studies to the subsequent radiation treat-ment machine.

To help with the definition of the tumor boundary, the CT and MRI image data sets are coregistered in a 3D

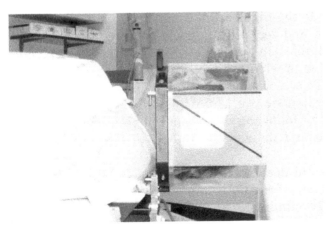

Figure 2 Patient undergoing CT scan with external fiducial system.

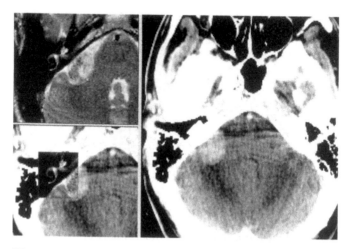

Figure 3 Co-registered axial images from a CT and MRI scans.

planning computer, which enables the reconstruction of the images in coronal, sagittal, or other defined planes (Fig. 3).

Conformal Treatment Planning and Delivery

Stereotactic radiation therapy may be delivered using either photons (most common) or charged particles. Due to its characteristic Bragg peak, a proton beam offers an advantage in dose reduction at depths greater than the target tumor. However, due to the high cost of construction and the considerable physics and technical support required, proton therapy is available in only a few centers worldwide. Conversely, due to wide availability of the linear accelerator (LINAC), SRT is more commonly delivered by high-energy photons generated from a LINAC modified for SRT application. Hence, the following discussion on treatment planning considerations and delivery is limited to the LINAC-based technology.

The minimal dose/fractionation that is required to prevent progression of an optic nerve astrocytoma or meningioma is 45 Gy administered in 25 fractions over 5 weeks. Therefore, the primary aim of treatment planning is to deliver this dose to the periphery of the tumor with the central maximum dose not exceeding 50 Gy in order to limit the risk of radiation optic neuropathy and retinopathy to less than 5%. Secondary considerations of treatment planning are to minimize the dose to the lens and the pituitary gland as damage to these organs, albeit correctable, has a low dose threshold. Lastly, minimizing the dose of radiation to the mesial temporal and orbitofrontal lobes of the brain would be prudent, as the threshold for damage to the limbic system is unknown and the effects are likely complex and long lasting.

Since a LINAC is originally designed to irradiate targets up to 40 cm in size, tertiary collimation is required to restrict the radiation beam down to a maximum size of approximately 4 cm for SRT use. As an optic nerve tumor is usually very elongated in shape, the most simple method is to use an array of multiple noncoplanar fixed beams, each of which conforms to the cross-section of the tumor in the "beam's eye view." Tertiary collimators fabricated from Cerrobend, a low melting point alloy consisting of 50% bismuth, 26% lead, 13% tin, and 10% cadmium, are the most cost-effective solution. However, because each collimator has to be manually mounted onto the treatment head of the LINAC before each beam is used, it is impractical to use more than 5–6 beams per treatment session. As a result, this leads to "dose peaks" along the entrance path of each beam (Fig. 4).

The introduction of the micro-multileaf collimator (mMLC) represents a big advancement in the technology of tertiary collimation. Depending on its manufacturer, an mMLC usually consists of 20–30 pairs of computer-controlled Tungsten leaves, each of which is usually 2–5 mm in width (Fig. 5).

Even in its most basic application, the mMLC allows for a rapid and automated deployment of a large number of static beams (Fig. 6). A more advanced application is the use of dynamic arc treatment—a dynamic shaping of the beam during gantry rotation, thus simulating an infinite number of static beams distributed in the most optimal distribution (Fig. 7). This results in greatly diminished entrance "dose peaks" compared to the dose distribution of Fig. 4.

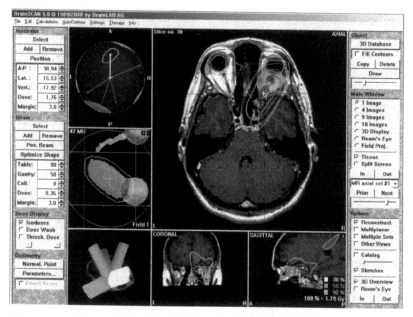

Figure 4 Dose distribution from a 5-beam radiation plan using cerrobend tertiary collimators.

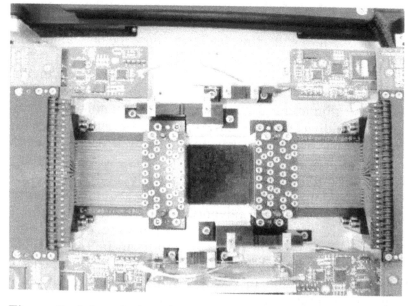

Figure 5 Internal view of a micro-multileaf collimator.

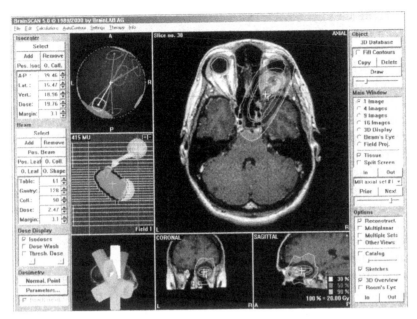

Figure 6 Dose distribution from a conformat 6-beam radiation plan using micro-multileaf collimator.

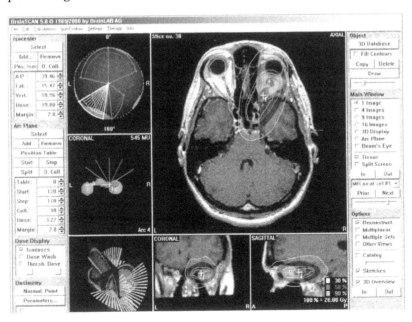

Figure 7 Dose distribution from a 6-sagittal dynamic arc radiation plan using micro-multileaf collimators.

FUTURE DEVELOPMENTS

An extension of conformal fixed beam technique is the use of the mMLC for intensity-modulated radiotherapy (IMRT). In IMRT, the movements of the Tungsten leaves into the beam's path modulate the photon fluence of the beam during irradiation. Therefore, if a critical structure resides within a beam's path and cannot be avoided, the application of IMRT can decrease the dose delivered in the portion of the field where the critical structure is located. The other fields then supplement additional dose to that portion of the tumor. Because of the complexity of IMRT planning, an inverse planning algorithm is used. This requires that the minimal dose to the tumor volume and maximum doses to the critical structures are first defined. Then, through multiple iterations, the planning algorithm deduces the optimal beam arrangements and intensity modulation within each field. As the dose prescription for the treatment of optic nerve neoplasms is relatively modest, it is unclear whether IMRT confers an advantage over the other non-IMRT conformal techniques discussed.

SUMMARY

Optic nerve neoplasm is ideally treated with SRT. With the advent of the mMLC, multiple conformal fixed beams and dynamic arc technique have become a reality for routine clinical treatment. The potential benefit of IMRT in the treatment of optic nerve neoplasms is promising and warrants research.

14

Pathogenesis of Graves' Ophthalmopathy

COLUM A. GORMAN

Mayo Clinic, Rochester, Minnesota, U.S.A.

ABSTRACT

The pathogenesis of Graves' ophthalmopathy remains unknown. While we clearly recognize the central importance of thyroid stimulating immunoglobulin (TSI) in causing thyroid gland overactivity, we have no corresponding clearly responsible agent for Graves' ophthalmopathy. In a proximate sense, we know that the clinical expressions of Graves' ophthalmopathy are caused by either swelling in the retrobulbar space or by restriction in the range of extraocular muscle motion. We understand that swelling occurs due to accumulation of inflammatory cells and of glycosaminoglycans (GAG), which bind water in the retrobulbar space. A variety of inflammatory cytokines stimulate GAG secretion from orbital fibroblasts. Although there is substantial evidence for an autoimmune process being responsible for Graves' ophthalmopathy, the case remains unproven and there is weak evidence in favor of an infectious etiology.

INTRODUCTION

All of the clinically significant eye symptoms and findings among patients with Graves' ophthalmopathy can be traced to one of two phenomena, swelling in the retrobulbar space or restriction of extraocular muscle motion (1). The former is due to retrobulbar deposition of glycosaminoglycans (GAG), which strongly bind water in both orbital muscle and connective tissue (2). The latter is due to swelling and later fibrosis of the extraocular muscles (3). These observations are no longer controversial and scientists are now preoccupied with the more fundamental questions of why GAG selectively accumulate in orbital tissue and why extraocular muscle fibrosis takes place (3–6). While we recognize some of the mechanisms that may contribute to these processes, a comprehensive awareness and understanding of the initiating factors remains elusive.

This paper will describe how GAG deposition and extraocular muscle fibrosis bring about the clinical features of Graves' ophthalmopathy. We will discuss how our knowledge of pathogenesis should inform our choice of measurements of change in Graves' ophthalmopathy (7), and we will briefly review some of the more fundamental but still unproven theories of pathogenesis.

HOW ARE THE CLINICAL FEATURES OF GRAVES' OPHTHALMOPATHY EVOKED?

Patients with Graves' eye disease typically complain of orbital or corneal pain, lacrimation, photophobia, blurring of vision, double vision, or impaired perception of color. On examination, they exhibit orbital congestion, proptosis, optic neuropathy, restricted gaze, divergent visual axes, corneal exposure, lid retraction, and periorbital edema. Early in the illness congestive features may predominate. Later, extraocular muscle fibrosis and restrictions of gaze are dominant (8).

Orbital congestive changes closely mimic the changes seen with inflammation. It is, therefore, difficult to define the extent to which redness, swelling, and pain are due to inflammation vs. congestion. The rapidity with which redness, swelling, and pain disappear after effective orbital decompression suggests that congestion is an important component in many patients (9).

CONSEQUENCES OF SWELLING IN THE RETROBULBAR SPACE

The bony orbit is shaped like a horizontally positioned cone with the globe occluding the anterior opening. The walls of the cone are relatively nondistensible. If soft tissues swell due to GAG deposition and water binding, then the globe is inevitably forced forward beyond the protective coverage of the eyelids. Patients will experience a sense of retrobulbar pressure. They will note a staring expression. The uncovered corneal surface is at risk of injury and offers a larger evaporative surface leading to dry eye complaints.

Increasing pressure in the retrobulbar space leads to impaired venous drainage, chemosis, and periorbital edema. Further pressure increase will impair optic nerve function with consequent loss of color vision, field defects, and reduced visual acuity. The complaint of visual blurring may be due to early diplopia, optic nerve pressure, or corneal changes (10,11).

CONSEQUENCES OF RESTRICTED EXTRAOCULAR MUSCLE MOTION

The motion of extraocular muscles may be restricted from engorgement alone or because over time they have become fibrosed. When the muscles that attach to the globe are involved, the consequence is restricted upward gaze with or without diplopia. When the eyelid retractors are affected, lid retraction is the result. Fibrosis or swelling of extraocular muscles is frequently asymmetric (12).

Fibrosis is often represented as the inactive or "burnt out" stage of Graves' ophthalmopathy. It should not be forgotten, however, that in another postulated autoimmune disease involving the thyroid, namely Riedel's thyroiditis, fibrosis is the visible indication of activity. Riedel's antibodies are presumed to induce fibrosis in the thyroid and many other tissues (13). Thus, the fibrotic stage of Graves' ophthalmopathy may indicate a shift in antibody type rather than the disappearance of antibodies or the lessening of an autoimmune process.

WHAT MEASUREMENTS REFLECT THE UNDERLYING PATHOLOGY IN GRAVES' OPHTHALMOPATHY?

Although most studies of Graves' ophthalmopathy in the past have relied on attempts to measure either patients' symptoms or the external consequences of the underlying processes, modem technology allows us to directly measure volume of extraocular muscles and retrobulbar fat on computerized tomographic scans and magnetic resonance images (1). Range of extraocular muscle motion can be reliably measured on a Goldman perimeter. Lid retraction is reflected in widening of the lid fissures, which can be recorded directly or on patient photographs. It is no longer necessary to aggregate largely subjective assessments of secondary external eye findings into clinical indices (14). All of the clinically significant expressions of Graves' ophthalmopathy can be measured objectively by determining volume of retrobulbar muscles and fat, defining range of motion and diplopia fields, and measuring lid fissure width and proptosis. From these primary changes, secondary consequences include corneal changes, periorbital edema, and optic nerve involvement.

WHY DO GAGS ACCUMULATE IN THE ORBIT IN GRAVES' DISEASE?

Glycosaminoglycan molecules are intensely hydrophilic and strongly bind water in the retrobulbar space. Orbital fibroblasts in culture secrete GAG (15), and the production of GAG is upregulated by a variety of cytokines, including leukoregulin, TGF Beta, and Interferon alpha (15,16). The same immunomodulatory molecules can be detected in fresh human orbital tissue removed during decompression for Graves' ophthalmopathy (17,18).

IS GRAVES' OPHTHALMOPATHY DEFINITELY AN AUTOIMMUNE DISEASE?

Bahn (6) has authoritatively reviewed this question. In brief, Witebsky et al. (19) defined criteria for showing that a particular human disease is autoimmune in nature. The criteria included: (1) demonstration of circulating or cell bound antibodies, (2) identification of the specific antigen against which the antibody is directed, (3) production of antibodies against the same antigen in experimental animals, and (4) reproduction of similar pathology in an actively sensitized experimental animal. According to these criteria, we cannot claim to have proven that Graves' ophthalmopathy is an autoimmune disease, since neither the autoantigen nor specific pathogenic antibodies have been definitively identified nor as yet an experimental animal exists that fully satisfies the postulates.

Recently, Rose and Bona (20) revised the criteria for autoimmune disease. They suggest that evidence that is direct, indirect, or circumstantial may be drawn upon to support the contention that a disease is autoimmune in nature. If the disease can be induced by passive transfer of pathogenic antibodies to a normal human being or an experimental animal, it would constitute direct evidence for autoimmunity. In accordance with these criteria, thyrotoxic Graves' disease fulfils the definition of an autoimmune process. Graves' ophthalmopathy does not so readily conform to the direct diagnostic requirements for autoimmunity.

Indirect evidence includes identification of the autoantigen and showing its immunogenic properties in vitro or in an experimental animal (20). This may have been accomplished in ophthalmopathy. One report exists of orbital changes consistent with active autoimmunity in mice genetically immunized with the TSH receptor. Splenocytes from the immunized mice were transferred to naive BALB/c mice, and 17/25 of the recipients showed lymphocytic and mast cell infiltration in the orbits together with adipose tissue accumulation and edema (21). This report has not yet been confirmed.

Finally, circumstantial evidence such as association with other autoimmune diseases or the demonstration of lymphocytes in the affected tissue or organ may be taken as suggestive of an autoimmune process (20). Graves' orbital tissue does contain lymphocytes, including retrobulbar T-cells that are CD8-positive and that specifically recognize autologous fibroblasts (22). Inflammatory cytokines are present (23). Immunohistochemical studies suggest the presence of a local autoimmune process (24).

The presence of the TSH receptor in orbital tissue suggests that it may be a significant orbital autoantigen (25). However, the clinical correlations between severity of Graves' ophthalmopathy and levels of the TSH receptor stimulating immunoglobulins are very weak in our own experience (30). Others have reported an association between TSI and the clinical activity score (26).

In summary, even with the more inclusive criteria offered by Rose and Bona (20), the case for autoimmunity as the cause of Graves' ophthalmopathy remains unproved although it remains a highly probable hypothesis.

COULD GRAVES' ORBITOPATHY BE AN INFECTIOUS DISEASE?

Involvement of the extraocular muscles in Graves' ophthalmopathy is frequently asymmetric. The inferior and medial recti are most frequently involved clinically. These are the muscles closest to the nasal sinuses, and the bone that separates them from the sinuses is porous. One might speculate that an as yet unidentified pathogen could infiltrate the orbit from the nasal sinuses. Some known pathogens carry TSH receptors on their surface (27–29). Antibodies to these bacteria or viruses could cross react with TSH receptors on orbital fibroblasts and then escape into the circulation to react with the thyroid TSH receptor and evoke Graves' hyperthyroidism. There is only weak supporting evidence for this hypothesis at present. While it would help to explain the asymmetry in extraocular muscle involvement and the preferential involvement of inferior and medial recti, the hypothesis lacks support in critical dimensions. Specifically, no such pathogens have been recognized or recovered from orbital tissues.

REFERENCES

1. Gorman CA, Garrity JA, Fatourechi V, Bahn RS, Bartley GB, Petersen IA, Stafford SL, Earle JD, Forbes GS, Kline RW, Bergstralh EJ, Offord KP, Rademacher DM, Stanley NM. A prospective, randomized, double blind, placebo-controlled study of orbital radiotherapy for Graves' ophthalmopathy. Ophthalmology 2001; 108:1523–1534.

2. Kahaly G, Forester G, Hansen C. Glycosaminoglycans in thyroid eye disease. Thyroid 1998; 8:429–432.

3. Bahn RS. Pathogenesis of Graves' ophthalmopathy. In: Rapoport B, McLachlan S, eds. Endocrine Updates Graves' Disease. Boston: Kluwer, 2000.

4. Smith TJ, Koumas L, Gagnon A, Bell A, Sempowski G, Phipps RP, Sorisky A. Orbital fibroblast heterogeneity may determine the clinical presentation of thyroid-associated ophthalmopathy. J Clin Endocrinol Metabol 2002; 87:385–392.

5. Akamizu T. Antithyroid receptor antibody: an update. Thyroid 2001; 11:1123–1134.

6. Bahn RS. Understanding the immunology of Graves' ophthalmopathy: is it an autoimmune disease? Endocrinol Metabol Clin North Am 2000; 29(2):287–296.

7. Gorman CA. The measurement of change in Graves' ophthalmopathy. Thyroid 1998; 8:539–543.

8. Jacobson DM. Dysthyroid orbitopathy. Semin Neurol 2000; 20(1):43–54.

9. Garrity JA, Fatourechi V, Bergstralh EJ, Bartley GB, Beatty CW, DeSanto LW, Gorman CA. Results of transantral orbital decompression in 428 patients with severe Graves' ophthalmopathy. Am J Ophthalmol 1993; 116(5):533–547.

10. Levine MR, Tomsak RL, El-Toukhy E. Thyroid related ophthalmopathy. Ophthalmol Clin North Am 1996; 4:645–658.

11. Burch BB, Wartofsky L. Graves' ophthalmopathy: current concepts regarding pathogenesis and management. Endocr Rev 1993; 14(6):747–793.

12. Feldon SE, Weiner JM. Clinical significance of extraocular muscle volumes in Graves' ophthalmopathy: a quantitative computed tomographic study. Arch Ophthalmol 1982; 100(8):1266–1269.

13. Schwaegerle SM, Bauer TW, Esselstyn CB Jr. Riedel's thyroiditis. Review of reported cases. Am J Clin Pathol 1988; 90(6):715–722.

14. Gorman CA. Clever is not enough: NOSPECS is form in search of function. Thyroid 1991; 1(4):353–355.

15. Imai Y, Ibaraki K, Odajima R, Shishiba Y. Analysis of proteoglycan synthesis by retroocular fibroblasts under the influence of interleukin 1 beta and transforming growth factor beta. Eur J Endocrinol 1994; 131(6):630–638.

16. Imai Y, Odajima R, Inoue Y, Shishiba Y. Effect of growth factors on hyaluronan and proteoglycan synthesis by retroocular tissue fibroblasts of Graves' ophthalmopathy in culture. Acta Endocrinol 1992; 126(6):541–542.

17. Heufelder AE. Involvement of the orbital fibroblast and TSH receptor in the pathogenesis of Graves' ophthalmopathy. Thyroid 1995; 5:331–340.

18. Heufelder AE, Spitzweg C. Immunology of Graves' ophthalmopathy. Dev Ophthalmol 1999; 30:24–38.

19. Witebsky E, Rose NR, Terplan K. Chronic thyroiditis and autoimmunization. JAMA 1957; 164:1439.

20. Rose NR, Bona C. Defining criteria for autoimmune diseases (Witebsky's postulates revisited). Immunol Today 1993; 14:426–430.

21. Many MC, Costagliola S, Detrait M, Denef F, Vassart G, Ludgate MC. Development of an animal model of autoimmune thyroid disease. J Immunol 1999; 162(8):4966–4974.

22. Grubeck-Loebenstein B, Trieb K, Sztankay A, Holter W, Anderl H, Wick G. Retrobulbar T-cells from patients with Graves ophthalmopathy are CD8+ and specifically recognize autologous fibroblasts. J Clin Invest 1994; 93(6):2738–2743.

23. De Carli M, D'Elios MM, Mariotti S, Marcocci C, Pinchera A, Ricci M, Romagnani S. Cytolytic T cells with Th1-like cytokine profile predominate in retroorbital lymphocytic infiltrates of Graves' ophthalmopathy. J Clin Endocrinol Metabol 1993; 77(5):1120–1124.

24. Lenderink T, Jager MJ, Bruijn JA, de Keltzer RJ. Immunohistology of eye muscles in idiopathic orbital inflammatory disease (pseudotumor), Graves' ophthalmopathy and healthy controls. Graefes Arch Clin Exp Ophthalmol 1993; 231(2):99–103.

25. Valyasevi RW, Erickson DZ, Harteneck DA, Dutton CM, Heufelder AE, Jyonouchi SC, Bahn RS. Differentiation of human orbital preadipocyte fibroblasts induces expression of functional thyrotropin receptor. J Clin Endocrinol Metabol 1999; 84(7):2557–2562.

26. Gerding MN, van der Meer JW, Broenink M, Bakker O, Wiersinga WM, Prummel MF. Association of thyrotropin receptor antibodies with the clinical features of Graves' ophthalmopathy. Clin Endocrinol 2000; 52(3):267–271.

27. Barteneva NS, Evstafieva AG, Gorelov VN, Wenzel BE. Identification and sequencing of a plasmid (pYV96)-encoded gene product of Yersinia enterocolitica recognized by antibodies in sera of patients with autoimmune thyroid disease. Ann NY Acad Sci 1994; 730:345–347.

28. Wenzel BE, Peters A, Zubaschev I. Bacterial virulence antigens and the pathogenesis of autoimmune thyroid diseases (AITD). Exp Clin Endocrinol Diabetes 1996; 104(suppl 4): 75–78.

29. Wenzel BE, Heesemann J, Heufelder A, Franke TF, Grammer-storf S, Stemerowicz R, Hopf U. Enteropathogenic Yersinia enterocolitica and organ-specific autoimmune diseases in man. Contrib Microbiol Immunol 1991; 12:80–88.

30. Gorman CA, Garrity JA, Fatourechi V, Bahn RS, Stafford SL, Earle JD, Forbes GS, Kline RW, Buettner H, Robertson DM, Bergstralh EJ, Offord KP, Rademacher DM, Stanley NM, Bartley GB. The aftermath orbital radiotheraphy for Graves' ophthalmopathy. Ophthalmopathy 2002 Nov; 109(11):2100–7.

15

Thyroid-Associated Ophthalmopathy: Principal Antigens and Significance of Corresponding Antibodies

IAN EPSTEIN, DONALD SMALLMAN, KATE LAZIER, and JACK R. WALL

Department of Medicine, Dalhousie University and Queen Elizabeth Health Science Centre, Halifax, Nova Scotia, Canada

STEPHEN BAKER

Department of Ophthalmology and Visual Sciences, Eye Care Centre, Dalhousie University, Halifax, Nova Scotia, Canada

MARIO SALVI

Institute of Endocine Sciences, Ospedale Maggiore IRCCS and University of Milan, Milan, Italy

ABSTRACT

Eye muscle antibody (EMAb) testing represents a possible means of diagnosing and characterizing thyroid-associated ophthalmopathy (TAO). In particular, antibodies against

157

flavoprotein (Fp), the "64 kDa protein" and G2s, the terminal fragment of the winged-helix transcription factor Fox p_1, may be markers of eye muscle damage in patients with Graves' hyperthyroidism. Here, we report upon the sensitivity and specificity of EMAb testing in patients with thyroid disorders with and without ophthalmopathy from a single center. Patient charts were reviewed and EMAb results correlated with clinical diagnosis and features of ophthalmopathy. A single endocrinologist assessed each patient and serum was tested for eye muscle antibodies and levels of free thyroxine (T4) and thyrotropin (TSH). Medical records, laboratory reports, and EMAb test results were reviewed and relevant clinical and biochemical findings extracted and entered into a database. One hundred and sixty-three EMAb tests were carried out on 99 patients. A statistically significant association between anti-G2s antibodies and clinical features of the ocular myopathy subtype of TAO, but not of the congestive ophthalmopathy subtype, was demonstrated. Anti-Fp antibody test results were not found to be significantly associated with any eye findings. We also report preliminary data on the first 15 patients with newly diagnosed Graves' hyperthyroidism treated with radioiodine or antithyroid drugs and followed for 1 year or more. In the first 15 patients followed for 1 year or more, serum antibodies against both Fp and G2s were found to be significantly associated with Graves' disease, but not other thyroid diagnoses. None of the four patients treated with antithyroid drugs developed autoantibodies or demonstrated features of extraocular disease. On the other hand, eye muscle antibodies were detected in eight of the nine patients treated with radioiodine, in five cases after therapy. Of the six patients who had eye muscle involvement as defined by increased intraocular pressure on upgaze, diplopia or restricted motility, all received radioiodine and had detectable serum autoantibodies. None of the results were statistically significant, possibly due to the small numbers of patients so far analyzed.

In conclusion, anti-G2s and anti-Fp antibodies are associated with clinical eye findings in patients with autoimmune thyroid disease and in patients with Graves' hyperthyroidism studied prospectively following treatment with radioiodine, but not antithyroid drugs. This suggests that EMAb testing may be of clinical use in evaluating ophthalmopathy in patients with thyroid autoimmunity and as markers for the eye disorder.

INTRODUCTION

Ophthalmopathy is a common manifestation of autoimmune thyroid disease. Periorbital swelling, exophthalmos, eyelid lag, and impaired vision may occur. From 25% to 50% of patients with Graves' hyperthyroidism will have some features of ophthalmopathy (1–3). Patients with Hashimoto's thyroiditis may also develop eye symptoms, although much less frequently. Thyroid-associated ophthalmopathy (TAO) may comprise two distinct subtypes, namely congestive ophthalmopathy and ocular myopathy (4–6). Congestive ophthalmopathy results from the swelling of the eyelid and surrounding orbital connective tissue (OCT). Clinically, this may result in a range of findings including eyelid lag and retraction, chemosis, conjunctival injection, orbital puffiness, redness and other signs of inflammation. Ocular myopathy results from autoimmune attack of extraocular muscle tissue. This results clinically in impaired extraocular muscle function and diplopia (4–6).

The mechanism for the development of the eye changes in patients with Graves' hyperthyroidism is still unclear. Congestive signs may be caused by an autoimmune attack against OCT antigens such as the TSH receptor and collagen type XIII, possibly in association with impaired venous drainage from the orbit (7). Ocular myopathy appears to be immune mediated (1,3,8) although the identity of the prime target antigen(s) is unclear. Several markers of immune-mediated damage to eye muscles have been identified. In particular, serum antibodies against 64 and 55 kDa eye muscle membrane proteins have been found in patients with TAO (5,8,9). The 64 kDa eye muscle protein has been identified as the flavoprotein (Fp) subunit of the mitochondrial enzyme succinate dehydrogenase (8). The novel thyroid and eye muscle shared 55 kDa eye muscle protein G2s has recently been identified as the terminal 141 amino acids of the winged-helix transcription factor Fox p_1.

Anti-Fp and anti-G2s antibodies are detected in the serum of the majority of patients with TAO (reviewed in Ref. 2). However, it has not yet been conclusively determined that a positive EMAb test is a useful clinical marker of TAO. The relationship between treatment of Graves' hyperthyroidism and ophthalmopathy is unclear. While some workers suggest that ophthalmopathy may worsen after radioiodine treatment, others have not found such an effect and the issue remains controversial (reviewed in Ref. 10). We are studying patients with newly diagnosed Graves' hyperthyroidism treated with antithyroid drugs or radioiodine in a 2 year prospective study. All patients undergo an eye examination each 3 months, at which time serum is taken for EMAb testing. Here, we report results on the first 15 patients after 1 year of follow-up. We have also determined how such EMAb testing is associated with clinical findings in a well-characterized group of patients with TAO from one center.

CLINICAL SUBJECTS AND METHODS

Patients

The *first study sample* consisted of patients seen at the thyroid clinic of the Queen Elizabeth II Health Sciences Centre in Halifax, Nova Scotia. The same endocrinologist (JRW) saw all patients between April 1999 and September 2001. Patients were assessed for thyroid diagnosis and eye symptoms. Serum was sent for EMAb testing and T4 and TSH measurements. Patients with no eye findings who were sent for EMAb testing were taken as a control group. For patients who were seen more than once, each EMAb test and concordant TAO status was recorded as a separate entry in the study. Overall, 163 EMAb tests were performed on 99 patients, 91 females and 8 males. Their ages ranged from 18 to 82 years with a mean

Table 1 Thyroid Diagnoses of Patients Tested for Eye Muscle Antibodies from One Center

Diagnosis*	Number	%
Graves' hyperthyroidism	48	48.5
Hashimoto's thyroiditis	18	18.2
Thyroid nodule, colloid goiter	14	1.6
"Thyrotoxicosis"	2	2.0
Hypothyroidism	5	5.1
Thyroiditis	3	3.0
Amiodarone induced hypothyroidism	2	2.0
"Thyroidectomy"	1	1.0
Euthyroid	4	4.0
Unknown abnormality	2	2.0

*As recorded in patient chart.

age of 43.9 ± 15.3 years. Patients were seen in the thyroid clinic for a range of thyroid diagnoses and clinical findings, as shown in Tables 1 and 2.

The *second study sample* consisted of a cohort of newly diagnosed patients with Graves' hyperthyroidism who are being studied prospectively. Clinical eye examination for congestive and ocular muscle involvement and serum EMAb testing was performed in these patients each 3 months, up to 24 months. Orbital computer tomographic (CT) scans were carried out at the initial visit and annually thereafter.

Table 2 Clinical Findings of Patients Tested for Eye Muscle Antibodies from One center

Clinical findings*	Number	%
Family history of thyroid disease	37	38
Goiter	49	50
Any eye findings	33	33.3
Extraocular muscle findings	13	13.1
Connective tissue eye findings	17	17.2
Both subtypes of eye findings	5	5.1

*As recorded in patient chart.

Treatment of the Graves' hyperthyroidism with antithyroid medications or radioactive iodine was initiated according to the discretion of the referring endocrinologist. Medical records were reviewed for relevant clinical findings including symptoms of thyroid disease, the presence or absence of a goiter, and the presence or absence of eye findings. Demographic data for each patient were extracted and relevant past medical history and family history of autoimmune or thyroid disease recorded. The presence of any other, nonthyroid, medical conditions was recorded, as was each patient's medications. In the case of positive eye findings, the type of finding was recorded. All available data were then entered into the study's database. Serum T4 and TSH serum levels were recorded for each patient. In most cases, T4 and TSH measurements and EMAb testing were performed on the same serum sample. Otherwise, the serum for the T4 and TSH values was drawn 1–3 days before or after the EMAb test serum.

Enzyme-Linked Immunosorbent Assay (ELISA)

This method has been described in previous publications from this laboratory (11,12). Concentrations of antigens used in these studies were Fp 1.25 µg/ml and G2s 0.25 µg/ml. G2s fusion protein was purified using a pFLAG ATS *Escherichia coli* expression system. Human recombinant Fp was kindly supplied by Dr. B.A.C. Ackrell (University of California, San Francisco). Serum dilution was 1:50. Second antibody was a rabbit antihuman IgG at a dilution of 1:2000. Results were expressed as optical density (OD). For the purposes of this study, a positive test was taken as an OD > mean (+2SD) for a panel of normal sera, for each antibody.

RESULTS

EMAb Studies from a Single Center

EMAb test results were compared with the thyroid diagnosis for each patient and analyzed by χ^2 testing. A statistically significant association, at 95% confidence, was found between both positive anti-Fp and positive anti-G2s results with the

Table 3   Correlation of Eye Muscle Antibodies with Thyroid Diagnoses from One Center

Diagnosis	p Value* with anti-Fp	p Value with anti-G2s
Graves' disease	0.046**	0.022**
Hashimoto's thyroiditis	0.479 NS	0.267 NS
Other thyroid diagnoses	0.201 NS	0.166 NS

*Pearson χ^2 p values.
**$p < 0.05$, NS = not significant.

diagnosis of Graves' disease. No statistically significant association was found between the EMAb test results and other thyroid diagnoses (Table 3). The clinical findings of goiter or positive family history were also compared to EMAb test results. No statistically significant associations were found (χ^2 tests, p = NS). EMAb test results were compared to each patient's clinical eye findings at the time of the test. No statistically significant associations were found between anti-Fp antibody results and eye findings (Table 4). A statistically significant association, at 95% confidence, was found between a positive anti-G2s antibody results and the presence of any eye findings. A positive anti-G2s antibody result was significantly associated with the ocular myopathy subtype of eye findings, but not with the congestive ophthalmopathy subtype (Table 4).

Table 4   Correlation of Eye Muscle Antibodies with Eye Findings from One Center

Eye findings	p Value* with anti-Fp	p Value* with anti-G2s
Present (any)	0.279 NS	0.027[a]
Presence of EOM[b] symptoms	0.306 NS	0.047[a]
Presence of CT symptoms	0.783 NS	0.065 NS

*Pearson χ^2 p values.
[a]$p < 0.05$, NS = not significant.
[b]EOM = extraocular muscle.

Table 5 Mean T4 and TSH Values for Each Group of Test Results from One Centre

EMAb Test Result	Mean (±SD) T4	Mean (±SD) TSH
Positive anti-Fp	20.6 ± 13.9 NS[a]	5.4 ± 16.6 NS
Nagative anti-Fp	17.5 ± 11.9	6.8 ± 18.2
Positive anti-G2s	22.5 ± 15.3 NS	3.5 ± 10.2 NS
Negative anti-G2s	17.4 ± 11.6	7.1 ± 19.1

NS = not significant.
[a]Difference between EMAB positive and EMAB negative groups, assessed using two-tailed Student's *t*-test.

Mean T4 level was slightly greater in EMAb-positive patients than in EMAb-negative patients, for both anti-Fp and anti-G2s antibodies (Table 5). Mean serum TSH was slightly lower in EMAb-positive patients compared to EMAb-negative patients. The differences in these means were not statistically significant (two-tailed Student's *t*-tests, $p = NS$).

Prospective Study of Graves' Disease Patients

Data on the first 15 patients with Graves' hyperthyroidism followed for 1 year or more are available. These comprise 12 females and 3 males, aged 18–56 (mean age 38), of whom 5 were smokers and 7 had a positive family history of thyroid or other autoimmune disease. Two of these patients were excluded from analysis due to insufficient follow-up. Of the remaining 13, 4 were being treated with antithyroid drugs and 9 received radioactive iodine. There were no differences in congestive or ocular muscle subtype between smokers and nonsmokers, or between patients with and without positive family history. None of the four medically treated patients developed EMAb or extraocular muscle involvement. On the other hand, anti-Fp or anti-G2s antibodies were detected in serum from eight of nine radio iodine-treated patients, in five cases following therapy. Six patients had eye muscle involvement as defined by increased intraocular pressure on upgaze, diplopia, or restricted motility, all of whom received radioiodine and had positive EMAb tests. None of these results were statistically significant, possibly due to the small numbers involved.

DISCUSSION

The objective of this study was to assess the association of EMAb test results with the clinical presentation of TAO in a single center. Firstly, we showed that both EMAb tests were associated with Graves' disease, with or without ophthalmopathy, but not with other thyroid diagnoses, in patients from a single center. A statistically significant association between positive anti-G2s results and the presence of clinical eye findings was demonstrated. Although a higher proportion of positive anti-Fp results was found in patients with TAO as compared to the controls, this difference did not achieve statistical significance.

While the pathogenesis of TAO is still debated, it does appear that autoimmune attack of extraocular muscle antigens plays an important role (2,5). In the current study, the association between EMAb test results and the clinical findings of TAO supports this hypothesis. In particular, the association between anti-G2s results and features of eye muscle disease suggests that these antibodies may play a role in the ocular myopathy subtype of TAO. However, a number of limitations in this study prohibit drawing any definitive conclusions. These include: a relatively small sample population, potential discrepancies in the description of eye findings reported, and little information available on other risk factors for TAO. Despite these limitations, this study did demonstrate some significant associations between EMAb testing and clinical findings. While not addressed in this study, positive EMAb test results in individuals without any signs of TAO may represent a risk factor for the development of future eye problems. If this were the case, many of the "false positives" found in this study may eventually develop into true positives, thereby improving the association found between the EMAb test results and the eye findings.

A major controversy over recent years concerns the putative effect of radioiodine treatment of Graves' hyperthyroidism on the ophthalmopathy (10). Here, in a preliminary study, we show that radioiodine treatment is associated with positive serum eye muscle antibodies, and the development of signs of eye muscle damage, but the result is not statistically significant. Further recruitment and follow-up should help characterize these associations.

In summary, we show that serum eye muscle antibodies are associated with the ocular myopathy subtype of TAO. In particular, anti-G2s results are significantly associated with eye findings. While further research on EMAb testing is needed, results from these studies suggest that EMAb testing may be of clinical use in assessing and characterizing TAO.

ACKNOWLEDGEMENTS

This work was supported by grant number MOP-37954 from the Canadian Institutes of Health Research (CIHR) and by a grant from the Queen Elizabeth II Research Foundation. We thank Dr. Brian A. C. Ackrell (University of California, San Francisco) for supplying us with human recombinant Fp, and Lisa Tramble, RN for coordinating the Graves' eye disease study.

REFERENCES

1. Burch H, Wartofsky L. Graves' ophthalmopathy: current concepts regarding pathogenesis and management. Endocr Rev 1993; 14:747–793.

2. Yamada M, Li AW, Wall JR. Thyroid-associated ophthalmopathy: clinical features, pathogenesis and management. Crit Rev Clin Lab Sci 2000; 37:523–549.

3. Weetman AP. Thyroid-associated eye disease: pathophysiology. Lancet 1991; 338:25–28.

4. Wall JR. Thyroid-associated ophthalmopathy: "in my view". Thyroid. Thyroid 2002; 12:35–36.

5. Gunji K, De Bellis AM, Kubota S, Swanson J, Wengrowicz S, Cochran B, Ackrell BA, Salvi M, Bellastella A, Bizzarro A, Sinisi A, Wall JR. Serum antibodies against the flavoprotein subunit of succinate dehydrogenase are sensitive markers of eye muscle autoimmunity in patients with Graves' hyperthyroidism. J Clin Endocrinol Metab 1999; 84:1255–1262.

6. Kasper M, Archibald C, De Bellis AM, Li AW, Yamada M, Wall JR. Orbital antibodies and subclass of ophthalmopathy. Proceedings of the International Symposium on Thyroid-Associated Ophthalmopathy, Kyoto, Japan, Oct 20–24, 2000. Thyroid 2002; 12:187–191.

7. Hudson HL, Levin L, Feldon SE. Graves' exophthalmos unrelated to extraocular muscle enlargement: superior rectus muscle inflammation may induce venous obstruction. Ophthalmology 1991; 98:1495–1499.

8. Kubota S, Gunji K, Ackrell BAC, Cochran B, Stolarski C, Wengrowicz S, Kennerdell JS, Hiromatsu Y, Wall JR. The 64-kilodalton eye muscle protein is the flavoprotein subunit of mitochondrial succinate dehydrogenase: the corresponding serum antibodies are good markers of an immune-mediated damage to the eye muscle in patients with Graves' hyperthyroidism. J Clin Endocrinol Metab 1998; 83:443–447.

9. Gunji K, De Bellis AM, Li AW, Yamada M, Kubota S, Ackrell B, Wengrowicz S, Bellastella A, Bizzarro A, Sinisi A, Wall JR. Cloning and characterization of the novel thyroid and eye muscle shared protein G2s: autoantibodies against G2s are closely associated with ophthalmopathy in patients with Graves' hyperthyroidism. J Clin Endocrinol Metab 2000; 85: 1641–1647.

10. Wartofsky L. Radioiodine therapy for Graves' disease: case selection and restrictions recommended to patients in North America. Thyroid 1997; 7(2):213–216.

11. Miller A, Sikorska H, Salvi M, Wall JR. Evaluations of an enzyme-linked immunosorbent assay for the measurement of

autoantibodies against eye muscle membrane antigens in Graves' ophthalmopathy. Acta Endocrinol 1986; 113:514–522.

12. Kapusta M, Salvi M, Triller H, Gardini E, Bernard N, Wall JR. Eye muscle membrane reactive antibodies are not detected in the serum of immunoglobulin fraction of patients with thyroid-associated ophthalmopathy using an ELISA and crude membranes. Autoimmunity 1990; 7:33–40.

16

Phenotypic Attributes of Orbital Fibroblasts Underlie Their Susceptibility in Graves' Disease

TERRY J. SMITH

Division of Molecular Medicine, Harbor-UCLA
Medical Center, Torrance, and School of
Medicine, University of California,
Los Angeles, California, U.S.A.

Thyroid-associated ophthalmopathy (TAO) involves a peculiar remodeling of the orbital connective tissues (1). Many components of this remodeling can be attributed to the activities of resident fibroblasts. Orbital contents, including muscle and connective tissue, occupy a greater volume than normal in many cases of TAO, a consequence at least in part of disordered glycosaminoglycan accumulation. The fatty tissue depot also enlarges and this may result from increased numbers and/or size of adipocytes as well as glycosaminoglycan infiltration. Tissues are often inflamed and become infiltrated with activated lymphocytes and mast cells (2). The factors driving connective tissue expansion and inflammation in TAO remain unidentified. It is currently believed that cytokines expressed by T-cells and mast cells directly or indirectly activate fibroblasts in the orbit. Recent evidence supports the concept that orbital fibroblasts differ from those inhabiting extraorbital tissue. A number of responses in these cells appear exaggerated when compared to those occurring in cells from other tissues and anatomic regions. I will briefly review the recent advances made in understanding the phenotype of orbital fibroblasts. We hypothesize that the unique attributes of these cells underlie both the targeting of the orbit for disease involvement and the unusual characteristics of the tissue remodeling associated with TAO.

COMPLEX ACTIVITIES OF HUMAN FIBROBLASTS ARE GENERALLY UNDERAPPRECIATED

Human fibroblasts serve diverse roles in the orchestration of tissue remodeling (3). They are capable of cross-talk with cellular components of the immune system by virtue of their synthesis of cytokines and other regulatory molecules (4). Moreover, they express many receptors for hormones, cytokines, and growth factors, strongly suggesting dynamic interplay between fibroblasts and bone-marrow-derived cells. Thus, they should be viewed as sentinels, participating in the initiating events of the inflammatory response, as well as sustaining processes that often culminate in fibrosis. When disease-related events persist and become chronic, they can lead to irreversible changes in tissue structure/function. Fibroblasts exhibit phenotypes that are defined by the tissues from which they derive (5–8). Of substantial potential relevance to Graves' disease is the set of attributes exhibited by orbital fibroblasts. These cells appear to express a number of genes and their products that might play direct roles in remodeling orbital tissues, such as occurs in TAO. That disease process is somehow related to Graves' disease of the thyroid gland, but the connections between the two are not obvious. The tissue changes occurring in the orbit are unlike those found in other anatomic regions. Thus, the suspicion exists that the peculiarities of resident cells might account for the selective involvement of the orbit in TAO. Prominent aspects of the orbital fibroblast phenotype include exaggerated responses to proinflammatory cytokines such as IL-1β, leukoregulin, and CD154 (9–11). Indeed, a large number of cytokine actions thus far documented in orbital fibroblasts appear greater in magnitude than those found in fibroblasts cultivated from other tissues. We hypothesize that these robust, over-determined responses found in orbital fibroblasts constitute the cellular basis for the manifestations of TAO. While the mechanisms underlying the recruitment of T-cells to the orbit and thyroid in Graves' disease are yet to be identified, it would appear that the consequences of their recruitment to the orbit can be attributed to the cellular attributes of orbital fibroblasts.

ORBITAL FIBROBLASTS ARE COMPRISED OF DISCRETE SUBPOPULATIONS OF CELLS

Heterogeneity among fibroblasts has been appreciated for several years in cultures derived from certain tissues, such as murine lung (12) and the female reproductive tract (13). In those organs, fibroblasts can be segregated on the basis of the surface display of Thy-1, a cell-surface glycoprotein with distinct signaling properties but an as yet undefined natural ligand (14). Thy-1$^+$ and Thy-1$^-$ lung fibroblasts in mouse lung express different profiles of IL-1, HLA-DR, and produce collagens differentially. With regard to reproductive fibroblasts, striking differences exist with regard to cyclooxygenase expression and prostaglandin synthesis (13). This precedent provided the rationale for examining whether subsets of human orbital fibroblasts also exist. Indeed, around 50% of cells in parental fibroblast strains display Thy-1 (15). The presence or absence of Thy-1 is stable and faithfully maintained. When individual cells are cloned and subcultured, daughter cells uniformly exhibit the Thy-1 status of the parent cell. Moreover, Thy-1 expression does not change despite extended periods of culture and serial passage. Thy-1$^+$ orbital fibroblasts express higher levels of IL-8 than do their Thy-1$^-$ counterparts (16). On the other hand, adipogenic potential following the ligation of PPARγ appears to be confined to Thy-1$^-$ subsets (17). All cells subjected to a differentiation medium and undergoing adipogenesis fail to display immunoreactive Thy-1 (17). Both subsets of orbital fibroblasts can express high levels of PGE$_2$ and the biosynthetic enzymes required for its synthesis following activation with IL-1β. A more complete and systematic inventory of the genes and proteins expressed differentially in Thy-1$^+$ and Thy-1$^-$ orbital fibroblast subsets is currently being undertaken. The observations made to date suggest that orbital fibroblasts are highly specialized and that subsets of these cells may participate in distinct processes associated with normal tissue homeostasis and in the pathogenesis of disease.

ORBITAL FIBROBLASTS SYNTHESIZE HIGH LEVELS OF PGE$_2$ WHEN TREATED WITH PROINFLAMMATORY CYTOKINES

When parental orbital fibroblast cultures and those subsetted on the basis of Thy-1 expression are treated with IL-1β, leukoregulin, or CD154, they synthesize large amounts of PGE$_2$ (9,10,18). Dermal fibroblasts cultured and treated under identical conditions exhibit a dramatically less robust upregulation in PGE$_2$ production (9,10). In orbital cultures, levels of PGE$_2$ increase up to 1000-fold above those observed in untreated fibroblasts. This production can be attributed to the induction of prostaglandin endoperoxide H synthase-2 (PGHS-2), the inflammatory cyclooxygenase (9,18). When treated with selective inhibitors of PGHS-2, the increase in PGE$_2$ synthesis provoked by IL-1β and leukoregulin was substantially blocked. The induction of this enzyme in orbital fibroblasts is a consequence of both increases in gene transcription and an enhanced stability of PGHS-2 mRNA

(9,10). Nuclear runon studies reveal that cytokine treatment increases gene transcription by 2- to 3-fold over baseline (9). Further, when constructs of the PGHS-2 gene promoter are fused to reporters and transfected into orbital fibroblasts, IL-1β increases their activities by a similar factor (19). The human PGHS-2 transcript is remarkably short-lived in most cell types, owing in part to the many AUUUA instability sequences in its 3′ untranslated region. While the impact of cytokine treatment on gene transcription is relatively modest, mRNA stability is enhanced dramatically, accounting for the substantial increase in steady-state transcript levels (10,19). Both the p38 and ERK components of the mitogen activated kinase pathways have been implicated in the upregulation by cytokines of PGHS-2 expression in orbital fibroblasts (19). Using both pharmacologic and molecular strategies for interrupting kinase expression or activity, studies to date strongly support the participation of both signaling pathways.

Recently, a terminal, glutathione-dependent PGE$_2$ synthase (PGES) family comprised of two enzymes has been found to be expressed in orbital fibroblasts (19). The microsomal localizing member, termed mPGES, has been found to be highly inducible in these cells (19). Moreover, the expression of this enzyme was found to depend at least in part on the activity of PGHS-2. Both PGHS-2 and mPGES are glucocorticoid-repressible enzymes, making them theoretically important targets for steroid therapy in TAO. In contrast, the cytosolic PGES (cPGES) is expressed at high levels in fibroblasts under basal conditions and its abundance is not influenced substantially by factors leading to increased PGE$_2$ production in these cells. Moreover, glucocorticoids fail to alter cPGES expression.

PROINFLAMMATORY CYTOKINES ENHANCE HYALURONAN SYNTHESIS IN ORBITAL FIBROBLASTS

A cardinal feature of the tissue remodeling associated with TAO is the accumulation of the linear polymer, hyaluronan

(1). This complex carbohydrate is comprised of alternating residues of n acetyl glucosamine and d-glucuronic acid (1). Hyaluronan is not sulfated and thus differs from the other abundant glycosaminoglycans. Moreover, it lacks a protein backbone. The rheologic properties of hyaluronan are similar to those exhibited by sulfated glycosaminoglycans. It is the extraordinary hydrophilic nature of hyaluronan that makes its accumulation in TAO so important to the function of the orbital contents. When fully hydrated, molecular hyaluronan occupies an extremely large volume and therefore can cause substantial anterior displacement of the eye.

With regard to hyaluronan production by orbital fibroblasts, treatment of cultured cells with IL-1β, leukoregulin, or CD154 results in large increases of net glycosaminoglycan synthesis (11,18,20). The effects observed in orbital fibroblasts are considerably greater than those in dermal fibroblasts (11). The cytokines fail to alter the abundance of sulfated glycosaminoglycans such as chondroitin, dermatan, and heparin sulfate (11,21). Pulse-chase studies reveal that hyaluronan accumulates in cultures as a consequence of increased synthesis and that degradation of the macromolecule is nil in cultured fibroblasts (22). In subsequent studies, it was found that expression of three members of the hyaluronan synthase (HAS) enzyme family was influenced by cytokine treatment (23). Of the three enzyme isoforms, HAS2 mRNA was the most abundant following exposure to IL-1β (23). The induction was blocked substantially by cycloheximide, an inhibitor of protein synthesis, suggesting that the effect might represent a secondary gene induction, dependent on the continued synthesis of an intermediate protein. The enzyme immediately upstream from HAS in the hyaluronan synthetic pathway, UDP-glucose dehydrogenase, was also found to be induced by IL-1β in orbital fibroblasts (20). Thus, it would appear that multiple levels of the pathway involved in cytokine-provoked hyaluronan synthesis in these cells might be upregulated by cytokines in the setting of inflammation. The physical/chemical properties of glycosaminoglycans are partially responsible for the mechanical embarrassment suffered by the eye in severe TAO. Clearly, the details surrounding disordered hyaluronan accumulation might prove instructive in the development of strategies for halting the progression of this disease.

ORBITAL FIBROBLASTS DISPLAY CELL-SURFACE CD40 AND RESPOND TO CD154

CD40, a member of the TNF-α receptor family, is highly expressed by orbital fibroblasts (4). Preliminary evidence suggests that the levels of CD40 expression may be higher in orbital fibroblasts than those found in several other types of cells. This expression is potentially important because CD40 is a critical antigenic molecule on B-cells and represents a major conduit through which B-lymphocytes are activated by T-cells. When CD40 is ligated by its natural ligand, CD154, expression of several orbital fibroblast genes is induced. Levels of PGHS-2, mPGES, IL-1α, IL-6, and IL-8 are increased (4,18). The demonstration of CD40 on orbital fibroblasts suggests that T-cells might directly influence the activity of these cells and thus may represent a direct route through which they could be activated. Interferon γ increases the levels of CD40 on fibroblasts and enhances the magnitude of fibroblast response to CD154 (18). Thus, a predominant Th1 immune response could condition the orbital fibroblast and facilitate the impact T-cells and mast cells might have on fibroblastic activity.

Widespread expression of CD40 on numerous cell types suggests that this receptor and its ligand(s) may be involved with the regulation of many metabolic events. Cells other than T-lymphocytes have now been shown capable of expressing CD154 (platelets and mast cells are examples) and thus the CD40/CD154 bridge may represent a particularly important conduit through which heterogeneous cells might cross-talk. With regard to Graves' disease, this pathway may represent an important therapeutic target, the interruption of which might allow attenuation of several aspects of the immune response.

FIBROBLASTS FROM SEVERAL ANATOMIC REGIONS CAN EXPRESS THE THYROTROPIN RECEPTOR

Cloning and characterization of the thyrotropin (TSH) receptor more than 10 years ago has been accompanied by substantial inquiry concerning its expression in extrathyroidal tissues. The earliest studies examined the presence of TSHR mRNA in tissues of the orbit using RT-PCR-based assays. Feliciello et al. (24) found the transcript in normal orbital tissues and those from patients with TAO. This important study was soon followed by several reports of orbital fibroblasts expressing TSHR mRNA (25–27). These studies used more reliable and somewhat quantitative methods of detecting low abundance mRNA, such as northern blot analysis, nuclease protection, and in situ hybridization. In addition, TSHR protein was found expressed by cultured orbital fibroblasts (28). Subsequently, extraorbital tissues and fibroblasts from some of those depots were found to also express TSHR (29,30). Among the first observations concerning TSHR expression occurring outside the thyroid gland were suggestions that the ectopic receptor might represent a truncated protein (31). The investigators believed it was inactive in that addition of TSH to the cultures of eye muscle-derived fibroblasts failed to enhance cAMP generation or to upregulate glycosaminoglycan production. Later studies have verified that a full-length receptor is expressed in extrathyroidal tissues. For instance, fat from infants expresses high levels of TSHR while lower levels were demonstrated in adipose tissue from adults (32). More recently, TSHR protein and mRNA have been found in fibroblasts/preadipocytes from omental and abdominal wall fat of adults (30). Moreover, the receptor is competent to signal through the p70^{s6k} pathway (30). At issue is whether TSHR is expressed widely by cells of the fibroblast lineage or only in the orbit. If the latter proved to be the case, it would be possible to implicate anatomically restricted TSHR expression as the basis for regional distribution of disease manifestations. Two reports have appeared recently suggesting that the transition from orbital fibroblasts incubated in a differentiation-provoking medium, into mature adipocytes resulted in enhanced TSHR expression (33,34). The claim was based on the increase in cAMP production elicited by TSH under those culture conditions. An important possibility, apparently not adequately controlled for in either study, relates to the theoretical contribution of cAMP enhancing components found in the medium. Thus, although these findings are consistent with earlier reports supporting the concept that adipogenic differentiation is accompanied by enhanced levels of TSHR, it remains a possibility that cell differentiation did not influence cAMP levels in those particular studies. In any event, it would appear that TSHR expression is not limited to orbital fibroblasts but rather may be widespread among the fibroblasts found in many connective/adipose tissue depots. The role of the TSHR in the pathogenesis of extra-thyroidal Graves' disease remains uncertain.

CONCLUSIONS

Orbital fibroblasts may play an important role in the pathogenesis of TAO. Unfortunately, most of the evidence supporting this concept is circumstantial and based on extensive studies conducted in cell culture. To date, these fibroblasts have been shown to exhibit phenotypic attributes that differ considerably from those of cells derived from other anatomic sites. Whether the differences found in vitro will ultimately prove relevant to human disease remains to be determined. Confirmation of their active participation in the disease will await the development of robust animal models for TAO.

ACKNOWLEDGEMENTS

The expert assistance of Ms Connie Madrigal is gratefully acknowledged. This work has been supported in part by National Institutes of Health grants DKOL3121, EY08976 and EY11708.

REFERENCES

1. Smith TJ, Bahn RS, Gorman CA. Connective tissue, glycosa-minoglycans, and diseases of the thyroid. Endocr Rev 1989; 10:366–391.

2. Huffnagel TS, Hickey WF, Cobbs WH, Jakobiec FA, Iwamoto T, Eagle RC. Immunohistochemical and ultra structural studies on the exenterated orbital tissues of a patient with Graves' disease. Ophthalmology 1984; 91:1411–1419.

3. Smith RS, Smith TJ, Blieden TM, Phipps RP. Fibroblasts as sentinel cells. Synthesis of chemokines and regulation of inflammation. Am J Pathol 1997; 151(2):317–322.

4. Sempowski GD, Rozenblit J, Smith TJ, Phipps RP. Human orbital fibroblasts are activated through CD40 to induce proin-flammatory cytokine production. Am J Physiol 1998; 274: C707–C714.

5. Young DA, Evans CH, Smith TJ. Leukoregulin induction of protein expression in human orbital fibroblasts: evidence for anatomical site-restricted cytokine–target cell interactions. Proc Natl Acad Sci USA 1998; 95:8904–8909.

6. Hogg MG, Evans CH, Smith TJ. Leukoregulin induces plasmi-nogen activator inhibitor type 1 in human orbital fibroblasts. Am J Physiol 1995; 269:C359–C366.

7. Berenson CS, Smith TJ. Human orbital fibroblasts in culture express ganglioside profiles distinct from those in dermal fibro-blasts. J Clin Endocrinol Metab 1995; 80:2668–2674.

8. Smith TJ, Kottke RJ, Lum H, Andersen TT. Human orbital fibroblasts in culture bind and respond to endothelin. Am J Physiol 1993; 265:C138–C142.

9. Wang H-S, Cao HJ, Winn VD, Rezanka LJ, Frobert Y, Evans CH, Sciaky D, Young DA, Smith TJ. Leukoregulin induction of prostaglandin-endoperoxide H synthase-2 in human orbital fibroblasts: an in vitro model for connective tissue inflammation. J Biol Chem 1996; 271:22718–22728.

10. Cao HJ, Smith TJ. Leukoregulin upregulation of prostaglan-din endoperoxide H synthase-2 expression in human orbital fibroblasts. Am J Physiol 1999; 277:C1075–C1085.

11. Smith TJ, Wang H-S, Evans CH. Leukoregulin is a potent inducer of hyaluronan synthesis in cultured human orbital fibroblasts. Am J Physiol 1995; 268:C382–C388.

12. Phipps RP, Baecher C, Frelinger JG, Penney DP, Keng P, Brown D. Differential expression of interleukin 1α by Thy-1$^+$ by Thy-1$^-$ lung fibroblasts subpopulations: enhancement of interleukin 1α production by tumor necrosis factor-α. Eur J Immunol 1990; 20:1723–1727.

13. Koumas L, King AE, Critchley HO, Kelly RW, Phipps RP. Fibroblast heterogeneity: existence of functionally distinct Thy1(+) and Thy1(–) human female reproductive tract fibroblasts. Am J Pathol 2001; 159:929–935.

14. Morris RJ, Ritter MA. Association of Thy-1 cell surface differentiation antigen with certain connective tissues in vivo. Cell Tissue Res 1980; 206:459–475.

15. Smith TJ, Sempowski GD, Wang H-S, Del Vecchio PJ, Lippe SD, Phipps RP. Evidence for cellular heterogeneity in primary cultures of human orbital fibroblasts. J Clin Endocrinol Metab 1995; 80:2620–2625.

16. Koumas L, Smith TJ, Phipps RP. Fibroblasts subsets in the human orbit: Thy-1+ and Thy-1– subpopulations exhibit distinct phenotypes. Eur J Immunol 2002; 32:477–485.

17. Smith TJ, Koumas L, Gagnon AM, Bell A, Sempowski GD, Phipps RP, Sorisky A. Orbital fibroblast heterogeneity may determine the clinical presentation of thyroid-associated ophthalmopathy. J Clin Endocrinol Metab 2002; 87: 385–392.

18. Cao HJ, Wang H-S, Zhang Y, Lin H-Y, Phipps RP, Smith TJ. Activation of human orbital fibroblasts through CD40 engagement results in a dramatic induction of hyaluronan synthesis and prostaglandin endoperoxide H synthase-2 expression. Insights into potential pathogenic mechanisms of thyrois-associated Ophthalopathy. J Biol Chem 1998; 273: 29615–29625.

19. Han R, Tsui S, Smith TJ. Up-regulation of prostaglandin E$_2$ synthesis by interleukin-1beta in human orbital fibroblasts involves coordination induction of prostaglandin endoperoxide H synthase-2 and glutathione-dependent pros-

taglandin E_2 synthase expression. J Biol Chem 2002; 277(19): 16355–16364.

20. Spicer AP, Kaback LA, Smith TJ, Seldin MF. Molecular cloning and characterization of the human and mouse UDP-glucose dehydrogenase genes. J Biol Chem 1998; 273:25117–25124.

21. Smith TJ, Bahn RS, Gorman CA, Cheavens M. Stimulation of glycosaminoglycan accumulation by interferon gamma in cultured human retroocular fibroblasts. J Clin Endocrinol Metab 1991; 72:1169–1171.

22. Smith TJ. *n*-Butyrate inhibition of hyaluronate synthesis in cultured human fibroblasts. J Clin Invest 1987; 79:1493–1497.

23. Kaback LA, Smith TJ. Expression of hyaluronan synthase messenger ribonucleic acids and their induction by interleukin-1β in human orbital fibroblasts: potential insight into the molecular pathogenesis of thyroid-associated ophthalmopathy. J Clin Endocrinol Metab 1999; 84:4079–4084.

24. Feliciello A, Porcellini A, Ciullo I, Bonavolonta G, Avvedimento EV, Fenzi G. Expression of thyrotropin-receptor mRNA in healthy and Graves' disease retro-orbital tissue. Lancet 1993; 342: 337–338.

25. Heufelder AE, Dutton CM, Sarkar G, Donovan KA, Bahn RS. Detection of TSH receptor RNA in cultured fibroblasts from patients with Graves' ophthalmopathy and pretibial dermopathy. Thyroid 1993; 3:297–300.

26. Wu S-L, Yang C-CJ, Wang H-J, Liao C-L, Chang T-J, Chang TC. Demonstration of thyrotropin receptor mRNA in orbital fat and eye muscle tissues from patients with Graves' ophthalmopathy by in situ hybridization. J Endocrinol Invest 1999; 22:289–295.

27. Spitzweg C, Joba W, Hunt N, Heufelder AE. Analysis of human thyrotropin receptor gene expression and immunoreactivity in human orbital tissue. Eur J Endocrinol 1997; 136:599–607.

28. Burch HB, Sellitti D, Barnes SG, Nagy EV, Bahn RS, Burman KD. Thyrotropin receptor antisera for the detection of immunoreactive protein species in retroocular fibroblasts obtained from patients with Graves' ophthalmopathy. J Clin Endocrinol Metab 1994; 78:1384–1391.

29. Crisp MS, Lane C, Halliwell M, Wynford-Thomas D, Ludgate M. Thyrotropin receptor transcripts in human adipose tissue. J Clin Endocrinol Metab 1997; 82:2003–2005.

30. Bell A, Gagnon A, Grunder L, Parikh SJ, Smith TJ, Sorisky A. Functional TSH receptor in human abdominal preadipocytes and orbital fibroblasts. Am J Physiol Cell Physiol 2000; 279:C335–C340.

31. Paschke R, Metcalfe A, Alcalde L, Vassart G, Weetman A, Ludgate M. Presence of non-functional thyrotropin receptor variant transcripts in retroocular and other tissues. J Clin Endocrinol Metab 1994; 79:1234–1238.

32. Janson A, Rawet H, Perbeck L, Marcus C. Presence of thyrotropin receptor in infant adipocytes. Pediatr Res 1998; 43: 555–558.

33. Valyasevi RW, Erickson DZ, Harteneck DA, Dutton CM, Heufelder AE, Jyonouchi SC, Bahn RS. Differentiation of human orbital preadipocyte fibroblasts induces expression of functional thyrotropin receptor. J Clin Endocrinol Metab 1999; 84:2557–2562.

34. Crisp M, Starkey KJ, Lane C, Ham J, Ludgate M. Adipogenesis in thyroid eye disease. Invest Ophthalmol Vis Sci 2000; 41:3249–3255.

17

Somatostatin Analogs in Ophthalmic and Orbital Disease: A Rationale for their Use

**STEVEN E. KATZ, MARKO I. KLISOVIC,
MARTIN LUBOW, and DINO D. KLISOVIC**
William H. Havener Eye Center, The Ohio State
University, Columbus, Ohio, U.S.A.

INTRODUCTION

Somatostatin (SST) is a cyclic neuropeptide that has diverse biological functions, the most important of which are neurotransmitter, antisecretory, and antiproliferative (1). SST-producing cells have been identified at high densities in a variety of normal human tissues, including endocrine, pancreas, gut, thyroid, adrenals, central and peripheral nervous systems, kidneys, prostate, placenta, and submandibular gland (1). Like many other protein hormones, SST is

183

synthesized as a propeptide, which undergoes tissue-specific processing to produce one of two isoforms, somatostatin-14 (SST-14) or somatostatin-28 (SST-28). The biological effects of SST peptides are mediated by high affinity membrane receptors (SSTRs), all of which bind SST-14 and SST-28 with nanomolar activity. SSTRs have a broad expression pattern and the individual receptors have both overlapping and tissue-specific patterns of expression, with SSTR2 usually being the most widely expressed subtype (1,2). There is a very high degree of amino acid homology among members of the SSTR family (overall approximately 50% amino acid homology) (1). The sequence differences, which reside primarily in the intracellular and extracellular domains, are responsible for their distinct signaling properties. SSTRs elicit their cellular responses through G-protein-linked modulation of various second-messenger systems including adenylyl cyclase, Ca^{2+} and K^+ ion channels, Na^+/H^+ antiporter, guanylate cyclase, phospholipase C, phospholipase A2, mitogen-activated protein (MAP) kinase and serine, threonine, and phosphotyrosyl protein phosphatase (1). Second messengers used by any SSTR are often cell, tissue, and species specific. The net result of activation of one or more of those signaling mechanisms, in any given tissue, is down-regulation of many synthetic and secretory processes including secretion of growth factors, cellular proliferation, and differentiation (1). Cloning of the five known receptor subtypes resulted in the development of highly specific agonists such as octreotide and lantreotide (SSTR-2 agonists).

Knowledge of SST production, its physiologic function, and the distribution of SSTR's in the human ocular and orbital tissues is very limited. To date, the distribution of SST-producing cells was only studied in human retinas. SST immunoreactive cells were detected in ganglion cell layer (GCL) and inner nuclear layer (INL) (amacrine cells) as well as on the cell processes in the inner plexiform layer (IPL) and nerve fiber layer (NFL) in fetal and adult human retinas (3–6). The exact function of SST positive cells in retina is poorly understood. No published data exist on the presence and distribution of SST-producing cells in other ocular, orbital, and related tissues.

SSTR agonists have been used for treatment of several hormone overproduction states and a variety of benign and malignant tumors (2). In spite of the lack of clear understanding of SSTR distribution in normal intraocular and intraorbital tissues, the antiproliferative and antiangiogenic properties of octreotide have been used in short clinical trials in the treatment of various diseases, including proliferative diabetic retinopathy (PDR), cystoid macular edema, thyroid orbitopathy, and pseudotumor cerebri in small numbers of patients (7–13).

We used reverse transcription polymerase chain reaction (RT-PCR) to study gene expression for all five SSTRs in cultured retinal pigment epithelium (RPE) cells and ocular tissues dissected from normal human eyes. In addition, we studied cell and tissue-specific distribution of SSTR1 and SSTR2 in normal human eyes, cultured RPE cells, extraocular muscles, orbital fat, arachnoid granulations (AG), and choroid plexus (CP) (14–16). Our results demonstrate that genes for SSTRs are expressed in all analyzed tissues with SSTR1 and SSTR2 genes being the most widely expressed, followed by SSTR4 gene (expressed in retina, choroids, and ciliary body/iris). SSTR3 and SSTR5 gene expression was detected only in the retina. Good correlation was detected in the distribution of SSTR1-ir and SSTR2-ir and SSTR1 and SSTR2 gene expression. Immunohistochemical data revealed SSTR1-ir and SSTR2-ir on most of cells derived from neural crest (i.e., stromal keratocytes, corneal endothelium, iris stroma, RPE cells, and choroidal melanocytes). These results are in concordance with the previously published data showing the presence of SSTR1 and SSTR2 (octreoscan, RT-PCR, immunohistochemical detection) on a variety of benign and malignant tumors originating from neural crest-derived cells (17). Although SSTR1 and SSTR2 are membrane-associated receptors, a significant amount of staining was also detected within the cytoplasm and in the perinuclear regions in many immunoreactive cells. Electron microscopic immunogold cytochemistry study done by Dournaud et al. (18) on rat brain neurons showed that the relative proportion of membrane-bound SSTR2 receptors (membrane versus intracytoplasmic receptor molecules) correlates inversely with the density of SST innervation of the same neurons. Those data suggest ligand-induced down-regulation of the receptor density on the cell membrane through the receptor internalization process.

This communication summarizes our results and provides rationale for the possible use of SSTR agonists for diagnosis and treatment of certain ocular and orbital diseases.

INTRAOCULAR TISSUES (Figs. 1 and 2)

Cornea

Corneal epithelium did not show immunoreactivity for either SSTR1 or SSTR2. Moderate SSTR1-ir and SSTR-2-ir were observed on cell membrane and cytoplasm of stromal keratocytes. On the other hand, corneal endothelial cells showed strong punctate SSTR1-ir and SSTR2-ir in all specimens. The exact function of SSTR1 and SSTR2 in human cornea, especially corneal endothelium, remains unknown. Considering the complex role of SSTRs in the processes of extracellular fluid formation and absorption (19) in human kidney and possibly CP, it is possible that SSTR1 and SSTR2 are involved in the fluid homeostasis in the cornea and anterior chamber provided by corneal endothelial cells.

Iris, Trabecular Meshwork, Schlemm's Canal, and Ciliary Body

Weak SSTR1-ir was detected in sphincter and dilator iris muscles. No other cells were found to be SSTR1 immunoreactive. However, strong SSTR2-ir was present on fibrocytes and clump cells present in iris stroma and sphincter and dilator muscles as well as on endothelial cells within iris blood vessels. SSTR1-ir or SSTR2-ir could not be reliably assessed for the posterior iris pigment epithelium and pigmented epithelium of the ciliary processes secondary to heavy pigmentation. We were the first to detect moderate SSTR1-ir and SSTR2-ir on trabecular endothelial cells in uveal and corneoscleral meshwork as well as on endothelial cells lining the Schlemm's

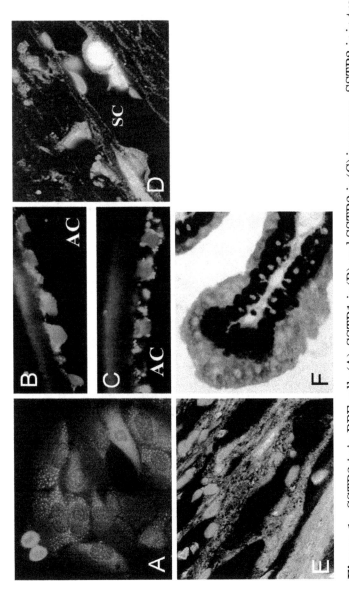

Figure 1 SSTR2-ir in RPE cells (A). SSTR1-ir (B) and SSTR2-ir (C) in cornea. SSTR2-ir in trabecular meshwork and Schlemm's canal (D), in ciliary muscle (E) and ciliary processes (F). AC, anterior chamber; SC, Schlemm's canal.

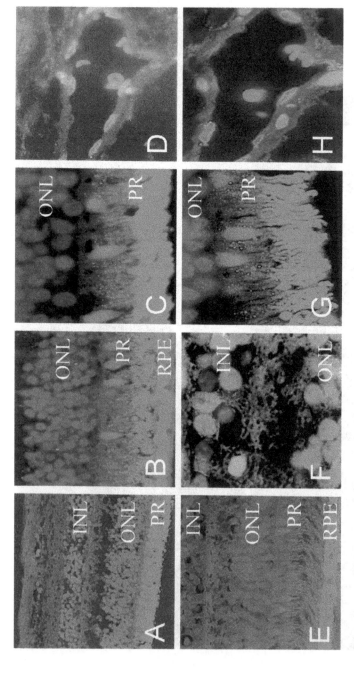

Figure 2 SSTR1-ir (A–D) and SSTR2-ir (E–H) in normal retina and retinal vessels (D, H). RPE, retinal pigment epithelium; PR, photoreceptors; ONL, outer nuclear layer; INL, inner nuclear layer.

canal in human eye. The potential role of these receptors in aqueous outflow is unknown at present.

Circular and longitudinal fibers of ciliary muscle showed intense cytoplasmic and membranous SSTR1-ir and SSTR2-ir. Intense SSTR1-ir and SSTR2-ir was detected in the non-pigmented epithelium and on the endothelium of marginal capillaries of ciliary processes. An RT-PCR study done by Mori et al. (20) showed SSTR2 and SSTR4 gene expression in rat iris/ciliary body complex. Several experimental studies showed SST regulation of biochemical processes that are involved in aqueous fluid production in the nonpigmented epithelium of ciliary processes in rabbit eyes, that is cyclic AMP production and concentration of intracellular Ca^{2+} (21–23). The exact function of SSTR1 and SSTR2 in ciliary body and outflow structures in the human eye is not known; however, based on animal studies, it seems likely that they may be involved in the aqueous fluid production and/or absorption in human eyes as well. SSTR1-ir and SSTR2-ir were also detected on nonpigmented ciliary epithelium (i.e., site of aqueous fluid production), marginal capillaries of ciliary processes, and on endothelial cells in trabecular meshwork and in Schlemm's canal (i.e., site of aqueous fluid absorption).

Retina, RPE, and Choroid

RT-PCR revealed gene expression for all five SSTRs in the retina. Expression of all five SSTRs in retina should not be surprising considering the complex cellular interactions among highly specialized cells present in the human retina. SSTR1-ir and SSTR2-ir were detected across all cell and fiber layers in retina. Both immunoreactivities were detected in the form of fine punctate staining on the membranes of outer and inner segments of rods and cones and individual cells in outer nuclear layer (ONL), INL, and GCL. Due to the high cell density within ONL and INL, morphology of individual cells could not be reliably assessed (i.e., amacrine cells, Muller cells, bipolar cells, etc.). Prominent SSTR1-ir and SSTR2-ir were also present in OPL, IPL, and NFL. Very intense SSTR1-ir and SSTR2-ir were abundantly present on the membranes and in the cytoplasm of RPE cells. SSTR1 and SSTR2 seem to be coexpressed on the same cell types across all retinal layers. In addition, distinct punctate SSTR1-ir and SSTR2-ir were present on the membrane and in the cytoplasm of endothelial cells in retinal vessels including arterioles, venules, and capillaries. The same pattern of SSTR1-ir and SSTR2-ir was present within small and large choroidal blood vessels. SSTR4 gene expression was detected in the choroid as well.

The exact physiologic role of SSTR1 and SSTR2 in visual signal processing in immunoreactive human retinal cells is currently unknown. In the rabbit eye, sst2A-ir (alternative splicing variant of SSTR2 molecule) was detected only on the plasma membrane of rod bipolar cells, suggesting very specific function of this receptor molecule in the signal processing in the rabbit eye (24). In monkey retina, SSTR2-ir was primarily observed on cone photoreceptors but also in cell bodies in the INL and on the processes in the IPL (25). The exact physiologic function of SST-ir cells in complex processing of visual information along the visual pathway in primates is poorly understood at present. The relatively small number of SST positive cells in primate retinas (25) suggests that SST influences the overall retinal circuitry by modulating the release and/or action of other retinal neurotransmitters (e.g., dopamine or acetylcholine) on retinal cells. Our results show that SSTR1-ir and SSTR2-ir is much more widely distributed in human retinas than would be expected based on the distribution and connectivity of SST-ir cells in the retina. There are two possible explanations for this phenomenon: (a) once released by SST-ir cells, SST could diffuse across retinal layers in a radial and tangential manner affecting the retinal cells that do not directly synapse with SST-ir cells, and (b) some of the widely distributed receptors could be binding another ligand(s) like cortistatin as suggested by Siehler et al.(26). In addition, SSTR1-ir and SSTR2-ir are present in the same retinal layers in which SST-ir was observed previously (3–6), that is, GCL and INL suggesting that SST may have an autocrine effect on retinal ganglion cells and amacrine cells.

Intense SSTR1-ir and SSTR2-ir were observed on cell membranes and in cytoplasm of individual RPE cells in culture. Actively dividing RPE cells showed increased cytoplasmic SSTR1-ir and SSTR2-ir compared to nondividing RPE cells. The role(s) of SSTR1 and SSTR2 on RPE cells remains speculative at present. Somatostatin could be involved in the modulation of a variety of biochemical processes involved in ion transport mechanisms as well as in synthesis and release of a variety of cytokines (e.g., IGF-I and VEGF). Increase in SSTR1-ir and SSTR2-ir by actively dividing RPE cells suggests that SST could be critically involved in the regulation of their cell cycle.

Strong SSTR1-ir and SSTR2-ir presence on endothelial cells within retinal and choroidal blood vessels may have critical implications for the development of future treatment modalities for conditions characterized by proliferation of endothelial cells in neovascularization processes, such as proliferative diabetic retinopathy and choroidal neovascularization in age-related macular degeneration. Experimental studies using SST and octreotide showed an inhibitory effect on the proliferation of human and murine endothelial cells in culture (cell lines HUV-EC-C and HECa10) (27). Whether this antiproliferative effect is directly mediated by one of the signaling pathways used by some of the SSTRs (presumably SSTR1 and/or SSTR2) or by modulating the synthesis and release of some of the paracrine trophic factors [e.g., vascular endothelial growth factor (VEGF), insulin-like growth factor-1 (IGF-1)] remains unknown. One of those processes, activation of phosphotyrosine phosphatases, seems to be crucial in mediating the direct antiproliferative activity of SST and its analogs in several normal and malignant cell lines. The antiproliferative effect of SST is further potentiated by SST-induced inhibition of biological activity of paracrine and autocrine growth factors, including basic fibroblast growth factor (bFGF) and IGF-1 (27).

Optic Nerve

Moderately strong SSTR1-ir and SSTR2-ir were observed in axons within the optic nerve (ON). No SSTR1-ir or SSTR2-ir could be detected on glial cells within the ON.

EXTRAOCULAR MUSCLES AND ORBITAL FIBROCYTES (Fig. 3)

SSTR analogs, such as octreotide, have been used for the diagnosis and treatment of thyroid ophthalmopathy (TO), again, mostly on an empirical basis without clear understanding of

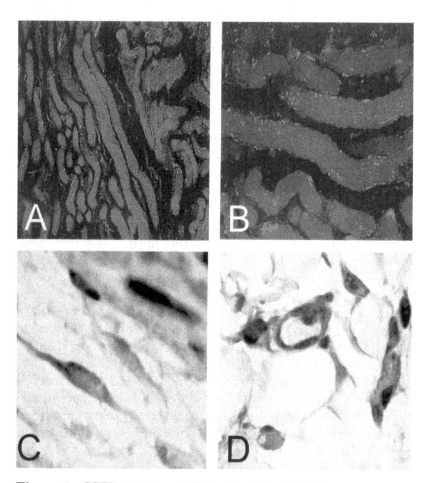

Figure 3   SSTR1-ir (A) and SSTR2-ir (B) in EOM. Immunoreactivity is present in the form of bright red punctate staining of the cell membrane, DAPI nuclear staining—bright blue. DAB-peroxidase immunohistochemistry; SSTR1-ir (C) and SSTR2-ir (D) in orbital fibrocytes.

the distribution of SSTRs in orbital tissues. Since the identification of SSTRs on lymphocytes, orbital infiltration with mononuclear cells in TO has provided a rationale for receptor imaging with octreotide scintigraphy. Patients with active TO have a two- to three-fold increase in uptake of indium-octreotide when compared to normals, which suggests that octreoscan could be used to monitor activity (stage) of the disease (28). Octreoscan seems to be particularly useful in moderately severe cases of TO in which it may be difficult to assess the activity of the disease by clinical examination. Consequently, octreoscan was also used to predict the response of TO to immunosuppressive treatment with corticosteroids. Patients with positive octreoscan (active disease) responded nicely to corticosteroid treatment, while those with negative scan did not (29). Several authors reported beneficial effects of octreotide or lantreotide treatment in TO (decrease in proptosis). The clinical effect could be explained by the fact that octreotide and other SST analogs inhibit IGF-1 action on orbital lymphocytes and fibrocytes, which may result in reduced glycosaminoglycan synthesis and collagen production (30). We detected very strong SSTR1-ir and SSTR2-ir on normal extraocular muscle (EOM) myocytes (all extraocular muscles analyzed), orbital fibroblasts, and lymphocytes. The exact function of those receptors on these cell types remains speculative. However, our results suggest that SSTRs could be involved in normal EOM physiology. In addition, the beneficial effect of SSTR analogs could be mediated at the level of individual muscle cells.

CHOROID PLEXUS AND ARACHNOID GRANULATIONS (Fig. 4)

The production of cerebrospinal fluid (CSF) by CP and its absorption by AG are complex and poorly understood phenomena in humans (31). Recent work has demonstrated synthesis of numerous peptides and their receptors in CP (32). Peptide molecules and their receptors involved in the process of CSF absorption that takes place in the AG are largely unknown.

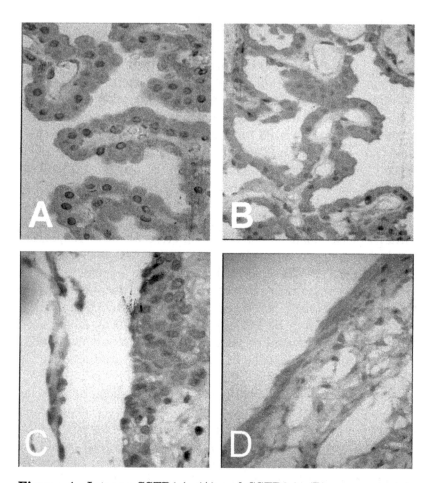

Figure 4 Intense SSTR1-ir (A) and SSTR2-ir (B) are present in the epithelial and vascular endothelial cells of CP in all samples analyzed. Strong SSTR1-ir (C) and SSTR2-ir (D) are evident on arachnoid cells, connective tissue, and dural layer cells in all analyzed A6 samples.

Octreotide has been used as an adjunctive treatment for idiopathic intracranial hypertension (IIH) without understanding its mechanism or site of action (33). By using immunohistochemistry, we detected intense membrane and cytoplasmic SSTR1 and SSTR2 immunoreactivity on all epithelial cells and vascular endothelial cells in capillaries within individual villi of CP. Equally strong SSTR1 and SSTR2-ir were observed in arachnoid cells, connective tissue, and dural layer cells in AG samples.

The exact function of SST and its receptors in CSF homeostasis in humans is unknown at present; however, the abundance of SSTRs on CP and AG implies their involvement in the processes of CSF production and absorption. Cerebrospinal fluid dynamics might be affected locally at the level of CP and AG through SSTRs or systemically by modulating the levels or activity of circulating hormones [i.e., growth hormone (GH), IGF-1, insulin, leptin, etc.]. In addition, SSTR1 and SSTR2 might modulate blood flow in CP capillaries and filtration in CP epithelium.

The SST axis has a role in ion transport, extracellular fluid production, and absorption in different mammalian and human tissues (1). Recent work has demonstrated SST effects in kidney and in the eye. Intravenous injection of SST modulates glomerular filtration rate, renal plasma flow, urine volume, and water clearance in normal human kidney (34,35). The recent work of Balster et al. (19) demonstrated SSTR1 and SSTR2 gene expression as well as orderly segmental distribution of SSTR1 and SSTR2-ir along the glomerular and tubular system in normal human kidney tissue. Such data offer us a reasonable theoretical model for a similar role of the SST axis in CSF dynamics.

In the rabbit eye, SST inhibits aqueous production by stimulating adenylyl cyclase activity and release of intracellular Ca^{2+} in nonpigmented epithelium of ciliary processes (22,23,36). The best studied activity of SST and its analogs in humans is the inhibition of the release of GH from pituitary, which in turn results in the reduction of circulating levels of IGF-1 (37). This is of special interest because it is now apparent that a side-effect of recombinant IGF-1 treatment in children with GH receptor deficiency is a transient increase of intracranial pressure (ICP) (38–48). The increased ICP resolves with complete cessation of IGF-1 treatment or reduction of IGF-1 dose by 50%. In this regard, it is important to recognize that CP epithelium has one of the highest densities of IGF-1R in the human brain (49,50). These data suggest a role for high plasma IGF-1 levels in the pathogenesis of increased ICP in these children. The IGF-1 axis also has a significant role in the pathogenesis of obesity. Obese patients often have numerous hormonal abnormalities including glucose intolerance, insulin resistance, hyperinsulinemia, low plasma levels of GH, and high levels of free IGF-1 due to overproduction of IGF-1 by adipocytes (51–53). It is well known that IIH is a disease that mostly affects obese women of childbearing age. Octreotide treatment in such patients might decrease levels of circulating IGF-1, but could also counteract its biological activity at the level of CP epithelium. In human retinal pigment epithelial cells (SSTR1 and 2 positive), SST and octreotide inhibit the biological effects of IGF-1 by inhibition of autophosphorylation of IGF-1R, thereby inhibiting the IGF-1 signaling cascade (54). Analogous to their demonstration and to their function in kidney and ocular tissues, SSTRs may be involved in the processes of CSF production and absorption in humans, and may play a role in the increased ICP in IIH.

ACKNOWLEDGMENT

This study was supported in part by the Ohio Lions Eye Research Foundation, The Bremer Fund, The George and Miriam Mikesell Research Fund, The Jacob and Florence Moses Fund (The Columbus Foundation), and ROI CA 64177.

REFERENCES

1. Patel YC. Somatostatin and its receptor family. Front Neuroendocrinol 1999; 20:157–198.

2. Reubi JC, Schaer JC, Markwalder R, Waser B, Horisberger U, Laissue A. Distribution of somatostatin receptors in normal and neoplastic human tissues: recent advances and potential relevance. Yale J Biol Med 1997; 70:471–479.

3. Tornqvist K, Ehinger B. Peptide immunoreactive neurons in the human retina. Invest Ophthalmol Vis Sci 1988; 29: 680–686.

4. Mitrofanis J, Robinson SR, Provis JM. Somatostatinergic neurons of the developing human and cat retinae. Neurosci Lett 1989; 104:209–216.

5. Li HB, Lam DM. Localization of neuropeptide-immunoreactive neurons in the human retina. Brain Res 1990; 522:30–36.

6. Jen PY, Li WW, Yew DT. Immunohistochemical localization of neuropeptide Y and somatostatin in human fetal retina. Neuroscience 1994; 60:727–735.

7. Lee HK, Suh KI, Koh CS, Min HK, Lee JH, Chung H. Effect of SMS 201-995 in rapidly progressive diabetic retinopathy. Diabetes Care 1988; 11:441–473.

8. Kirkegaard C, Norgaard K, Snorgaard O, Bek T, Larsen M, Lund-Andersen H. Effect of one year continuous subcutaneous infusion of a somatostatin analog, octreotide, on early retinopathy, metabolic control and thyroid function in Type I (insulin-dependent) diabetes mellitus. Acta Endocrinol (Copenh) 1990; 122:766–772.

9. McCombe M, Lightman S, Eckland DJ, Hamilton AM, Lightman SL. Effect of a long-acting somatostatin analogue (BIM23014) on proliferative diabetic retinopathy: a pilot study. Eye 1991; 5:569–575.

10. Mallet B, Vialettes B, Haroche S. Stabilization of severe proliferative diabetic retinopathy by long-term treatment with SMS 201-995. Diabetes Metab 1992; 18:438–444.

11. Antaraki A, Piatides G, Vergados J, Andreou A, Chlouverakis C. Octreotide in benign intracranial hypertension. Lancet 1993; 342:1170.

12. Kuijpers RW, Baarsma S, van Hagen PM. Treatment of cystoid macular edema with octreotide. N Engl J Med 1998; 338:624–626.

13. Nocaudie M, Bailliez A, Itti E, Bauters C, Wemeau JL, Marchandise X. Somatostatin receptor scintigraphy to predict the clinical evolution and therapeutic response of thyroid-associated ophthalmopathy. Eur J Nucl Med 1999; 26:511–517.

14. Klisovic D, O'Dorisio MS, Katz SE, Sall JW, O'Dorisio T, Balster D, Craig E, Lubow M. Somatostatin receptor (SSTR)

gene expression in human ocular tissues: RT-PCR and immunohistochemical study. Invest Ophthalmol Vis Sci 2001; 42:
2193–2201.

15.   Katz S, Klisovic D, O'Dorisio MS, Lynch R, Lubow M. Expres-
      sion and distribution of somatostatin receptors 1 and 2 in human
      choroid plexus and arachnoid granulations: implications for
      idiopathic intracranial hypertension. Arch Ophthalmol 2002;
      120:1540–1543.

16.   Klisovic DD, Katz SE, O'Dorisio MS, O'Dorisio T, Balster D,
      Craig E, Lubow M. Distribution of somatostatin receptors
      (SSTR) 1 and 2 in normal human extraocular muscles (EOM)
      and orbital fibrocytes (OF). Neuro-Ophthalmology 2000; 23:
      233.

17.   Eriksson B, Oberg K. Summing up 15 years of somatostatin
      analog therapy in neuroendocrine tumors: future outlook.
      Ann Oncol 1999; 10:31–38.

18.   Dournaud P, Boudin H, Schonbrunn A, Tannenbaum GS,
      Beaudet A. Interrelationship between somatostatin sst2A
      receptors and somatostatin-containing axons in rat brain: evi-
      dence for regulation of cell surface receptors by endogenous
      somatostatin. J Neurosci 1998; 18:1056–1071.

19.   Balster DA, O'Dorisio MS, Summers MA, Turman MA. Seg-
      mental expression of somatostatin receptor subtypes sst(1)
      and sst(2) in tubules and glomeruli of human kidney. Am J
      Physiol Renal Physiol 2001; 280:F457–F465.

20.   Mori M, Aihara M, Shimizu T. Differential expression of
      somatostatin receptors in the rat eye: SSTR4 is intensely
      expressed in the iris/ciliary body. Neurosci Lett 1997; 223:
      185–188.

21.   Bauscher LP, Horio B. Neuropeptide Y and somatostatin inhibit
      stimulated cyclic AMP production in rabbit ciliary processes.
      Curr Eye Res 1990; 9:371–378.

22.   Wax MB, Barret DA. Regulation of adenylyl cyclase in rabbit
      iris ciliary body. Curr Eye Res 1993; 12:507–520.

23.   Xia SL, Fain GL, Farahbakhsh NA. Synergistic rise in Ca^{2+}
      produced by somatostatin and acetylcholine in ciliary body
      epithelial cells. Exp Eye Res 1997; 64:627–635.

24. Johnson J, Wong H, Walsh JH, Brecha NC. Expression of the somatostatin subtype 2A receptor in the rabbit retina. J Comp Neurol 1998; 393:93–101.

25. Johnson J, Rickman DW, Brecha NC. Somatostatin and somatostain subtype 2A expression in the mammalian retina. Microsc Res Tech 2000; 50:103–111.

26. Siehler S, Seuwen K, Hoyer D. [^{125}I]Tyr^{10}-cortistatin14 labels all five somatostatin receptors. Naunyn Schmiedebergs Arch Pharmacol 1998; 357:483–489.

27. Grant MB, Caballero S, Millard WJ. Inhibition of IGF-1 and b-FGF stimulated growth of human retinal endothelial cells by the somatostatin analogue, octreotide. A potential treatment for ocular neovascularization. Regul Pept 1993; 48:267–278.

28. Forster GJ, Krummenauer F, Nickel O, Kahaly GJ. Somatostatin-receptor scintigraphy in Graves' disease: reproducibility and variance of orbital activity. Cancer Biother Radiopharm 2000; 15:517–525.

29. Colao A, Lastoria S, Ferone D, Pivonello R, Macchia PE, Vassallo P, Bonavolonta G, Muto P, Lombardi G, Fenzi G. Orbital scintigraphy with [111In-diethylenetriamine pentaacetic acid-D-phe1]-octreotide predicts the clinical response to corticosteroid therapy in patients with Graves' ophthalmopathy. J Clin Endocrinol Metab 1998; 83:3790–3794.

30. Pasquali D, Vassallo P, Esposito D, Bonavolonta G, Bellastella A, Sinisi AA. Somatostatin receptor gene expression and inhibitory effects of octreotide on primary cultures of orbital fibroblasts from Graves' ophthalmopathy. J Mol Endocrinol 2000; 25:63–71.

31. Speake T, Whitwell C, Kajita H, Majid A, Brown PD. Mechanisms of CSF secretion by the choroid plexus. Mircrosc Res Tech 2001; 52:49–59.

32. Chodobski A, Szmydynger-Chodobska J. Choroid plexus; target for polypeptides and site of their synthesis. Mircrosc Res Tech 2001; 52:65–82.

33. Antaraki A, Piadites G, Vergados J, Andreou A, Chlouverakis C. Octreotide in benign intracranial hypertension. Lancet 1993; 342:1170.

34. Vora JP, Owens DR, Ryder R, Atiea J, Luzio S, Hayes TM. Effect of somatostatin on renal function. Br Med J 1986; 292: 1701–1702.

35. Tulassay T, Tulassay Z, Rascher W, Szucs L, Seyberth HW, Nagy I. Effect of somatostatin on kidney function and vasoactive hormone systems in healthy subjects. Klin Wochenschr 1991; 69:486–490.

36. Bausher LP, Horio B. Regulation of cyclic AMP production in adult human ciliary processes. Exp Eye Res 1995; 60:43–48.

37. Brazeau P, Vale W, Burgus R. Hypothalamic polypeptide that inhibits the secretion of immunoreactive pituitary growth hormone. Science 1973; 179:77–79.

38. Otten BJ, Roettvel JJ, Ruysberg JRM. Pseudotumor cerebri following treatment with growth hormone. Horm Res 1992; 37:16.

39. Malozowski S, Tanner LA, Wysowski DK, Fleming GA. Growth hormone, insulin-like growth factor I and benign intracranial hypertension [letter]. N Engl J Med 1993; 329:665–666.

40. Lordereau-Richard I, Roger M, Chaussain JL. Transient bilateral papilloedema in a 10-year-old boy treated with recombinant insulin-like growth factor I for growth hormone receptor deficiency. Acta Pediatr Suppl 1994; 399:152.

41. Guevara-Aguire J, Vasconez O, Martinez V. A randomized, double blind, placebo-controlled trial on safety and efficacy of recombinant human insulin-like growth hormone receptor deficiency. J Clin Endocrinol Metab 1995; 80:1393–1398.

42. Malozowski S, Tanner LA, Wysowski DK, Fleming GA, Stadel BV. Benign intracranial hypertension in children with growth hormone deficiency treated with growth hormone. J Pediatr 1995; 126:996–999.

43. Price DA, Clayton PE, Loyd IC. Benign intracranial hypertension induced by growth hormone treatment [letter]. Lancet 1995; 345:458–459.

44. Wingenfeld P, Schmidt B, Hoppe B. Acute glaucoma and intracranial hypertension in a child on long-term peritoneal dialysis treated with growth hormone. Pediatr Nephrol 1995; 9:742–745.

45. Francois I, Casteels I, Silberstein J, Casaer P, de Zegher F. Empty sella, growth hormone deficiency and pseudotumour cerebri: effect of initiation, withdrawal and resumption of growth hormone therapy. Eur J Pediatr 1997; 156:69–70.

46. Koller EA, Stadel BV, Malozowski SN. Papilledema in 15 renally compromised patients treated with growth hormone. Pediatr Nephrol 1997; 11:451–454.

47. Azcona C, Preece MA, Rose SJ. Growth response to rhIGF-I 80 mg/kg twice daily in children with growth hormone insensitivity syndrome: relationship to severity of clinical phenotype. Clin Endocrinol 1999; 51:787–792.

48. Rogers AH, Rogers GL, Bremer DL, McGregor ML. Pseudotumor cerebri in children receiving recombinant human growth hormone. Ophthalmology 1998; 106:1186–1190.

49. Lai ZN, Emtner M, Rood, Nyberg F. Characterization of putative growth hormone receptors in human choroid plexus. Brain Res 1991; 546:222–226.

50. De Keyser J, Wilczak N, De Backer JP, Herroelen L, Vaquelin G. Insulin-like growth factor-I receptors in human brain and pituitary gland: an autoradiographic study. Synapse 1994; 17:196–202.

51. Frystyk J, Vestbo E, Skjaerbaek C, Mogensen CE, Orskov H. Free insulin-like growth factors in human obesity. Metabolism 1995; 44(10 suppl 4):37–44.

52. Frystyk J, Skjaerbaek C, Vestbo E, Fisker S, Orskov H. Circulating levels of free insulin-like growth factors in obese subjects: the impact of type 2 diabetes. Diabetes Metab Res Rev 1999; 15:314–322.

53. Nam SY, Marcus C. Growth hormone and adipocyte function in obesity. Horm Res 2000; 53(suppl 1):87–97.

54. Sall JW, Klisovic DD, O'Dorisio MS, Katz SE. Somatostatin inhibits IGF-1 mediated induction of VEGF in human retinal pigment epithelial cells. Exp Eye Res 2004; 79(4):465–476.

18

Predictors of Disease Severity in Thyroid-Related Orbitopathy

PETER J. DOLMAN and JACK ROOTMAN

Department of Ophthalmology and Visual Sciences and Department of Pathology, University of British Columbia and the Vancouver General Hospital, Vancouver, British Columbia, Canada

JUGPAL ARNEJA

The Faculty of Medicine, University of Manitoba, Winnipeg, Manitoba, Canada

INTRODUCTION

Most patients suffering from thyroid orbitopathy (TO) develop mild disease with lid retraction and proptosis; however, a minority may have a more aggressive presentation with greater inflammatory features, progressive restriction of ocular motility, and possible optic neuropathy (1–3).

To date, there are only a few known prognostic variables concerning disease severity, with smoking, male gender, and age increasing the likelihood of progression to a severe level requiring aggressive therapy (4,5).

This study compared retrospectively the demographic, historic, and clinical variables on first presentation and on the consecutive visit in 50 patients with mild and 50 patients with severe disease to determine possible prognosticators of severity in TO.

METHODS

This was a retrospective case–control study using chart review. The charts from 340 new patients consecutively referred to the University of British Columbia Thyroid Orbitopathy Clinic between 1993 and 1996 were separated into two groups based on therapy during the active phase of their disease. At our clinic, we grade the inflammatory activity of thyroid orbitopathy using a clinical activity index similar to that described by Mourits et al. (Table 1). We categorize patients with inflammatory scores less than 4 (out of a possible 8), with no progressive strabismus, and without optic neuropathy, as having mild disease and treat them conservatively with observation, lubricant eye drops, or cool compresses. We define severe disease as including those patients with an inflammatory score of 4 or greater out of 8, with progressive ocular motility restriction, or with optic neuropathy. These patients are offered more aggressive

Table 1 Thyroid Orbitopathy Inflammatory Score (UBC Thyroid Orbitopathy Clinic)

Clinical finding	Score
Orbital pain (none, at rest, movement)	0–2
Chemosis	0–2
Eyelid edema	0–2
Conjunctival injection	0–1
Eyelid injection	0–1
Total	0–8

therapy including systemic anti-inflammatories and/or orbital radiation.

From each of the two groups, 50 patients were randomly selected using a computer-generated sequence and their charts reviewed for differences in symptoms, signs, rate of disease onset, and progression between their first and subsequent visit. Statistical analysis was applied using Student's t-test, χ^2-test, and Mann–Whitney U-test.

RESULTS

Demographics

Of the 340 patients initially reviewed, we classified 119 (35%) as having severe disease and 221 (65%) with mild disease. The randomly selected groups of 50 patients each were compared for age, sex, race, family history, and smoking history (Table 2).

The mean age at presentation of patients in the severe group was 55.4 years and in the mild group 39.3 years; this difference was statistically significant ($p < 0.0001$, Student's t-test).

The severe group included 73.8% females and 26.2% males, while the mild group had 83% females and 17% males;

Table 2 Demographic Comparison Between Disease Severity Groups (Student's t- and χ^2-tests)

Category	Severe disease	Mild disease	p Value
Age (years)			
Mean	55.4	39.3	$p < 0.00001$
Standard deviation	12.2	11.8	
Gender	73.8% F	83.0% F	$p > 0.05$
	26.2% M	17.0% M	
Race	90.5% white	66.0% white	$p < 0.006$
	9.5% other	34.0% other	
Smokers	57.1%	44.7%	$p > 0.05$
Family history	33.3%	27.7%	$p > 0.05$

these gender distributions were statistically insignificant ($p > 0.05$).

A significant difference ($p < 0.006$) was present with regard to racial distribution, with the severe group comprised of 90.5% white and 9.5% other races (Chinese, Indian, Native American Indian, and African) and the mild group comprised of 66% white and 34% others.

A positive smoking history was present in 57.1% of the severe group and 44.7% of the mild group, which was found to be not statistically different ($p > 0.05$).

A positive family history of thyroid orbitopathy was present in 33.3% of the severe group and 27.7% of the mild group, statistically not different ($p > 0.05$).

Historical Features

Symptoms of thyroid orbitopathy and systemic thyroid disease were recorded at the initial presentation (Table 3).

Diplopia and lid and conjunctival swelling were reported more frequently in the severe group than in the mild group and found to have a statistically significant difference ($p < 0.0005$). Orbital pain (including both deep orbital aching as well as foreign body irritation) was reported equally commonly in both groups ($p > 0.05$).

Table 3 Comparison of Symptoms Between Disease Severity Groups (χ^2-test)

Symptom	Severe disease (%)	Mild disease (%)	p Value
Orbit symptoms			
Diplopia	59.5	19.1	$p < 0.0001$
Lid swelling	85.7	38.2	$p < 0.00001$
Orbit pain	61.9	53.2	$p > 0.05$
Proptosis	52.4	87.2	$p < 0.0004$
Thyroid symptoms			
Weight change	69.0	70.2	$p > 0.05$
Palpitations	33.3	38.3	$p > 0.05$
Heat intolerance	21.4	51.1	$p < 0.004$

All patients on their first visit were asked if their ocular complaints were worsening, stable, or improving in the past few weeks. Fifty percent of the severe group had reported worsening in their symptoms on their first visit compared with 12% of the mild group, which was highly statistically significant different ($p < 0.0001$).

Systemic thyroid symptoms of weight change and palpitations were not statistically different between the severe and mild groups.

Most patients (85.7% of the severe group and 87.2% of the mild group) presented with a history of hyperthyroidism. There was no significant difference between the type of primary thyroid disease nor the type of systemic thyroid treatment received between the two groups.

Tempo of Disease Onset

On their initial visit, all patients were asked to categorize the tempo of onset of their orbital and systemic thyroid symptoms as either acute (onset from 0 to 4 weeks) or chronic (onset greater than 4 weeks). There was a significant difference ($p = 0.0001$) between the severe and mild groups with respect to orbitopathy onset rate, with the severe group having 54.8% acute and 45.2% chronic onset and the mild group having 12.8% acute and 87.2% chronic onset.

There was no significant difference ($p > 0.05$) between the mild and severe groups with respect to thyroid disease onset rate. The severe group had 30.9% acute onset and 66.7% chronic while the mild group had 19.1% acute onset and 68.1% chronic onset.

Clinical Features

Five parameters were recorded from the charts at both the initial and the subsequent follow-up visits: soft-tissue inflammatory features, proptosis, corneal exposure, motility, and optic neuropathy (Table 4).

Eyelid edema and chemosis scores were significantly higher in the severe group.

Table 4 Comparison of Clinical Measurements Between Disease Severity Groups at First Visit and Change Documented Between Visits (Mann–Whitney U-test)

	First visit measurements			Difference between visits		
Clinical signs	Severe	Mild	p Value	Severe	Mild	p Value
Inflammatory						
Lid edema (0–2)	1.60	0.34	p < 0.001	0.14	−0.40	p < 0.004
Chemosis (0–2)	1.42	0.23	p < 0.001	0.14	−0.20	p < 0.004
Proptosis (mm)	21.1	19.9	NS	1.0	−0.4	p < 0.001
Exposure						
Corneal staining	9%	7%	NS	−3%	−4%	NS
Motility						
Primary diplopia	17%	8%	p < 0.001	0%	−4%	NS
Gaze diplopia	25%	9%	p < 0.0001	−4%	−2%	NS
Ductions (degrees)						
Horizontal	32.8	44.2	p < 0.005	−4.2	1.1	p < 0.003
Vertical	20.2	35.7	p < 0.005	−3.4	3.6	p < 0.001

The mean globe proptosis was 1.2 mm higher in the severe group, not statistically significant. The incidence of corneal punctate stain or ulcers was not significantly different between the groups.

The incidence of diplopia in up- and horizontal gazes, and restricted ocular ductions in upgaze and abduction from the worst eye was more common in the severe group. We found no statistical difference between the groups in downgaze measurements.

Optic neuropathy was documented in none of the mild group and 10% of the severe group.

Progress and Duration of Inflammatory Features

Differences in average clinical measurements between the initial and subsequent visits were recorded and compared between the two groups.

Soft-tissue inflammatory signs of chemosis and lid edema worsened between the two visits in the severe group but improved in the mild group. This difference was statistically significant ($p < 0.04$).

Proptosis measurements worsened on average in the severe group and improved slightly in the mild group, a statistically significant difference ($p < 0.003$).

Degrees of duction in the most restricted direction of the most affected eye worsened on average 3–5° in the severe group and improved very slightly in the mild group, again statistically significant ($p < 0.003$).

There was no significant change in optic neuropathy status nor corneal exposure signs between the two visits in either group.

The duration of clinic management (from the first to final visit at the orbitopathy clinic when no further medical or surgical intervention was required) was significantly longer in the severe group (26.62 months) compared to the mild group (9.57 months), $p < 0.00001$.

DISCUSSION

Sixty-five percent of patients referred to our thyroid orbitopathy clinic in the 3-year study period were treated conservatively during their inflammatory phase, while 35% received more aggressive intervention, including systemic anti-inflammatories or radiotherapy. This figure is much higher than those reported elsewhere (6), possibly because of the referral center bias; patients with mild thyroid orbitopathy are often not recognized or not referred.

Demographic characteristics of our two groups correspond well with those of other studies. In our mild group, the racial distribution reflected our referral city's racial make-up, with 65% white, 20% Chinese, 10% Indian, and 5% other. The severe group had a much higher proportion of whites (92% compared with other races 8%), a finding noted in other studies (7).

Thyroid orbitopathy occurs most typically in the third to fifth decade (1). We found that patients with severe disease were on average 13 years older than those with mild disease, agreeing with previous observations.

While females outnumber males almost 4:1 in TO, it has been observed that males are more likely to present with severe disease (8); in our study, the severe group contained 78% females and 22% males while the mild group contained 84% females and 16% males, an insignificant difference.

The association between smoking and thyroid orbitopathy and other immune-mediated diseases has been well documented (9,10). The prevalence of smokers in the Canadian general population is 33% in 1992. A higher percentage of patients with severe orbitopathy were smokers in our study (54%) compared with those with milder disease (44%); although suggestive, this difference did not meet statistical significance.

The clinical symptoms and signs of soft-tissue inflammation and impaired ocular motility were significantly worse in the severe, treated group compared with the mild, nontreated group. This is an expected finding since at our clinic, medical intervention is only offered for significant soft-tissue inflammatory signs, progressive ocular motility restriction, or optic neuropathy.

Proptosis is not a criterion for medical intervention, but was on average 1.2 mm worse in the severe group (not statistically significant). Interestingly, more patients with mild disease complained of proptosis than those in the severe group, presumably because lid swelling, orbital pain, and diplopia were a bigger priority for the latter group, while lid retraction may have increased the perceived prominence in the mild group.

The course of disease documented by both patient and clinician is in our opinion another indication for anti-inflammatory intervention, although not often recognized as a deciding factor. In other words, the clinician should consider anti-inflammatory medications or radiotherapy for those patients who have progressive orbitopathy symptoms or signs. This study confirms that patients who were ultimately treated had shown significant worsening in soft-tissue inflammation and ocular motility compared to the mild, untreated group.

This study also identified that patients with severe disease requiring treatment are more likely to have an acute onset (over several weeks) of their symptoms and signs compared with patients having a mild course whose onset may occur over several months, even based on historical observations at their first clinical visit. Patients with severe disease were four times more likely to have an acute onset compared with those with mild disease. Therefore, patients with a rapid development of symptoms (less than 4 weeks) should be considered early for medical intervention rather than waiting for further worsening. Also, patients with an indolent course and mild symptoms on their first visit may be reassured that they are less likely to develop serious disease. We have not seen this observation recorded elsewhere, but feel that it is a useful predictive variable of orbitopathy severity.

As well, patients with mild disease stabilize rapidly with regard to management, while those with serious disease on average have a more protracted course. Patients with severe disease require on average 2 years of management before reaching a stable state where no further follow-up or intervention is required.

These differences between the mild and severe orbitopathy groups may help guide the clinician to advise and manage patients with TO, even on the first visit. Younger female patients with an indolent course and mild inflammatory features can be reassured that they are less likely to develop severe orbital sequelae. Older patients, those who report recent progression, and those with an acute onset of orbital symptoms and signs (including eyelid and conjunctival edema, progressive ocular restriction, and proptosis) should be followed closely and advised to watch for progression. These patients have a statistically higher risk of developing severe clinical findings, and treatment might be discussed and offered as early as the first office visit. Patients with mild disease can be told that on average all management will be completed within 9 months, while those with more severe features can plan for medical and surgical treatments lasting up to 2 years. All patients should be encouraged to stop smoking.

REFERENCES

1. Perros P, Kendall-Taylor P. Natural history of thyroid eye disease. Thyroid 1998; 8:423–425.

2. Kendall-Taylor P, Perros P. Clinical presentation of thyroid associated orbitopathy. Thyroid 1998; 8:427–428.

3. Perros P, Kendall-Taylor P. Natural history of thyroid associated ophthalmopathy. Clin Endocrinol 1995; 42:45–50.

4. Bartley GB, Gatourechi V, Kadrmas EF, et al. Long-term follow-up of Graves ophthalmopathy in an incidence cohort. Ophthalmology 1996; 103:958–962..

5. Gorman CA. The measurement of change in Graves' ophthalmopathy. Thyroid 1998; 8:539–543.

6. Char DH. Thyroid Eye Disease. 3rd ed. Boston: Butterworth-Heinemann, 1997.

7. Tellez M, Cooper J, Edmonds C. Graves' ophthalmopathy in relation to cigarette smoking and ethnic origin. Clin Endocrinol 1992; 36:291–294.

8. Kendler DL, Lippa J, Rootman J. The initial clinical characteristics of Graves' orbitopathy vary with age and sex. Arch Ophthalmol 1993; 111:197–201.

9. Brix TH, Hansen PS, Kyvik KO, Hegedus L. Cigarette smoking and risk of clinically overt thyroid disease: a population-based twin case–control study. Arch Int Med 2000; 160: 661–666.

10. Walfish PG, Wall JR, Volpe R. Autoimmunity and the Thyroid. Orlando: Academic Press, 1985.

19

Prognostic Factors

CLAUDIO MARCOCCI, MICHELE
MARINÒ, ROBERTO ROCCHI,
BARBARA MAZZI, FRANCESCA
MENCONI, EUGENIA MORABITO, and
ALDO PINCHERA
Dipartimento di Endocrinologia e
Metabolismo, Universita' di Pisa,
Varese, Italy

LUIGI BARTALENA
Cattedra di Endocrinologia,
Universita' dell'Insubria, Varese, Italy

The natural history of Graves' orbitopathy (GO) is incompletely understood but it is well established that severe forms of the disease are encountered in no more than 35% of patients (1). Genetic predisposition to GO, extensively studied especially for human leukocyte antigen associations, has so far been poorly characterized, and discrepant results have been reported (2). The disease tends to be more severe in older patients, and men tend to be more severely affected than women. The overall age-adjusted incidence rate in a population-based cohort study in Minnesota was 16 cases per

100,000 population/year for women, 2.9 cases per 100,000 population/year for men (3). Most interestingly, the disease seems less common and severe than in the past. Perros and Kendall-Taylor (4) reviewed the clinical records of the first 100 consecutive patients diagnosed as having Graves' disease at the beginning of each decade (1960–1990) at their large thyroid clinic. They found a significant decrease in the prevalence of relevant eye manifestations from 57% in 1960 to 35% in 1990; likewise, there was also a decline in the prevalence of the severe forms of the disease. The reason for this trend is unclear but it is conceivable that, on one hand, the earlier diagnosis of hyperthyroidism and its prompter correction by the endocrinologist, and, on the other hand, the increased attention of the ophthalmologist to the possible link between initial and mild ocular changes and thyroid dysfunction, may account for this variation.

Several risk factors have been identified, which may favor the development or worsening of GO (Table 1).

Graves' orbitopathy may occur before, concomitantly with, but also after the onset of hyperthyroidism (5). Thus, in many instances, the onset of eye disease follows the institution of treatments aimed at controlling or curing hyperthyroidism, making it difficult to establish whether the occurrence, amelioration, or aggravation of the ophthalmopathy is related to the natural history of the disease or is treatment-induced. Thyroid status per se, or, more likely, TSH-receptor activation, which occurs in both hyperthyroidism (via TSH-receptor antibody) and hypothyroidism

Table 1 Risk Factors for the Development/Worsening of Graves' Ophthalmopathy

---

Recurrence of hyperthyroidism
Severe hyperthyroidism
Elevated TSH-receptor antibodies
Elevated TSH levels
Radioiodine
Late correction of hypothyroidism
Preexisting orbitopathy
Smoking

(via TSH), can influence the course of the ophthalmopathy (1). In a series of 87 patients with ophthalmopathy, 54 were euthyroid at the time of referral and did not show any substantial modification of ocular involvement over the next 5 months, while the remaining 33 patients (slightly hyperthyroid or hypothyroid at the time of referral), showed a substantial improvement of the ophthalmopathy over the same period of time upon restoration of the euthyroid state (6). In another study, in which patients were subgrouped according to the increasing severity of the ophthalmopathy, a greater prevalence of patients with abnormal thyroid function was found in the subgroups with more severe ophthalmopathy (7). On the other hand, Karlsson et al. (8) noted that among 30 patients referred for severe ophthalmopathy, eye disease occurred in nine cases after radioiodine therapy (associated with a rise in TSH-receptor antibody levels), in three cases after a temporary withdrawal of thionamides (associated with a rebound of abnormal thyroid stimulation), but in 15 cases it manifested following a period with elevated serum TSH levels. Thus, the above studies suggested that both hyper- and hypothyroidism may account for progression of GO.

The information on the effect of treatment of hyperthyroidism on GO is, therefore, often conflicting, contradictory, and unclear. DeGroot et al. (9) found that the chance of having a progression of the ophthalmopathy was significantly higher in patients who required two or more doses of radioiodine than in those becoming hypothyroid after the first dose, suggesting that persistent hyperthyroidism may worsen the course of eye disease.

If abnormal thyroid status can affect the course of GO, what therefore is known about the effects of different treatment modalities for hyperthyroidism? Restoration of euthyroidism by thionamides was reported to be associated with an amelioration of eye disease (6,10). In a recent randomized and prospective study on the effect of radioiodine and methimazole on nonsevere ophthalmopathy, we found that among 148 patients treated with methimazole, 3 of the 74 patients with preexisting ophthalmopathy (4%) showed improvement and 4 patients in the whole group (3%) had a worsening of their eye disease (11). The large majority of available studies indicate that antithyroid drug therapy does not substantially affect the course of the ophthalmopathy and should not be considered a disease-modifying treatment. The major problem posed by antithyroid drug therapy is represented by the large number of recurrences after drug withdrawal. Recurrence of hyperthyroidism due to Graves' disease is accompanied by a reactivation of thyroid autoimmunity and it is conceivable that the exacerbation of thyroid autoimmune reactions may adversely affect the course of the ophthalmopathy.

Likewise, thyroid surgery does not seem to be associated with variations of the natural history of GO. Among other studies (11), a recent case–control prospective study of a relatively large cohort of patients submitted to near-total thyroidectomy showed no differences between the outcome of thyroid surgery and that of antithyroid drug treatment in terms of progression of the ophthalmopathy, since worsening of eye disease occurred only in 1 out of 30 patients (3.3%) submitted to surgery (12).

Radioiodine therapy is a well-established method of treatment of hyperthyroidism due to Graves' disease (13). The relationship between radioiodine therapy and GO course is a matter of controversy (14,15). In a randomized study, we treated a small cohort of patients with Graves' hyperthyroidism and mild or no ophthalmopathy with either radioiodine alone or radioiodine associated with a 3-month course of oral prednisone (0.4–0.5 mg/kg/day, initial dose) (16). Progression of ophthalmopathy was observed in 9 of 26 patients (35%) with eye involvement prior to radioiodine therapy; in the group also receiving prednisone, progression did not occur and preexisting ophthalmopathy improved in most cases. In a subsequent randomized, controlled study, Tallstedt et al. (17) found that the frequency of ophthalmopathy development or progression was similar in patients treated with thionamide or with thyroidectomy, but significantly higher in those receiving radioiodine therapy. The same group subsequently reported that the prompt administration of levothyroxine and the avoidance of untreated postradioiodine hypothyroidism were associated with a decrease in GO development

after radioiodine (18). The few available randomized and controlled studies suggest that radioiodine carries a small but
definite risk of causing GO progression, especially if GO
preexists or the patient smokes (10). However, this undue
outcome can effectively be prevented by concomitant glucocorticoid therapy (16). The GO progression after radioiodine
might be due to thyroid antigen release following radiation
injury and to subsequent exacerbation of autoimmune reactions directed towards antigens shared by thyroid and orbit
(13).

Progression of ophthalmopathy after radioiodine does
not occur in the majority of patients. This suggests that other
risk factors or cofactors for the progression of eye disease
must cooperate to this outcome: smoking (19), high pretreatment T3 values (17), high serum TSH-receptor antibody
(20), and thyrotropin (8) levels, and preexisting ophthalmopathy (11,16) are recognized risk factors for deterioration of eye
disease after radioiodine. A search for and identification of
other risk factors should allow a better coordinated treatment
of high-risk patients (1).

The effects of radioiodine on GO may have modified the
attitude of many endocrinologists. In a recent European survey, with regard to the treatment of recurrent hyperthyroidism after antithyroid drug therapy, thyroidectomy was
selected by 43% of respondents, a second course of antithyroid
drugs by 32%, and radioiodine by only 25% (21). Thus, when
ablative therapy was selected, the preference went to surgery
rather than radioiodine. We do not share the view that radioiodine therapy should be avoided in GO patients because GO
progression does not occur in the majority of cases and can be
prevented by concomitant glucocorticoid therapy. In addition,
thyroid ablation may prove useful for the long-term outcome
of GO.

In a prospective, randomized study, we assigned 450
patients with hyperthyroidism due to Graves' disease and
mild or no ophthalmopathy to treatment with either radioiodine alone, methimazole, or radioiodine followed by treatment
with oral prednisone. Among the 150 patients treated with
radioiodine alone, progression of the ophthalmopathy was

observed in 23 cases (15%), and this was persistent only in 8 (5%) who subsequently required treatment for ophthalmopathy. Progression of eye disease was not observed in the group treated also with prednisone, in which preexisting eye disease improved in two-thirds of cases. Treatment with methimazole did not influence the course of the ophthalmopathy. Admittedly, progression of ophthalmopathy after radioiodine does not occur in the majority of patients.

An increased prevalence of smokers has been reported in patients with Graves' hyperthyroidism, particularly when associated with orbitopathy (22–24). In a case–control study, the odds ratio for smoking was 7.7 (95% CI 4.3–13.7) (23). Indeed, among patients with Graves' ophthalmopathy and Graves' hyperthyroidism, 64% are smokers, which is a significantly higher proportion than the 48% smokers among Graves' hyperthyroid patients without clinically apparent GO; the figure of 48% in its turn is higher than the 31% smokers in control populations (10). The odds ratio of smoking for Graves' hyperthyroidism without eye changes is 1.9 (95% CI 1.1–2.7) (23). Thus, smoking is a risk factor for Graves' hyperthyroidism too, but the odds are much higher for GO. Indeed, the odds increase progressively with more severe eye disease.

Some but not all studies observe a dose–response relationship between smoking and GO. Pfeilschifter and Ziegler (24) report among current smokers a relative risk (RR) for diplopia of 1.8 (95% CI 0.8–4.3) at a dose of 1–10 cigarettes per day; the RR is 3.8 (95% CI 1.9–7.7) for 11–20 cigarettes per day, and 7.0 RR (95% CI 3.0–16.5) for greater than 20 cigarettes per day. They report similar figures for proptosis. Most importantly, among ex-smokers who smoked more than 20 cigarettes per day the RR for diplopia is 1.9 (95% 0.5–7.7), which is no longer significant. The disappearance of excess risk in heavy smokers who quit smoking constitutes positive evidence that to stop smoking prevents GO.

Other circumstantial evidence for a causal relationship between smoking and development of GO is derived from incidence rates. A questionnaire study among 84 physicians from the European Thyroid Association indicated that 43% of respondents thought the incidence of GO had fallen in the last decade: 42% thought the incidence had remained the same, 12% noticed an increased incidence, and 4% had no opinion (21). The respondents who thought the incidence had fallen were mainly from Western European countries (United Kingdom, The Netherlands, and France) in which tobacco consumption has declined in the last decade. In contrast, the 12% of respondents who saw a rising incidence of GO came mainly from Poland and Hungary, countries where tobacco consumption is on the increase since the fall of the wall.

We recently reviewed the outcome of mild ophthalmopathy after radioiodine therapy and the response of severe ophthalmopathy to orbital radiotherapy and systemic glucocorticoids in relation to smoking habits. Among patients with mild ophthalmopathy, we found that after radioiodine therapy, eye disease progressed in 4 of 68 nonsmokers (5%) and in 19 of 32 smokers (23%, $p = 0.007$) the combination of radioiodine therapy with a short course of oral prednisone was associated with an improvement of ophthalmopathy in 37 of 58 nonsmokers (64%) and 13 of 87 smokers (15%, $p < 0.001$). Among patients with severe ophthalmopathy treated with orbital radiotherapy and high-dose glucocorticoids, a response to treatment was observed in 61 of 65 nonsmokers (94%) and 58 of 85 smokers (68%, $p < 0.001$).

Thus, it seems evident that cigarette smoking can profoundly influence the occurrence and the course of eye disease, and also impair its response to orbital radiotherapy and glucocorticoids. Smoking might do this by direct irritative actions on the eyes; however, this might account for inflammatory changes but not for the increased volume of the extraocular muscles and retrobulbar fibroadipose tissue (25). Smoking might affect immunological reactions possibly involved in the pathogenesis of eye disease by altering the structure of the TSH receptor and making it more immunogenic, hampering restoration of tolerance to autoantigens shared by the thyroid and the orbit, or sensitizing the orbital tissue to whatever substance or antibody that can trigger GO. The mechanisms by which cigarette smoking affects GO remain a matter of argument but the relationship between smoking and eye disease appears to be well established. Accordingly, patients should be strongly urged to stop smoking. Although some data suggest that refraining from smoking might favorably influence the course of ophthalmopathy, this remains to be established by appropriate prospective studies.

In conclusion, several risk factors have been identified that may favor the occurrence and worsening of GO. Future research should include among its goals the identification of other currently unknown environmental risk factors for the development of GO, as well a better definition of its genetic background. This should help to understand why only a minority of Graves' patients develop severe ocular manifestations.

REFERENCES

1. Burch HB, Wartofsky L. Graves' ophthalmopathy: current concepts regarding pathogenesis and management. Endocr Rev 1993; 14:747–793.

2. Farid NR, Balazs C. The genetics of thyroid associated ophthalmopathy. Thyroid 1998; 8:407–409.

3. Bartley GB. The epidemiological characteristics and clinical course of ophthalmopathy associated with autoimmune thyroid disease in Olmsted County, Minnesota. Trans Am Ophthalmol Soc 1994; 92:477–588.

4. Perros P, Kendall-Taylor P. Natural history of thyroid eye disease. Thyroid 1998; 8:423–425.

5. Marcocci C, Bartalena L, Bogazzi F, Panicucci M, Pinchera A. Studies on the occurrence of ophthalmopathy in Graves' disease. Acta Endocrinol (Copenh) 1989; 120:473–478.

6. Prummel MF, Wiersinga WM, Mourits MP, Koornneef L, Berghout A, van der Gaag R. Amelioration of eye changes of Graves' ophthalmopathy by achieving euthyroidism. Acta Endocrinol (Copenh) 1989; 121(suppl 2):185–189.

7. Prummel MF, Wiersinga WM, Mourits MP, Koornneef L, Berghout A, van der Gaag R. Effect of abnormal thyroid function on the severity of Graves' ophthalmopathy. Arch Intern Med 1990; 150:1098–1101.

8. Karlsson AF, Westermark K, Dahlberg PA, Jansson R, Enoksson P. Ophthalmopathy and thyroid stimulation. Lancet 1989; 2:691.

9. DeGroot LJ, Mangklabruks A, McCormick M. Comparison of RA^{131}I treatment protocols for Graves' disease. J Endocrinol Invest 1990; 13:111–118.

10. Bartalena L, Pinchera A, Marcocci C. Management of Graves' ophthalmopathy: reality and perspectives. Endocr Rev 2000; 21:168.

11. Bartalena L, Marcocci C, Bogazzi F, Manetti L, Tanda ML, Dell'Unto E, Bruno-Bossio G, Nardi M, Bartolomei MP, Lepri A, Rossi G, Martino E, Pinchera A. Relation between therapy for hyperthyroidism and the course of Graves' ophthalmopathy. N Engl J Med 1998; 338:73–78.

12. Marcocci C, Bruno-Bossio G, Manetti L, Tanda ML, Miccoli P, Iacconi P, Bartolomei MP, Nardi M, Pinchera A, Bartalena L. The course of Graves' ophthalmopathy is not influenced by near-total thyroidectomy: a case–control study. Clin Endocrinol (Oxf) 1999; 51:503–508.

13. Marcocci C, Bartalena L, Pinchera A. Ablative or non-ablative therapy for Graves' hyperthyroidism in patients with ophthalmopathy? J Endocrinol Invest 1998; 21:468–471.

14. Gorman CA. Radioiodine therapy does not aggravate Graves' ophthalmopathy. J Clin Endocrinol Metab 1995; 80:340–342.

15. Pinchera A, Bartalena L, Marcocci C. Radioiodine may be bad for Graves' ophthalmopathy, but .... J Clin Endocrinol Metab 1995; 80:342–345.

16. Bartalena L, Marcocci C, Bogazzi F, Panicucci M, Lepri A, Pinchera A. Use of corticosteroids to prevent progression of Graves' ophthalmopathy after radioiodine therapy for hyperthyroidism. N Engl J Med 1989; 321:1349–1352.

17. Tallstedt L, Lundell G, Torring O, Wallin G, Ljunggren J-G, Blomgren H, Taube A. Thyroid Study Group. Occurrence of ophthalmopathy after treatment for Graves' hyperthyroidism. N Engl J Med 1992; 326:1733–1738.

18. Tallstedt L, Lundell G, Blomgren H, Bring J. Does early administration of thyroxine reduce the development of Graves'

ophthalmopathy after radioiodine treatment? Eur J Endocrinol 1994; 130:494–497.

19. Bartalena L, Marcocci C, Tanda ML, Manetti L, Dell'Unto E, Bartolomei MP, Nardi M, Martino E, Pinchera A. Cigarette smoking and treatment outcomes in Graves' ophthalmopathy. Ann Intern Med 1998; 129:632–635.

20. Kung AWC, Yau CC, Cheng A. The incidence of ophthalmopathy after radioiodine therapy for Graves' disease: prognostic factors and the role of methimazole. J Clin Endocrinol Metab 1994; 79:542–546.

21. Weetman A, Wiersinga WM. Current management of thyroid-associated ophthalmopathy in Europe. Results of an international survey. Clin Endocrinol (Oxf) 1998; 49:21–28.

22. Bartalena L, Martino E, Marcocci C, Bogazzi F, Panicucci M, Velluzzi F, Loviselli A, Pinchera A. More on smoking habits and Graves' ophthalmopathy. J Endocrinol Invest 1989; 12:733–737.

23. Prummel MF, Wiersinga WM. Smoking and risk of Graves' disease. JAMA 1993; 269:479–482.

24. Pfeilschifter J, Ziegler R. Smoking and endocrine ophthalmopathy: impact of smoking severity and current vs lifetime cigarette consumption. Clin Endocrinol (Oxf) 1996; 45: 477–481.

25. Bartalena L, Bogazzi F, Tanda ML, Manetti L, Dell'Unto E, Martino E. Cigarette smoking and the thyroid. Eur J Endocrinol 1995; 133:507–512.

20

Relationship Between Thyroid Disorders and Orbitopathy, Including Management Factors

WILMAR M. WIERSINGA

Department of Medicine, Academic Medical
Center, University of Amsterdam,
Amsterdam, The Netherlands

Graves' disease is a multisystem disorder, which can manifest itself as Graves' hyperthyroidism, Graves' ophthalmopathy (GO), localized myxedema, and thyroid acropachy. Graves' hyperthyroidism is the most prevalent phenotype with a female to male ratio of 8:1. Graves' ophthalmopathy is less prevalent with a sex ratio of 5.5:1, occurring mostly in association with Graves' hyperthyroidism but hyperthyroidism is absent in about 20% of patients presenting with GO. Localized myxedema is rare with a sex ratio of 3.5:1, almost always occurring together with Graves' hyperthyroidism

223

and to a lesser extent with GO. Thyroid acropachy is a very rare condition with an equal sex distribution of 1:1, seen almost exclusively in patients who also express the other phenotypes of Graves' disease. When present, GO usually manifests itself in the first year after the onset of Graves' hyperthyroidism, localized myxedema in the second year and thyroid acropachy in the third year. Serum concentrations of thyroid stimulating immunoglobulins (TSI), the hallmark of Graves' disease, are generally higher in Graves' hyperthyroid patients with GO than in Graves' hyperthyroid patients without GO, and are even higher in patients who also have the other two phenotypes. The question arises whether the differential expression of phenotypes in Graves' disease patients just reflects the severity of the autoimmune attack, or that the phenotypes constitute different albeit closely related disease entities.

GRAVES' HYPERTHYROIDISM AND GRAVES' OPHTHALMOPATHY: ONE OR TWO DISEASE ENTITIES?

Not all patients with GO have hyperthyroidism, and not all Graves' hyperthyroid patients have clinically apparent GO. The question whether Graves' hyperthyroidism and GO belong to one disease entity or that they must be viewed as two different entities, can be approached from either the population of GO patients or from the population of Graves' hyperthyroid patients.

Among 125 consecutive patients referred because of GO, Graves' hyperthyroidism—past or present—was found in 77% and Hashimoto's hypothyroidism in 3%; the remaining patients (20%) were clinically euthyroid (1). Taking together several large series of patients with both GO and Graves' hyperthyroidism, it appears that the onset of GO occurred before the onset of Graves' hyperthyroidism in 19.6%, concurrent with Graves' hyperthyroidism in 39.4%, and after Graves' hyperthyroidism in 41% (2). Thus, the vast majority of GO patients develop the eye disease in conjunction with

Graves' hyperthyroidism, that is, in the presence of TSH receptor stimulating antibodies (TSI). The rare patients with hypothyroid GO have serological evidence of Hashimoto's thyroiditis as evident from the presence of serum thyroid peroxidase antibodies (TPO-Ab). They usually also have antibodies directed against the TSH receptor, which may be of the blocking type thereby contributing to the hypothyroid state. A switch from blocking to stimulating TSH receptor antibodies has been described in such patients, associated with evolvement of the hypothyroid state towards hyperthyroidism (3). A typical case history in this respect is that of a 53-year-old man presenting in our clinics with mild GO and goitrous Hashimoto's hypothyroidism, which was treated with thyroxine. Three months later GO deteriorated, necessitating treatment with prednisone. Two months thereafter the dose of thyroxine had to be decreased because of weight loss and tachycardia. Subsequently, the patient appeared hyperthyroid without any thyroxine medication, and methimazole was instituted. Patients with euthyroid GO do not differ from those with hyperthyroid GO with regard to sex, age at onset of the eye disease, or clinical presentation of GO as judged from a similar frequency distribution of eye changes in the various NO SPECS classes (4). In 90% of patients with euthyroid GO, thyroid abnormalities are found, as evident from discrete changes in the hypothalamus-pituitary-thyroid axis (e.g., an abnormal serum TSH, TRH stimulation test, or T3-suppression test) and from the presence of thyroid autoimmunity (e.g., TPO-Ab, TSI) (2). A fair proportion of these patients progress to develop hyperthyroidism ($\sim$13%) or hypothyroidism ($\sim$15%). Thus, although thyroid function remains normal in many patients with euthyroid GO, the vast majority has evidence of coexisting autoimmune thyroid disease.

Among Graves' hyperthyroid patients without clinically apparent GO, evidence for subclinical orbital involvement can be found in the vast majority if not all patients. The evidence includes: (a) a shift to higher proptosis values as compared to healthy controls and patients with Hashimoto's disease (5), (b) an abnormal elevation of intraocular pressure with upward gaze in 61% of patients (6), and (c) enlarged extra-ocular muscles on echography or CT scan in 70% to 100% (7).

The close temporal relationship between onset of GO and hyperthyroidism, the subclinical eye involvement in Graves' hyperthyroidism without clinically apparent GO, and the thyroid involvement in euthyroid GO all argue in favor of the view that we are dealing with one disease entity (namely Graves' disease) rather than with two separate disease entities.

GENETIC AND ENVIRONMENTAL FACTORS INVOLVED IN PHENOTYPIC APPEARANCE OF GRAVES' DISEASE

If one accepts the view that GO and Graves' hyperthyroidism belong to one and the same disease, then which factors determine the expression of both phenotypes? Reasons for differences in phenotypic appearance of Graves' disease could be related to differences in genetic background and in exposure to environmental factors.

Numerous studies have been done searching for genetic differences between Graves' hyperthyroid patients with or without GO. Results have been mainly conflicting, explained largely by a too small sample size in most studies. Besides, improvement in the accuracy of genotyping plays a role; whereas older studies used the mixed lymphocyte reaction and antibodies for HLA typing, nowadays the more reliable polymerase chain reaction is applied using allele-specific oligonucleotide probes. The only undisputed locus so far, both in Caucasian and Japanese patients, seems to be in the HLA-DP region: HLA-DPBI*201 is less prevalent in GO patients (3%) than in Graves' hyperthyroid patients without GO (21%) or controls (30%) (8). The protection against GO by the presence of HLA-DPBI*201 is, however, weak. CTLA-4 alleles are associated with Graves' disease in Caucasians and in Japanese. One study reports that the biallelic polymorphism CTLA-4 A/G at codon 17 confers susceptibility to GO (9). The strength of the G allele with GO increases with the severity of the eye disease: odds ratios are 1.49 for classes 1 and 2, 1.67 for classes 3 and 4, and 3.06 for classes 5 and 6 eye changes compared to Graves' hyperthyroid patients without GO. Other studies do not confirm a specific association between CTLA-4 polymorphism and GO (10,11). The obtained results so far have not demonstrated a powerful association of a specific genotype with the phenotype of GO.

The situation is different with respect to environmental factors, as smokers among Graves' disease patients have a clearly higher risk to develop GO than nonsmokers. As compiled from 10 studies, the proportion of smokers is 65% in Graves' hyperthyroid patients with GO, 43% in Graves' hyperthyroid patients without GO, and 34% in controls. The risk to develop Graves' hyperthyroidism in relation to smoking is small: the reported odds ratio in a large case–control study is 1.9 (95% CI 1.1–3.2). The odds for developing GO are much higher: 7.7 (95% CI 4.3–13.7) for current smokers including those who had stopped smoking in the last 5 years (12). The odds increase with increasing severity of the eye disease. A dose–response relationship between smoking (number of cigarettes per day or pack-years) and GO is observed in some but not all studies. The biologic explanation for the association between smoking and GO is incompletely understood, but exposure to hypoxia and tobacco glycoprotein enhances the production of IL-1 and glycosaminoglycans by orbital fibroblasts in culture. Of special interest is a study demonstrating a relative risk of 7.0 (95% CI 3.0–16.5) for the development of diplopia in current smokers (> 20 cigarettes per day), whereas the relative risk was 1.9 (95% CI 0.5–5.7) in ex-smokers who also had smoked > 20 cigarettes per day (13). This finding constitutes positive evidence that refraining from smoking prevents to a certain extent the development of GO.

INFLUENCE OF THYROID FUNCTION ON GRAVES' OPHTHALMOPATHY

One may ask if it matters for the eyes whether the patient is euthyroid or still has an abnormal thyroid function. To answer this question, we evaluated the severity of untreated GO in relation to thyroid function in a series of consecutive patients referred because of GO, in whom the hyperthyroid state had already been treated by the referring physicians. Still, a slightly abnormal thyroid function existed in 36 patients. As compared to the 54 patients who were euthyroid at the time of referral, the dysthyroid patients had more severe GO as indicated by a higher total eye score (8.6 ± 6.6 vs. 10.6 ± 6.6, p = 0.009) (14). While awaiting specific treatment for GO, the eye changes remained stable in the euthyroid patients during a mean follow-up of 20 weeks. Restoration of euthyroidism in the dysthyroid patients by adjusting the dose of antithyroid drugs and/or thyroxine ameliorated the eye changes, as evident from a significant fall in their total eye score (15). Improvements were mainly in classes 2 and 4 of the NO SPECS system. Restoration and maintenance of the euthyroid state thus appear to have a beneficial albeit small effect on the ophthalmopathy.

EFFECT OF ANTITHYROID DRUGS, THYROIDECTOMY, AND RADIOACTIVE IODINE ON GRAVES' OPHTHALMOPATHY

The next obvious question is whether it matters for the eyes how the hyperthyroid state is treated. The topic has been the subject of heavy dispute. In view of the existing controversy around this issue, the most appropriate way to proceed is to go by the results of randomized clinical trials (RCTs).

An RCT by Tallstedt et al.(16) found that the frequency of developing or worsening of GO was similar in Graves' hyperthyroid patients treated with thionamides (10%) or with thyroidectomy (16%), but significantly higher after ^{131}I therapy (33%). The authors concluded that a pretreatment serum T3 of > 5 nmol/L and ^{131}I therapy are risk factors for developing or worsening of GO. Their study has been criticized because the prevalence of smokers was higher in the radioiodine group than in the other groups, and because thyroxine was not prescribed in ^{131}I treated patients until hypothyroidism had developed whereas thyroxine was given routinely to the surgical and medical groups. Indeed a subsequent study by the same authors indicated developing or worsening of GO after ^{131}I therapy in 18% when thyroxine administration was delayed until hypothyroidism had occurred, but in 11% (a significantly lower proportion) when thyroxine was administered routinely after radioactive iodine (17). Another study also observed that an elevated serum TSH after ^{131}I therapy was a risk factor for developing or worsening of GO (18).

The risk of ^{131}I therapy has been confirmed in a large RCT by Bartalena et al.(19). Developing or worsening of GO occurred in 3% of 148 Graves' hyperthyroid patients randomized to receive methimazole, in 15% of 150 patients treated with ^{131}I, and in 0% of 145 patients treated with ^{131}I and prednisone. The data on prednisone merely confirm the beneficial effect of glucocorticoids on eye changes in Graves' disease; the relevant comparison is between the methimazole and ^{131}I group. In view of the absence of an untreated control group, one may argue that 15% of patients with developing or worsening ophthalmopathy after ^{131}I therapy reflect the natural course of Graves' disease. If so, one must then conclude that methimazole favorably affects the natural history, as the frequency of 3% ophthalmopathy in this group is significantly lower than 15% after [131]I. However, there are good reasons to believe that 3% reflects the natural history, and that the excess of 15% is really caused by ^{131}I therapy because a plausible biologic explanation is at hand (20). Specifically,[131]I therapy is followed by activation of peripheral blood T-cells (21) and a long-lasting increase in concentration and activity of TSH-receptor antibodies, which does not happen after antithyroid drugs (22). Serum TSI in GO patients is directly related to quantitative measures of the eye disease such as proptosis and the clinical activity score (23), and a functional TSH receptor is expressed in orbital adipose/connective tissue of GO patients (24). Development or progression of GO after ^{131}I therapy might thus be due to release of thyroid antigens caused by radiation injury and to subsequent autoimmune reactions directed toward shared antigens (possibly the TSH receptor) between the thyroid and the orbit (25).

The risk on eye changes after ^{131}I therapy is fortunately small. Eye changes when they occur, develop in the first 6 months and are transient, lasting for 2–3 months in two-thirds of patients; the eye changes persist in one-third of patients, mainly in those who had pre-existing ophthalmopathy. The occurrence of eye changes after ^{131}I therapy is four times more common in smokers than in nonsmokers. Determinants of developing or worsening of eye changes after ^{131}I therapy are thus smoking, pre-existent ophthalmopathy, pretreatment serum T3 > 5 nmol/L, elevated serum TSH posttreatment, and high serum TSI. Rather than exposing all patients selected for ^{131}I therapy to prednisone in order to prevent eye changes in a small subset, one may restrict preventive administration of glucocorticoids to high-risk patients, who are identifiable by the mentioned determinants of postradioiodine eye changes (26). An alternative course might be to treat Graves' hyperthyroidism with antithyroid drugs until treatment of the ophthalmopathy has been completed. This may take 1–2 years, and there is a risk of a flare-up of the eye disease upon recurrent Graves' hyperthyroidism after discontinuation of antithyroid drugs. However, deterioration or development of eye changes after a relapse seems to be a rare event (22).

Based upon the results of RCTs, it seems that antithyroid drugs and thyroidectomy are neutral with respect to eye changes.^{131}I is not contraindicated in Graves' hyperthyroid patients without GO. In patients with mild pre-existent GO,^{131}I therapy carries a small risk of developing or worsening of (mostly transient) eye changes; preventive use of glucocorticoids in this setting should be restricted to high-risk patients. There are no RCTs on treatment of Graves' hyperthyroidism in patients with severe pre-existent GO; our own preference in this group is treatment with antithyroid drugs. It can be argued that complete ablation of thyroid tissue is important for the removal of both thyroid-orbit cross-reacting antigens and thyroid autoreactive T-lymphocytes, and thus of benefit for the ophthalmopathy (27). Indeed, a retrospective study in surgically treated Graves' hyperthyroid patients showed less ophthalmopathy after total thyroidectomy (6%) than after subtotal thyroidectomy (16%) (28). The extent of thyroid surgery, however, had no substantial effect on GO (29). A carefully executed case–control study demonstrated an equal frequency of 3.3% for development or worsening of eye changes after near-total thyroidectomy and after treatment with methimazole (30). Whether or not total thyroid ablation is useful in preventing or ameliorating GO remains an unresolved issue.

The adverse effects of ^{131}I therapy on ophthalmopathy have apparently changed medical practice. In a questionnaire among European endocrinologists regarding treatment of recurrent Graves' hyperthyroidism, radioiodine was the preferred option in 64% and surgery in 8% of respondents in the absence of GO; in case of coexistent GO, there was a clear shift away from radioiodine (now preferred by only 25%) toward surgery (preferred by 43%) (31).

PREVENTION OF GRAVES' OPHTHALMOPATHY BY EARLIER DIAGNOSIS AND TREATMENT OF GRAVES' HYPERTHYROIDISM?

Graves' ophthalmopathy seems to a certain extent a preventable event. Most important in the primary prevention of GO appears to be to refrain from smoking (13). Discontinuation of smoking might also lower the chance of a relapse of Graves' hyperthyroidism (and thereby of GO) as the recurrence rate is higher in smokers than in nonsmokers (49% vs. 21%) (32). If one accepts the view that subclinical GO is already present in Graves' hyperthyroid patients without apparent eye changes, early diagnosis and appropriate treatment of Graves' hyperthyroidism might have value in the secondary prevention of GO. The introduction of a sensitive TSH assay in the late 1980s and its wide accessibility to family physicians certainly have facilitated the early diagnosis of hyperthyroidism, and the impression is that hyperthyroidism is indeed diagnosed at an earlier stage than in former times. In agreement with this line of thinking are the results of a European survey on GO: 43% of respondents said the prevalence of GO had decreased in the last decade, 42% said the prevalence was unchanged, and 12% had noted an increased prevalence (but these latter respondents came all from Eastern European countries where the prevalence of smoking has greatly risen since the fall of the wall). A decline in the prevalence of GO among referred patients with Graves' hyperthyroidism is also reported by one large thyroid clinic in the United Kingdom, from 57% in 1960 to 35% in 1990; this group also noted a decline in the severity of GO (33). Although the evidence for the efficacy of secondary prevention of GO is less solid, it would be of great utility to know which patients with just Graves' hyperthyroidism would progress to develop full-blown GO. If the determinants of developing GO were known more precisely, an accurate prediction of the development of GO could be made. Preventive intervention in such patients at risk might then become feasible.

REFERENCES

1. Wiersinga WM, Smit T, van der Gaag RD, Koornneef L. Temporal relationship between onset of Graves' ophthalmopathy and onset of thyroidal Graves' disease. J Endocrinol Invest 1988; 11:615–619.

2. Burch HB, Wartofsky L. Graves' ophthalmopathy: current concepts regarding pathogenesis and management. Endocr Rev 1993; 14:747–793.

3. Takasu N, Yamada T, Sato A, Nakagawa M, Komiya I, Naga-sawa Y, Asawa T. Graves' disease following hypothyroidism due to Hashimoto's disease: studies of eight cases. Clin Endo-crinol 1990; 33(6):687–698.

4. Wiersinga WM, Smit T, van der Gaag RD, Mourits MPh, Koornneef L. Clinical presentation of Graves' ophthalmopathy. Ophthalmic Res 1989; 21:73–82.

5. Amino N, Yuasa T, Yaba Y, Miyai K, Kumahaza Y. Exophthal-mos in autoimmune thyroid disease. J Clin Endocrinol Metab 1980; 51:1232–1234.

6. Gamblin GT, Harper DG, Galentine P, Buck DR, Chernow B, Eil C. Prevalence of intraocular pressure in Graves'

disease—evidence of frequent subclinical ophthalmopathy. New Engl J Med 1983; 308:420–424.

7. Forrester JV, Sutherland GR, McDougall IR. Dysthyroid ophthalmopathy: orbital evaluation with B-scan ultrasonography. J Clin Endocrinol Metab 1977; 45:221–224.

8. Weetman AP, Zhang L, Webb S, Shine B. Analysis of HLA-DQB and HLA-DPB alleles in Graves' disease by oligonucleotide probing of enzymatically amplified DNA. Clin Endocrinol 1990; 33:65–71.

9. Vaidya B, Imrie H, Perros P, Dickinson J, McCarthy MI, Kendall-Taylor P, Pearce SH. Cytokine T lymphocyte antigen-4 (CTLA-4) gene polymorphism confers susceptibility to thyroid associated orbitopathy. Lancet 1999; 354(9180):743–744.

10. Kotsa K, Watson PF, Weetman AP. A CTLA-4 gene polymorphism is associated with both Graves' disease and autoimmune hypothyroidism. Clin Endocrinol 1997; 46:551–554.

11. Donner H, Rau H, Walfish PG, Braun J, Siegmund T, Finke R, Herwig J, Usadel KH. CTLA 4 alanine-17 confers genetic susceptibility to Graves' disease and to type 1 diabetes mellitus. J Clin Endocrinol Metab 1997; 82(1):143–146.

12. Prummel MF, Wiersinga WM. Smoking and risk of Graves' disease. JAMA 1993; 269:479–482.

13. Pfeilschifter J, Ziegler R. Smoking and endocrine ophthalmopathy: impact of smoking and current vs lifetime cigarette consumption. Clin Endocrinol (Oxf) 1996; 45:477–481.

14. Prummel MF, Wiersinga WM, Mourits MPh, Koornneef L, Berghout A, van der Gaag RD. Effect of abnormal thyroid function on the severity of Graves' ophthalmopathy. Arch Intern Med 1990; 150:1098–1101.

15. Prummel MF, Wiersinga WM, Mourits MPh, Koornneef L, Berghout A, van der Gaag RD. Amelioration of eye changes of Graves' ophthalmopathy by achieving euthyroidism. Acta Endocrinologica 1989; 121(suppl 2):185–189.

16. Tallstedt L, Lundell G, Torring O, Wallin G, Ljunggren J-G, Blomgren H, Taube A, Thyroid Study Group. Occurrence of ophthalmopathy after treatment for Graves' hyperthyroidism. N Engl J Med 1992; 326:1733–1738.

17. Tallstedt L, Lundell G, Blomgren H, Bring J. Does early administration of thyroxine reduce the development of Graves' ophthalmopathy after radioiodine treatment? Eur J Endocrinol 1994; 130:494–497.

18. Kung AWC, Yau CC, Cheng A. The incidence of ophthalmopathy after radioiodine therapy for Graves' disease: prognostic factors and the role of methimazole. J Clin Endocrinol Metab 1994; 79:542–546.

19. Bartalena L, Marcocci C, Bogazzi F, Manetti L, Tanda ML, Dell'Unto E, Bruno-Bossio G, Nardi M, Bartolomei MP, Lepri A, Rossi G, Martino E, Pinchera A. Relation between therapy for hyperthyroidism and the course of Graves' ophthalmopathy. N Engl J Med 1998; 338:73–78.

20. Wiersinga WM. Preventing Graves' ophthalmopathy. N Engl J Med 1998; 338:121–122.

21. Teng W-P, Stark R, Munro AJ, Young SM, Borysiewicz LK, Weetman AP. Peripheral blood T cell activation after radioiodine treatment for Graves' disease. Acta Endocrinol (Copenh) 1990; 122(2):233–240.

22. Törring O, Tallstedt L, Wallin G, Lundell G, Ljunggren JG, Taube A, Saaf M, Hamberger B. Graves' hyperthyroidism: treatment with antithyroid drugs, surgery, or radioactive iodine—a prospective, randomized study. Thyroid Study Group. J Clin Endocrinol Metab 1996; 81(8):2986–2993.

23. Gerding MN, van der Meer JWC, Broenink M, Bakker O, Wiersinga WM, Prummel MF. Association of thyrotropin receptor antibodies with the clinical features of Graves' ophthalmopathy. Clin Endocrinol 2000; 52(3):267–271.

24. Valyasevi RW, Erickson DZ, Harteneck DA, Dutton CM, Heufelder AE, Jyonouchi SC, Bahn RS. Differentiation of human orbital preadipocyte fibroblasts induces expression of functional thyrotropin receptor. J Clin Endocrinol Metab 1999; 84(7):2557–2562.

25. Wiersinga WM, Prummel MF. Pathogenesis of Graves' ophthalmopathy; current understanding. J Clin Endocrinol Metab 2001; 86:501–503.

26. Wiersinga WM. Preventing Graves' ophthalmopathy. N Engl J Med 1998; 338:121–122.

27. Bartalena L, Pinchera A, Marcocci C. Management of Graves' ophthalmopathy: reality and perspectives. Endocr Rev 2000; 21:168–199.

28. Winsa B, Rastad J, Akerstrom G, Johansson H, Westermark K, Karlsson FA. Retrospective evaluation of subtotal and total thyroidectomy in Graves' disease with and without endocrine ophthalmopathy. Eur J Endocrinol 1995; 132:406–412.

29. Miccoli P, Vitti P, Rago T, Iacconi P, Bartalena L, Bogazzi F, Fiore E, Valeriano R, Chiovato L, Rocchi R, Pinchera A. Surgical treatment of Graves' disease: subtotal or total thyroidectomy? Surgery 1996; 120(6):1020–1024.

30. Marcocci C, Bruno-Bossio G, Manetti L, Tanda ML, Miccoli P, Iacconi P, Bartolomei MP, Nardi M, Pinchera A, Bartalena L. The course of Graves' ophthalmopathy is not influenced by near-total thyroidectomy: a case–control study. Clin Endocrinol (Oxf) 1999; 51:503–508.

31. Weetman A, Wiersinga WM. Current management of thyroid-associated ophthalmopathy in Europe. Results of an international survey. Clin Endocrinol 1998; 49:21–28.

32. Glinoer D, de Nayer P, Bex M. Belgian Collaborative Study Group on Graves' Disease. Effects of L-thyroxine administration, TSH-receptor antibodies and smoking on the risk of recurrence in Graves' hyperthyroidism treated with antithyroid drugs: a double-blind prospective randomized study. Eur J Endocrinol 2001; 144(5):475–483.

33. Perros P, Kendall-Taylor P. Natural history of thyroid eye disease. Thyroid 1998; 8:423–425.

21

Monitoring Activity of Graves' Ophthalmopathy

WILMAR M. WIERSINGA

Department of Medicine, Academic Medical
Center, University of Amsterdam,
Amsterdam, The Netherlands

CLINICAL UTILITY OF MEASURING DISEASE ACTIVITY IN GRAVES' OPHTHALMOPATHY

The best description of the natural history of Graves' ophthalmopathy (GO) is given by Rundle (1–3). He performed sequential quantitative measurements of eye changes in patients who did not receive any specific treatment of GO. From their studies, a curve can be constructed reflecting the natural course of the severity of GO (Fig. 1A). An initial dynamic phase is followed by a late static phase. The dynamic phase starts with a stage of increasing severity. Exophthalmos develops in conjunction with restriction of

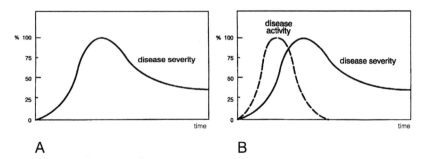

A   B

Figure 1 Natural history of Graves' ophthalmopathy, depicted as changes in severity of the eye disease according to Rundle (A) and as changes in activity of the eye disease as hypothesized by ourselves (B). (Reproduced with permission from Ref. 7.)

eye muscle motility and widening of the lid aperture. In general, for every increase of proptosis of 1 mm, elevation is restricted by 4–5°. After having reached the peak of disease severity, the eye changes spontaneously improve to a certain extent, the stage of reconvalescence. When the eye changes remain stable, the disease has come in its end-stage, the static phase. Note that in 75% of patients, the eye changes have not completely resolved, and remaining eye changes may still be disfiguring and incapacitating. Histologic examination of orbital tissues in the early stages demonstrate lymphocytic infiltration, activated fibroblasts, and edema in extraocular muscles and orbital fat. In the late stages, there is dense collagen, fibrosis, and fat accumulation (4–6). The findings in the early stages reflect the active ongoing inflammation caused by the autoimmune reaction, whereas findings in the late stages indicate the inactive, fibrotic, burnt-out end-stage of the disease. We hypothesized that upon spontaneous resolution of the eye changes at the stage of reconvalescence, the activity of the eye disease must already be on the decline. Consequently, we propose an additional curve describing the natural history of GO in terms of disease activity (Fig. 1B) (7).

It is likely that immunosuppressive treatment of GO will have no effect when applied in the inactive fibrotic stage of the disease, but will be effective when administered in the active inflammatory stage. As can been seen in Fig. 2, the severity of the eye changes by themselves are not good predictors of the response to immunosuppression: similar eye changes may indicate different outcomes. For example, half maximal disease severity can be associated with either no response or a good response depending on the timing of treatment in the inactive or active stage, respectively. Duration of the eye disease is also not very reliable, as the time interval to reach the static phase varies considerably between patients. Probably, the best predictor of a response to immunosuppression is the assessment of disease activity. Cumulative clinical experience tells us that in general one out of every three patients with GO does not respond to immunosuppression (be it oral prednisone, retrobulbar irradiation, or intravenous immunoglobulins), whereas two out of every three patients do respond (8). The one-third nonresponders are likely in the inactive stage of the disease. The clinical utility of measuring disease activity in GO is then mainly to predict the response to immunosuppression and, if accurate, would save the expense and exposure to the adverse effects of immunosuppression in one-third of the patients. If one accepts this reasoning, it follows that validation of any measurement of disease activity must be by the accuracy of that measurement to predict the response to immunosuppression, for the gold standard of disease activity—histology of orbital tissues—cannot usually be obtained.

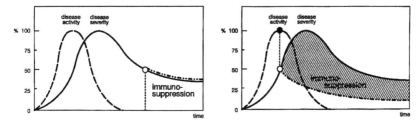

Figure 2 Outcome of immunosuppression of Graves' ophthalmopathy as a function of the activity of the eye disease at the time of treatment. (Reproduced with permission from Ref. 7.)

Table 1 Methods to Assess Disease Activity in Graves'
Ophthalmopathy

Clinical	Observation over time
	Clinical activity score
Radiological	A-mode echography
	Octreoscan
	Magnetic resonance imaging
Chemical	Urinary glycosaminoglycans
	Serum cytokines
	Serum thyroid stimulating immunoglobulins

METHODS TO ASSESS DISEASE ACTIVITY IN GRAVES' OPHTHALMOPATHY

There are several ways in which the activity of GO can be assessed, as listed in Table 1. The time-honored method has been to observe the patient; if the eye changes remain stable over a period of 6–8 months, the eye disease is most probably inactive and rehabilitative surgery can be done. If not, the eye disease is probably still active, and rehabilitative surgery is then better postponed because improvement of eye changes obtained from surgery may be lost after a few months due to ongoing inflammatory reactions in the orbital tissues.

CLINICAL ACTIVITY SCORE

The clinical activity score (CAS) was designed by Mourits et al. (9) based on the classical signs of inflammation, pain, redness, swelling, and impaired function. The score assigns one point each for the presence of the following items: painful oppressive feeling on or behind the globe during the last 4 weeks; pain on attempted up-, side or downgaze; redness of the eyelid(s); diffuse redness of the conjunctiva covering at least one quadrant; swelling of the eyelid(s); chemosis; swollen caruncle; increase in proptosis of 2 mm or more during a period of 1–3 months; decrease of eye movements in any duration equal to or greater than 5° during a period of 1–3 months, and decrease of visual acuity of 1 or more lines on the Snellen chart using a pinhole during a period of 1–3 months. The maximal score is thus 10. Patients with a high CAS are supposedly more likely to respond to immunosuppression and indeed as tested in a prospective manner, a CAS of 4 or higher had a positive predictive value (+ve PV) of 80% in this respect, whereas a CAS of less than 4 had a negative predictive value (−ve PV) of 64% (10). The disadvantage of the CAS is that it is still largely subjective in nature, with consequently a large interobserver variation. To improve observer agreement, a recently published color atlas depicting grading of the various signs can be of much help (11). The advantage of the CAS is that it is inexpensive and can be done instantaneously in a few minutes. Omitting the last three items of the CAS (i.e., the changes in proptosis, eye muscle motility, and visual acuity over the last few months, thereby decreasing the maximal score to 7) is also useful and has been recommended by a committee of the four international thyroid associations (12).

ORBITAL ECHOGRAPHY

Ultrasound is a noninvasive method to visualize orbital contents and has been used to measure the thickness of eye muscles. It can also depict the internal echogenicity of eye muscles, which is best done using two-dimensional A-mode echography. The sound beam is directed perpendicular to the axis of the rectus muscles, and reflectivity is determined at the muscle belly. The eye muscle reflectivity is calculated from Polaroid pictures by measuring the distance from the baseline to the mean of the tops of all spikes within the anterior and posterior muscle sheaths and expressed as a percentage of the initial scleral spike, which is set at 100%. Due to the orbital configuration, it is difficult to obtain a reproducible image of the inferior rectus muscles. Therefore, reflectivity is assessed only in the superior, medial, and lateral rectus muscles. The intra- and interobserver coefficients of repeatability are 10.2% and 11.9%, respectively, in GO patients (13).

It was hypothesized that the internal reflectivity of the sound beam would be low in patients with active eye disease due to muscle edema, and high and irregular in inactive eye disease due to muscle fibrosis. Indeed, pretreatment reflectivity of < 30% in the eye muscle with lowest reflectivity occurred more frequently in 28 responders than in 28 nonresponders to retrobulbar irradiation (39% vs. 7%, $p = 0.004$) (14). Using the cut-off value of 30%, the +ve PV was 85% and the − ve PV 60%. No correlation was found between eye muscle reflectivity and CAS. The advantage of A-mode ultrasonography is its noninvasive nature. Disadvantages are the rather low −ve PV and that the precision of the technique is very much operator-dependent. The low −ve PV might be due to the inability to reliably assess the inferior rectus muscle, which happens to be the most frequently involved eye muscle in GO clinically.

ORBITAL OCTREOSCAN

Somatostatin receptors are expressed on activated T-lymphocytes and on orbital fibroblasts, even to a greater extent in fibroblasts derived from GO patients than from controls (15). By radiolabeling the long-acting somatostatin analogue octreotide, tissues that express somatostatin receptors can be visualized. This provides the rationale for applying [^{111}In-DTPA-D-Phe1] octreotide scintigraphy (Octreoscan®) in GO patients.

The orbital uptake of radiolabeled octreotide is specific, as peak activity in the orbit 5 hr after injection (set at 100%) decreases to 40% at 24 hr, significantly different from the decrease in blood pool radioactivity (from 100% at 5 hr to 15% at 24 hr) (16). Whereas some but not all studies report a direct relationship between orbital uptake and the severity of GO, all studies observe a higher uptake in active than in inactive eye disease (16–18). The orbital uptake is directly related to other parameters of disease activity, like the CAS (16,19) and the T2 relaxation time on magnetic resonance imaging (MRI) (20). Successful immunosuppression is associated with a fall in the orbital uptake (17,19).

There are, however, wide differences between the various studies in the administered dose of radiolabeled octreotide, in the time interval after injection for determining the uptake, in the selection of orbital slices for quantification of orbital uptake, and in the methods of correction for background radioactivity (21). For accurate prediction, a standardization of the technique is required. In correcting for background radioactivity, we observed that uptake in the occipital area of the skull had less variability than uptake in the temporal skull area. Moreover, a substantial part of the temporal uptake is due to uptake in the parotid gland (22). Consequently, we calculate the orbital to occipital uptake ratio in fixed rectangular regions of interest, selecting the four slices with maximal orbital uptake in the transverse plane, using the pituitary gland as the anatomical reference. Eight orbital images are analyzed per patient, and the number of counts is averaged. By doing so, we observed that the orbital to occipital uptake ratio 4 hr after a mean dose of 111 MBq-radiolabeled octreotide was significantly higher in patients who subsequently responded to orbital radiotherapy than in nonresponders (22). Using a cut-off value of the uptake ratio of 1.85, the +ve PV was 92% and the −ve PV 70%.

The advantage of the orbital octreoscan is that it provides a rather good prediction of outcome of immunosuppression. Limitations are, however, manifold: it is a demanding technique in terms of accuracy for prediction; expensive; has a non-negligible radiation burden (of 16 mSv at a dose of 222 MBq); nonspecific (positive scans are also seen in meningioma, lymphoma, and inflammatory disorders); and provides no imaging of orbital structures (computed tomographic or MR scans are still required). It thus remains to be seen if orbital octreotide scintigraphy will become a widely applied tool in the management of GO patients.

ORBITAL MAGNETIC RESONANCE IMAGING

Orbital MRI may discriminate between active and inactive eye disease by its ability to distinguish between edema and fibrosis; an increased water content of tissues will result in a longer T2 relaxation time. Indeed, T2 relaxation times of extraocular muscles were found to be longer in GO patients than in controls, decreasing to near-normal values after immunosuppression (23). Hiromatsu et al.(24) measured STIR based signal intensity ratios on MR images and observed a higher signal in GO patients than in controls. Using a cut-off value of 1.9 for the signal intensity ratio of eye muscles, he reports a +ve PV of 69% and a −ve PV of 86% for the outcome of treatment with intravenous pulses of methylprednisolone. Another study in a small number of patients found the response to steroids better correlated to the clinical activity than to the T2 relaxation time (25).

We also measured longer T2 relaxation times in all extraocular muscles (except the lateral recti) of GO patients than in controls (26). The longest T2 relaxation time observed in any of six extraocular muscles (excluding the lateral muscles for technical reasons) was longer in patients than in controls (160 ± 38 vs. 102 ± 12 msec, $p < 0.001$). Using a cut-off value of 130 msec (derived from a receiver–operator characteristics curve), the longest T2 relaxation time observed in any of six extraocular muscles had a +ve PV of 64% and a −ve PV of 92% for the outcome of retrobulbar irradiation (26). Our results are thus in good agreement with those of Hiromatsu et al.(24). In contrast to other parameters of disease activity in GO, MRI has a higher negative than positive PV. Apparently, orbital MRI is more reliable in detecting the inactive stage of GO than the active edematous stage. This property may be of special advantage when combined with other disease activity parameters having a high +ve PV. Other advantages of MRI are its lack of ionizing irradiation and its clear delineation of orbital structures. However, the MRI scanning protocol will need adjustment in most centers in order to calculate the T2 time in eye muscles, since the method to measure the signal intensity varies with the MRI equipment.

URINARY GLYCOSAMINOGLYCANS

The cytokine-induced accumulation of hydrophilic glycosaminoglycans (GAGS) and its fractions chondroitin sulphate A, dermatan sulphate, and hyaluronic acid in retrobulbar tissues lead to edema. An increased GAG excretion in the urine might thus reflect the activity of the eye disease. Indeed, higher levels of urinary GAG have been found in patients with GO compared to controls and to patients with Graves' hyperthyroidism without eye changes (27). The data allowed discrimination between active and inactive GO, which, however, could not be confirmed by other investigators (28). When comparing responders and nonresponders to radiotherapy, we found no significant difference in pretreatment levels of urinary GAG excretion, or in its fractions measured by HPLC (29). We conclude that measuring urinary GAG has very little relevance in predicting outcome of immunosuppression in GO. It could be, however, that measurement of plasma GAG levels still has some prognostic value (30), although no relation exists between plasma GAG and orbital tissue GAG concentrations in GO patients (31).

SERUM CYTOKINES

Infiltrating lymphocytes of orbital tissues produce a variety of cytokines. Some (such as IFNγ, TNFβ, and IL-1) stimulate GAG production by fibroblasts, others (like IL-1RA) inhibit GAG production (32–34). We measured serum concentrations of IL-1RA, sIL-2R, IL-6, sIL-6R, TNFαRI, TNFαRII, and sCD30 in patients with untreated GO. All cytokine levels were significantly elevated compared with healthy controls, except for IL-1RA, which was similar in both groups (35). Cytokine levels did not correlate with duration, activity, or severity of GO. However, backward logistic regression indicated that IL-6, sCD30, and TNFαRI together had some value for predicting therapeutic outcome to orbital irradiation. As determined from a receiver–operator characteristics curve of these three cytokines combined, the area under the curve has a disappointing low-value of 0.69. The contribution of measuring these cytokines to prediction is thus low, and probably not worth the effort. Hofbauer et al. (36) reported lower IL-1RA serum concentrations in smokers than in nonsmokers among GO patients, and higher baseline IL-1RA levels were associated with a response to radiotherapy. We could not confirm these findings.

Cytokines may also induce the expression of adhesion molecules on orbital fibroblasts (37). Serum concentrations of sICAM, sVCAM, and sELAM are indeed higher in GO patients than in controls, but again have a too low predictive value for the outcome of immunosuppression to warrant their measurements (38).

SERUM THYROID STIMULATING IMMUNOGLOBULINS

The full-length thyrotropin (TSH) receptor is being expressed at the mRNA and at the protein level in Graves' orbital adipose/connective tissues (39). The TSH receptor is thus a potential autoantigen in GO, and TSH receptor antibodies may play a role in the immunopathogenesis of the eye disease. Some but not all studies report a direct relationship between the serum concentration of TSH receptor antibodies and the severity of GO. In a series of patients with untreated moderately severe GO who had been euthyroid for at least 2 months, we found a highly significant correlation between the CAS and serum concentrations of TSH receptor antibodies measured either in a competitive binding assay (TBII, $r = 0.54$) or in a cAMP assay (TSI, $r = 0.50$) (40). In view of the observed relationship, we evaluated if TSH receptor antibodies might have predictive value for the outcome of immunosuppression. There were, however, no baseline differences in serum TBII and thyroid stimulating immunoglobulins (TSI) between responders and nonresponders to radiotherapy. The receiver–operator characteristics curves had a disappointingly low area under the curve (0.59 for TBII and 0.53 for TSI) (41).

CONCLUSION

It is clear that none of the discussed parameters of disease activity in GO has sufficient predictive value on its own to warrant routine application in the selection of suitable patients for immunosuppression. Measurement of urinary GAGs, serum cytokines, or TSH receptor antibodies does not contribute to an accurate prediction. In our opinion, the disadvantages of orbital octreoscan outweigh its advantages, precluding its routine application as a predictive tool. This leaves us with the CAS and orbital ultrasonography and MRI. When applied to a large series of consecutive patients with moderately severe GO, the combination of duration of the eye disease (cut-off value < 18 months), CAS (cut-off value ≥ 4), and orbital A-mode echography (cut-off value of < 30% for the eye muscle with the lowest reflectivity) provided a rather accurate prediction for the outcome of radiotherapy with a +ve PV of 79% and −ve PV of 89% (14). It is precisely in the group of patients with moderately severe GO that accurate prediction is most needed, because the patients with very severe GO characterized by optic neuropathy almost by definition will have active ophthalmopathy. It could well be that exchanging ultrasonography for quantitative MRI will further enhance the accuracy of prediction in view of the high −ve PV of MRI, whereas duration of GO and CAS have higher positive than negative PVs (26). The combination of duration, CAS, and MRI is also attractive in terms of cost-effectiveness: duration and CAS are assessed very quickly without expense, and MRI will also provide images depicting the extent of muscle and fat enlargement. Prediction, as always, remains a difficult topic, and a 100% accuracy rate will unlikely ever be reached.

REFERENCES

1. Rundle FF. Development and course of exophthalmos and ophthalmoplegia in Graves' disease with special reference to the effect of thyroidectomy. Clin Sci 1945; 5:177–194.

2. Rundle FF. Management of exophthalmos and related ocular changes in Graves' disease. Metabolism 1957; 6:36–48.

3. Rundle FF. Ocular changes in Graves' disease. QJM 1960; 29:113–126.

4. Naffziger HC. Pathologic changes in the orbit in progressive exophthalmos. Arch Ophthalmol 1933; 9:1–12.

5. Dunnington JH, Berke RN. Exophthalmos due to chronic orbital myositis. Arch Ophthalmol 1943; 30:446–466.

6. Brain RW. Exophthalmic ophthalmoplegia. QJM 1938; 31: 293–323.

7. Wiersinga WM. Advances in medical therapy of thyroid-associated ophthalmopathy. Orbit 1996; 15:177–186.

8. Prummel MF, Wiersinga WM. Medical management of Graves' ophthalmopathy. Thyroid 1995; 5:231–234.

9. Mourits MP, Koornneef L, Wiersinga WM, Prummel MF, Berghout A, van der Gaag R. Clinical criteria for the assessment of disease activity in Graves' ophthalmopathy: a novel approach. Br J Ophthalmol 1989; 73(8):639–644.

10. Mourits MP, Prummel MF, Wiersinga WM, Koornneef L. Clinical activity score as a guide in the management of patients with Graves' ophthalmopathy. Clin Endocrinol 1997; 47:9–14.

11. Dickinson JA, Perros P. Controversies in the clinical evaluation of active thyroid-associated orbitopathy: use of a detailed protocol with comparative photographs for objective assessment. Clin Endocrinol 2001; 55:283–303.

12. Wiersinga WM, Prummel MF, Mourits MP, Koornneef L, Buller HR. Classification of eye changes of Graves' disease. Thyroid 1991; 1(4):357–360.

13. Prummel MF, Suttorp-Schulten MSA, Wiersinga WM, Verbeek AM, Mourits MPh, Koornneef L. A new ultrasonographic method to detect disease activity and predict response to immunosuppressive treatment in Graves' ophthalmopathy. Ophthalmology 1993; 100:556–561.

14. Gerding MN, Prummel MF, Wiersinga WM. Assessment of disease activity in Graves' ophthalmopathy by orbital ultrasonography and clinical parameters. Clin Endocrinol 2000; 52:641–646.

15. Pasquali D, Vassalo P, Esposito D, Bonavolonta G, Bellastella A, Sinisi AA. Somatostatin receptor gene expression and inhibitory effects of octreotide on primary cultures of orbital

fibroblasts from Graves' ophthalmopathy. J Mol Endocrinol 2000; 25:63–71.

16. Postema PTE, Krenning EP, Wijngaarde R, Kooy PP, Oei HY, van den Bosch WA, Reubi JC, Wiersinga WM, Hooijkaas H, van der Loos T, Poublon RML, Lamberts SWJ, Hennemann G. [^{111}In-DTPA-D-Phe] octreotide scintigraphy in thyroidal and orbital Graves' disease: a parameter for disease activity? J Clin Endocrinol Metab 1994; 79(6):1845–1851.

17. Kahaly G, Dinz M, Haka K, Beyer J, Bockisch A. Indium-111-pentetreotide scintigraphy in Graves' ophthalmopathy. J Nucl Med 1995; 36:550–554.

18. Durak I, Durak H, Ergin M, Yürekli Y, Kaynak S. Somatostatin receptors in the orbit. Clin Nucl Med 1995; 20:237–242.

19. Moncayo R, Baldnisera I, Decristoforo C, Kendler D, Donnemiller E. Evaluation of immunological mechanisms mediating thyroid-associated ophthalmopathy by radionuclide imaging using the somatostatin analog ^{111}In-octreotide. Thyroid 1997; 7:21–29.

20. Kahaly G, Diaz M, Just M, Beyer J, Lieb N. Role of octreoscan and correlation with MR imaging in Graves' ophthalmopathy. Thyroid 1995; 5:107–111.

21. Wiersinga WM, Gerding MN, Prummel MF, Krenning EP. Octreotide scintigraphy in thyroidal and orbital Graves' disease. Thyroid 1998; 8:433–436.

22. Gerding MN, van der Zant FM, van Royen EA, Koornneef L, Krenning EP, Wiersinga WM, Prummel MF. Octreotide-scintigraphy is a disease-activity parameter in Graves' ophthalmopathy. Clin Endocrinol 1999; 50(3):373–379.

23. Just M, Kahaly G, Higer HP, Rosler HP, Kutzner J, Beyer J, Thelen M. Graves' ophthalmopathy: role of MR imaging in radiation therapy. Radiology 1991; 179(1):187–190.

24. Hiromatsu Y, Kojima K, Ishisaka N, Tanaka K, Sato M, Nonaka K, Nishimura H, Nishida H. Role of magnetic resonance imaging in thyroid-associated ophthalmopathy: its predictive value for therapeutic outcome of immunosuppressive therapy. Thyroid 1992; 2(4):299–305.

25. Polito E, Leccisotti A. MRI in Graves' orbitopathy: recognition of enlarged muscles and prediction of steroid response. Ophthalmologica 1995; 209:182–186.

26. Prummel MF, Gerding MN, Zonneveld FW, Wiersinga WM. The usefulness of quantitative orbital magnetic resonance imaging in Graves' ophthalmopathy. Clin Endocrinol 2001; 54:205–209.

27. Kahaly G, Schuler M, Sewell AC, Bernhard G, Beyer J, Krause U. Urinary glycosaminoglycans in Graves' ophthalmopathy. Clin Endocrinol 1990; 33(1):35–44.

28. Martinez-Bru C, Ampudia X, Castrillo P, Gonzalez-Sastre F. Urinary glycosaminoglycans in active Graves' ophthalmopathy. Clin Chem 1992; 38(11):2341.

29. Gerding MN, van der Meer JWC, Broenink M. Urinary glycosaminoglycans do not correlate with disease activity in Graves' ophthalmopathy. In: Gerding MN, ed. Assessment of Disease Activity in Graves' Ophthalmopathy. Ph.D. thesis. Amsterdam: University of Amsterdam, 1999: 57–66.

30. Kahaly G, Hansen C, Beyer J, Winand R. Plasma glycosaminoglycans in endocrine ophthalmopathy. J Endocrinol Invest 1994; 17:45–50.

31. Pappa A, Jackson P, Stone J, Munro P, Fells P, Pennock C, Lightman S. An ultrastructural and systemic analysis of glycosaminoglycans in thyroid-associated ophthalmopathy. Eye 1998; 12:237–244.

32. Korducki JM, Loftus SJ, Bahn RS. Stimulation of glycosaminoglycan production in cultured human retroocular fibroblasts. Invest Ophthalmol Vis Sci 1992; 33:2037–2042.

33. Heufelder AE, Bahn RS. Modulation of Graves' orbital fibroblast proliferation by cytokines and glucocorticoid receptor agonists. Invest Ophthalmol Vis Sci 1994; 35:120–127.

34. Tan GH, Dutton CM, Bahn RS. Interleukin-I (IL-1) receptor antagonist and soluble IL-1 receptor inhibit IL-1-induced glycosaminoglycan production in cultured human orbital fibroblasts from patients with Graves' ophthalmopathy. J Clin Endocrinol Metab 1996; 81:449–452.

35. Wakelkamp IMMJ, Gerding MN, van der Meer JWC, Prummel MF, Wiersinga WM. Both Th1- and Th2-derived cytokines in serum are elevated in Graves' ophthalmopathy. Clin Exp Immunol 2000; 121:453–457.

36. Hofbauer LC, Muhlberg T, Konig A, Heufelder G, Schworm HD, Heufelder AE. Soluble interleukin-1 receptor antagonist serum levels in smokers and nonsmokers with Graves' ophthalmopathy undergoing orbital radiotherapy. J Clin Endocrinol Metab 1997; 82(7):2244–2247.

37. Heufelder AE, Bahn RS. Graves' immunoglobulins and cytokines stimulate the expression of intercellular adhesion molecule-1 (ICAM-1) in cultured Graves' orbital fibroblasts. Eur J Clin Invest 1992; 22:529–537.

38. Wakelkamp IMMJ, Gerding MN, van der Meer JW, Prummel MF, Wiersinga WM. Smoking and disease severity are independent determinants of serum adhesion levels in Graves' ophthalmopathy. Clin Exp Immunol 2002; 127:316–320.

39. Bahn RS, Dutton CM, Natt N, Joba W, Spitzweg C, Heufelder AE. Thyrotropin receptor expression in Graves' orbital adipose/connective tissues: potential autoantigen in Graves' ophthalmopathy. J Clin Endocrinol Metab 1998; 83:998–1002.

40. Gerding MN, van der Meer JWC, Broenink M, Bakker O, Wiersinga WM, Prummel MF. Association of thyrotropin receptor antibodies with the clinical features of Graves' ophthalmopathy. Clin Endocrinol 2000; 52:267–271.

41. Gerding MN. TSH-receptor autoantibodies as predictors of outcome of immunosuppression in Graves' ophthalmopathy. In: Gerding MN, ed. Assessment of Disease Activity in Graves' Ophthalmopathy. Ph.D. thesis. Amsterdam: University of Amsterdam, 1999:99–102.

22

VISA Classification for Thyroid-Related Orbitopathy

PETER J. DOLMAN and JACK ROOTMAN

Department of Ophthalmology and Visual
Sciences, and Department of Pathology, University
of British Columbia , Vancouver General Hospital,
Vancouver, British Columbia, Canada

BACKGROUND

One of the challenges in thyroid-related orbitopathy (TO) is
how to classify and grade its various clinical manifestations.
Over the past few decades, numerous classifications have
been devised (1), including Werner's NO SPECS classification
(1969) that graded symptoms and signs associated with the
disease (2), Bahn and Gorman's focus on measuring objective
and reproducible criteria (3), and Mourits et al.'s clinical
activity score for grading the inflammatory phase of the
disease (4).

These three concepts were amalgamated in 1992 into a set of guidelines by a Working group of delegates from various international thyroid associations (5). The group recommended retaining NO SPECS as a mnemonic; using objective measurements for proptosis, extraocular movements, cornea, and optic nerve; using the clinical activity scale or a recorded change in objective measures to document the disease activity, and lastly, documenting the patient's perception of their disease status.

Since then, no one has organized these ideas into a clinical form that can be used in the office setting to record changes and to guide and assess therapy. We have developed such a classification based on the Working Group's suggestions.

VISA CLASSIFICATION

Our system is based on four disease endpoints: vision, inflammation, strabismus, and appearance/exposure and can be remembered by the acronym, "VISA." Each section records subjective and measurable objective inputs as well as plans ancillary testing.

Figure 1 shows the follow-up examination sheet with the four separate VISA sections, with historical symptoms recorded on the left, signs documented on the right, and a summary grade for each of the four categories. The first visit history differs in that it includes the date and rate of onset of both the orbital and systemic symptoms (since this may help predict the ultimate severity of the inflammatory phase). The layout is designed to simplify data recording and possible later research data collation.

INDIVIDUAL SECTION MEASUREMENTS

Vision

The primary goal of this section is to rule out TO optic neuropathy. The history includes visual blurring or color desaturation and the progress and duration of symptoms. Objective measures include best-corrected visual acuity, color vision, pupil responses, and optic nerve appearance. Ancillary

UBC THYROID ORBITOPATHY CLINIC – Follow-Up   Patient: _____
                                                  Date: _____

HISTORY

Thyroid status: Orbital therapy:

Thyroid therapy: Medications:

SUBJECTIVE	OBJECTIVE		OD	OS	

VISION
Vision: n / abn
	Central Vision sc/cc		20/	20/	W: ____ + ____ x ____
					    ____ + ____ x ____
					M: ____ + ____ x ____
					    ____ + ____ x ____

		cM	20/	20/	
Color vis: n / abn Progress: s / b / w	Color Vision errors (AO) Pupils (afferent defect)		y / n	y / n	normal < 4

INFLAMMATORY
Retrobulbar pressure/
discomfort
    at rest: y / n
    with gaze: y / n
Lid edema: y / n
 	
Progress: s / b / w
	Chemosis (0-2)
	Conjunctival injection (0-1)
	Lid injection (0-1)
	Lid edema [upper] (0-2)
	         [lower] (0-2)
					Inflammatory Index (worse)
					Chemosis (0-2):
					Conjunctival injection (0-1):
					Lid injection (0-1):
					Lid edema (0-2):
					Rest pain (0-1):
					Movement pain (0-1):
					TOTAL (8):

STRABISMUS / MOTILITY
Diplopia –   none
    intermittent
    with gaze
    constant
 	
Progress: s / b / w
	Ductions - Hirschberg (degrees)		+	+	Strabismus: y / n
					Prism measurement:

APPEARANCE / EXPOSURE
Lid retraction   y / n
 	
Proptosis   y / n
Tearing   y / n
FB sensation   y / n
 	
Progress: s / b / w
	Fat prolapse (draw & label)
	Interpalpebral fissure
	Lid retraction (upper) - MRD__
	        (upper scleral show)
	        (lower scleral show)
	Levator function
	Lagophthalmos
	Exophthalmometry (Hertel)
			y / n
			mm
			mm
			mm
			mm
			mm
			mm
			mm
				y / n
				mm
				mm
				mm
				mm
				mm
				mm
				mm
					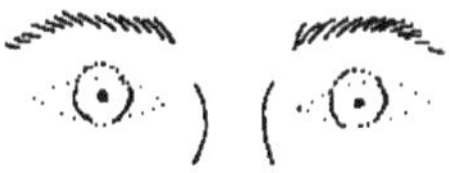

BIOMICROSCOPY	Corneal erosions IOP - Straight Up Other		y / n mmHg mmHg	y / n mmHg mmHg	
FUNDUS	Optic nerve Edema Pallor		y / n y / n	y / n y / n	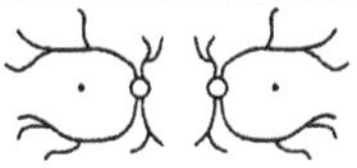

DISEASE PROGRESS / RESPONSE

MANAGEMENT   Follow-up:

Figure 1   Examination sheet with VISA sections.

testing includes computed tomographic (CT) scans to confirm crowding of the orbital apex, standardized visual fields, and possibly VEP (visual evoked potentials) or optic nerve head photos. As a summary grade, we either list optic neuropathy as present or absent.

Our usual management for Graves' optic neuropathy is high dose oral or intravenous steroids, adjunctive radiotherapy, followed by orbital decompression if neuropathy persists or recurs. Success of therapy from both a clinical or research standpoint would be based on specific improved measurements for central vision, color vision, and visual fields.

Inflammation

Symptoms of soft-tissue inflammation include orbital aching at rest or with movement, and eyelid or conjunctival swelling and redness.

The clinical activity score described and validated by Mourits and the Amsterdam Orbitopathy group assigns one point for each of the following: orbital pain at rest, orbital pain with movement, chemosis, caruncular edema, eyelid edema, conjunctival injection, and eyelid injection (4).

We use a slightly modified scale that eliminates caruncular edema as a separate sign (since we feel it is part of chemosis) but which grades chemosis and lid edema with a 0–2 scale (Table 1). Chemosis is graded as 1 if the conjunctiva lies behind the grey line of the lid and as 2 if it extends beyond the grey line. Lid edema is graded as 1 if it is present but not causing overhang of the tissues, and as 2 if it causes a roll in the lid skin (festoons in the lower lid). We have found this classification to be reproducible both inter- and intra-observer and to allow for documentation of more subtle changes in inflammatory features beyond simple absence or presence of chemosis or lid edema.

Table 1 UBC Clinic Thyroid Orbitopathy Inflammatory Score

Clinical finding	Score
Orbital pain (none, at rest, movement)	0–2
Chemosis	0–2
Eyelid edema	0–2
Conjunctival injection	0–1
Eyelid injection	0–1
Total	0–8

At our clinic, management of active inflammation in TO depends on the grade and evidence of progression. If the grade is less than 4 out of 8, and there is no deterioration based on history or sequential clinical examination, we would manage conservatively with cool compresses, head elevation with sleeping, and nonsteroidal anti-inflammatories. In general, if the inflammatory grade is 5 or more, or if there is subjective or objective evidence of progression in the inflammation, we would offer more aggressive therapy, including oral or intravenous steroids, immunosuppressive agents, or radiotherapy.

Strabismus

The symptoms for strabismus include a progression from no diplopia, intermittent diplopia, diplopia with horizontal or vertical gaze, and diplopia in straight gaze.

Ocular ductions can be graded from 0° to 45° in three directions (abduction, adduction, and infraduction) using the Hirschberg principle (upgaze is usually measured from 0° to 30°). The patient is asked to look as far as possible up, down, right, and left while the observer studies the light reflex on the surface of the eye. If the light reflex hits the edge of the pupil, the eye has moved 15°, between the pupil edge and the limbus, 30°, and at the limbus, 45°. These points can be used as grading points for research purposes or to quantify response to therapy.

Strabismus can be measured objectively by prism cover testing in different gaze directions.

Ancillary testing includes using the Goldmann perimeter to quantify ocular ductions in four directions (6).

Management of strabismus depends on whether the orbitopathy is actively inflamed (measured in the previous section) or with evidence of progression in symptoms and signs. If inflammation is present, this is managed first, either with conservative treatment or with anti-inflammatories or radiotherapy. During this stage, the strabismus can be managed with patching one eye or with Fresnel prisms. Once the inflammatory score has dropped to 0 and there is no evidence of progression, management of strabismus might include prisms or surgical alignment with adjustable sutures.

Appearance/Exposure

Symptoms in this category include bulging of the eyes, eyelid retraction, and fat pockets in the lid, as well as exposure complaints of foreign body sensation, glare, dryness, or secondary tearing.

Objective measures of appearance change include lid retraction (measured in millimetres), proptosis (measured with the Hertel exophthalmometer), and documentation of redundant skin and fat prolapse. Measures of exposure include corneal staining or ulceration.

Photographs can document the appearance changes.

Management of appearance and exposure changes depend on the inflammatory stage of the disease. During the inflammatory phase, lubricant drops and ointments can relieve ocular irritation. Rarely a tarsorrhaphy or emergency orbital decompression may be required for severe exposure or corneal ulceration. Once the inflammatory phase has settled, management for proptosis might include orbital decompression and for eyelid retraction may include upper lid müllerectomy or lower lid elevation with spacer materials. These surgical measures often relieve many of the exposure complaints.

DISCUSSION

This classification system clusters the four functions disrupted by TO in a logical sequence for recording and management. Subjective input and reproducible objective measurements are recorded for each section and a global severity grade can be assigned for each function. The subjective and objective progress and tempo of disease can be documented to reflect disease activity. All of these factors meet the Working Group's criteria for a classification system for thyroid orbitopathy. The layout of the form is designed to organize measurements to help in clinical management or for research purposes. Although the forms store a lot of information, they may be completed in as much or little detail as the clinician chooses.

The sequence of the sections (V-I-S-A) reflects the order in which the problems should be managed. Vision dysfunction from optic neuropathy is the first priority, and depending on whether inflammation is present, might be treated with steroids, radiotherapy, and/or orbital decompression. Inflammation, graded by the inflammatory score (a derivative of Mourits et al.'s clinical activity score), is the next priority, and is treated with steroids, immunosuppressives, and/or radiotherapy. Strabismus and appearance changes are usually managed medically and expectantly until the signs of inflammation and disease activity have subsided. Once the inflammation has settled, strabismus can be managed with prisms or surgery while proptosis, lid retraction, and dermatochalasia can be managed surgically.

REFERENCES

1. Bartley GB. Evolution of classification systems for Graves' ophthalmopathy. Ophthalmic Plastic Reconstr Surg 1995; 11:229–237.

2. Werner SC. Classification of the eye changes of Graves' disease. Am J Ophthalmol 1969; 68:646–648.

3. Bahn RS, Gorman CA. Choice of therapy and criteria for assessing treatment outcome in thyroid-associated ophthalmopathy. Endocrinol Metab Clin North Am 1987; 16:391–407.

4. Mourits MP, Koorneef L, Wiersinga WM, et al. Clinical criteria for the assessment of disease activity in Graves' ophthalmopathy: a novel approach. Br J Ophthalmol 1989; 73:639–644.

5. Pinchera A, Wiersinga W, Glinoer D, et al. Classification of eye changes of Graves' disease. Thyroid 1992; 2:235–236.

6. Dolman P, Kendler D, Rootman J. Measuring ocular excursions in thyroid-related orbitopathy (Abst). International Congress of Ophthalmology, 1994.

23

Current Medical Management of Thyroid Orbitopathy

CLAUDIO MARCOCCI, MICHELE MARINÒ, ROBERTO ROCCHI, BARBARA MAZZI, FRANCESCA MENCONI, EUGENIA MORABITO, and ALDO PINCHERA

Dipartimento di Endocrinologia e Metabolismo, Universita' di Pisa, Varese, Italy

LUIGI BARTALENA

Cattedra di Endocrinologia, Universita' dell'Insubria, Varese, Italy

INTRODUCTION

The majority of Graves' patients have a mild and nonprogressive ocular involvement that does not require any specific treatment. Furthermore, nonsevere Graves' orbitopathy (GO) often tends to improve spontaneously (1). In its severe expression, GO is a disfiguring and invalidating disease that profoundly influences and impairs the quality of life of affected individuals (2).

261

The decision of whether the ophthalmopathy must be treated should rely on the assessment of two different features, the severity and activity of the disease. Severity and activity of GO are not synonymous. If the ophthalmopathy is nonsevere, no aggressive medical or surgical treatment is required, although the disease shows some signs of activity. If the patient has severe ocular involvement, assessment of the degree of activity is important, because patients with active orbital disease are likely to respond to medical treatment (especially glucocorticoids and/or orbital radiotherapy), whereas such a treatment is unlikely to be of benefit in patients with inactive GO, who are then candidates to surgical treatment (orbital decompression or rehabilitative surgery) (4). The present discussion will focus on the current medical management of GO.

NONSEVERE GRAVES' OPHTHALMOPATHY

Most patients with Graves' disease have mild ocular manifestations that do not require any aggressive treatment. In these cases, local supportive measures are usually sufficient to obtain symptomatic relief until the eye disease becomes inactive, for example, photophobia can be alleviated by the use of sunglasses, and a foreign body, gritty sensation is usually controlled by the use of lubricating eye drops. If lagophthalmos is present, taping the eyelids shut during the night is useful to prevent nocturnal corneal drying. Prisms may be beneficial for correction of mild diplopia, if they are tolerated by the patient.

Thus, in patients with nonsevere ophthalmopathy, the most important therapeutic measure is probably reassuring the patient that the chance of his/her ophthalmopathy progressing to more severe forms is very low. Elimination of controllable risk factors for progression of ophthalmopathy (e.g., smoking) is also very important.

SEVERE GRAVES' OPHTHALMOPATHY

Management of severe GO represents a difficult task that does not consistently provide favorable results. The recent years have seen the proposal of novel treatments that add to the list of established treatments (glucocorticoids, orbital radiotherapy, and orbital decompression).

Glucocorticoids

Glucocorticoids represent a well-established method of treatment for GO, owing to anti-inflammatory and immunosuppressive actions (3). In addition, they reduce the synthesis and secretion of glucosaminoglycans (GAG) by orbital fibroblasts.

Glucocorticoids have been used in GO through different routes, oral, local (retrobulbar or subconjunctival), and more recently, intravenous (IV) (4). Oral glucocorticoids have usually been employed at high doses (prednisone 60–100 mg/day, or equivalent doses of other steroids) and for prolonged periods of time (several months). Many studies have documented a high effectiveness of high-dose oral glucocorticoids on soft tissue changes and optic neuropathy, whereas the decrease in proptosis and improvement in ocular motility were not always impressive. Recurrence of active disease is a rather frequent problem with oral glucocorticoid therapy, not only when the drug is withdrawn but also when its dose is tapered. Interestingly, in one study the rate of recurrence was abated when cyclosporine was administered concomitantly with and after glucocorticoid therapy (5). In summary, favorable effects of high-dose oral glucocorticoids are reported in slightly more than 60% of cases (range, 40–100%).

In the last 10 years or so, glucocorticoids have also been used intravenously by the acute administration of high doses of methylprednisolone acetate (0.5–1.0 g) at different intervals (4). In general, favorable effects have been observed on inflammatory signs and optic nerve involvement, whereas the effects on extraocular muscle involvement and, especially, proptosis have not been constantly impressive. The available results seem to indicate a higher percentage of favorable results in patients treated with IV glucocorticoids, compared to patients treated with oral glucocorticoids. In a randomized prospective study, we recently shown that IV glucocorticoids combined with orbital radiotherapy are more effective, and that oral glucocorticoids combined with orbital radiotherapy are better tolerated and associated with a lower rate of side effects (6).

A major drawback of systemic glucocorticoid therapy is represented by the rather high rate of its side effects and complications. In addition to transient cushingoid features, adverse effects, such as diabetes, depression, reactivation of chronic diseases, infections, hypertension, osteoporosis, increased body weight, peptic ulcer, hirsutism, and cataract, have been reported during prolonged glucocorticoid therapy for GO, although their precise prevalence is uncertain. This prompted us compare in a prospective study the effectiveness of local (retrobulbar or subconjunctival) glucocorticoid therapy combined with orbital irradiation (7). The overall results of local glucocorticoid therapy were less satisfactory than those obtained with the systemic administration of steroids. Side effects were limited to transient ocular discomfort or pain and few cases of conjunctival hemorrhages. Thus, local glucocorticoid therapy may be considered in patients with active ophthalmopathy and with major contraindications to the systemic administration of glucocorticoids.

Orbital Radiotherapy

The rationale for the use of radiotherapy for GO resides both in its nonspecific anti-inflammatory effect and in the high radiosensitivity of lymphocytes infiltrating the retroorbital space (8). In addition, radiotherapy might also reduce GAG production by orbital fibroblasts. Whether the reported effectiveness of orbital radiotherapy in GO is related to its nonspecific anti-inflammatory action, to specific immunosuppressive effects, or to both remains to be elucidated.

Most centers today utilize linear accelerators delivering 4–6 MeV and use a 4×4-cm lateral field slightly angled posteriorly to avoid as much as possible irradiation to the contralateral lens (8). The use of higher energy sources did not prove particularly advantageous. The commonest cumulative dose is 20 Gy per eye, fractionated in 10 daily doses over a 2-week period. Recently, Kahaly et al. (9) reported that 1 Gy per week over a 20-week period is equally effective and better tolerated than the 2-week scheme. The use of higher cumulative doses (30 Gy vs. 20 Gy) does not improve the results. With few exceptions, favorable effects of orbital radiotherapy are observed in approximately 60% of cases, especially on soft tissue inflammatory changes, recent extraocular muscle involvement, and optic neuropathy. Recently, one study by Mourits et al.(10) confirmed the effectiveness of irradiation, although mainly confined to extraocular muscle motility. Another paper by Gorman et al. (11) reported substantially unfavorable results, although biases in patients' selection may have influenced the results.

Orbital radiotherapy is usually well tolerated. It may be associated with a transient exacerbation of inflammatory eye signs and symptoms, but this is unlikely to occur if glucocorticoids are concomitantly administered. Cataract is a possible complication of irradiation to the lens, but fractionation of the dose should maintain the radiation exposure of the lens below the threshold dose for radiation-induced cataract. Radiation retinopathy is an extremely rare complication of radiotherapy. A major concern relates to the possibility that orbital radiotherapy may be carcinogenic. To date, no case of secondary tumor following orbital radiotherapy for GO has been reported in the literature. Nevertheless, it seems prudent to avoid irradiation in young patients.

Orbital Radiotherapy Combined with Glucocorticoids

Orbital radiotherapy and systemic glucocorticoids can be used for GO either alone or in combination. In addition to these synergistic effects, the combined regimen exploits the more prompt effects of glucocorticoids and the more sustained action of irradiation. The inclusion of glucocorticoids prevents radiation-associated transient exacerbation of ocular manifestations, while the inclusion of orbital radiotherapy probably reduces the prevalence of recurrences of eye disease, which is not infrequently observed when glucocorticoids are withdrawn. Thus, we suggest that this combined therapeutic regimen should be employed in patients with severe GO if conservative therapy, rather than orbital decompression, is selected (1).

Immunosuppressive Drugs

Cyclosporine is the immunosuppressive drug that has been more thoroughly evaluated in the management of GO (12). Several studies have reported favorable results but only two were randomized and controlled. Thus, the favorable effects of cyclosporine reported in most uncontrolled studies must be interpreted with caution. Prummel et al. (13) indicated a lower efficacy of cyclosporine compared to prednisone as a single-agent treatment, but both Prummel et al. (13) and Kahaly et al.(5) suggested that a combination of cyclosporine and prednisone may be more effective than either treatment alone. Thus, the use of cyclosporine might be maintained, in association with glucocorticoids, in patients who are resistant to glucocorticoids alone and in whom the persistent activity of the disease warrants a continuing medical intervention. Side effects of cyclosporine cannot be neglected; some of them can be severe, calling for caution in the use of this drug. Doses lower than 7.5 mg/kg/day probably should be employed. Another immunosuppressive agent that is currently being evaluated in patients with GO is methotrexate. However, it has not systematically been evaluated in the management GO.

Plasmapheresis

The rationale for the use of plasmapheresis in the treatment of GO is based on the assumption that this procedure might remove either immunoglobulins or immune complexes possibly involved in the pathogenesis of the disease. The use of plasmapheresis provided conflicting results, since both favorable effects and treatment failures were reported (1). No study on the effects of plasmapheresis was randomized and controlled, and the interpretation of results is made even more difficult by the frequent concomitant (or subsequent) treatment with glucocorticoids or immunosuppressive drugs (azathioprine or cyclophosphamide). In addition, recurrences of eye disease that required further courses of plasmapheresis were relatively frequent. Thus, plasmapheresis should be regarded as a "desperate" treatment for severe GO, when other therapies have failed (4).

Somatostatin Analogues

Expression of different subtypes of somatostatin receptors was demonstrated in the various cellular components of orbital tissue (14). Somatostatin receptors can be visualized in vivo in orbital tissue of Graves' patients by octreoscan. Patients with active GO have a higher orbital uptake of the tracer than those with inactive eye disease. These findings led to the idea of using somatostatin in the management of GO (15).

A few uncontrolled studies of patients treated with 0.1 mg subcutaneous octreotide three times daily for 3 months have shown an improvement in soft tissue inflammatory changes and extraocular muscle impairment. These beneficial effects were achieved in patients who had positive octreoscans prior to treatment.

A major limitation of octreotide is its short half-life, which requires multiple daily injections. Krassas (15) has reported that lanreotide, a long-acting analogue (40 mg every other week for 3 months) was also effective in most patients, with no differences between the subgroup treated with octreotide and the subgroup treated with lanreotide.

In summary, the available data indicate favorable effects of somatostatin analogues in approximately 80% of patients. However, the number of patients thus far treated is too limited and it is therefore difficult to draw definite and sound conclusions on the real effectiveness of somatostatin analogues. Properly controlled studies enrolling a larger number of patients are warranted.

Intravenous Immunoglobulins

High-dose intravenous immunoglobulins (IVIG) have been used effectively in a number of autoimmune diseases. In a randomized study, the effects of IVIG either alone or in association with orbital radiotherapy were evaluated in a small series of GO patients and the results compared with a "historical" group of patients previously treated with oral glucocorticoids and orbital radiotherapy (16). Favorable results were reported in the three groups, with no significant differences among them. In a subsequent randomized trial, the effect of IVIG was compared with that of oral prednisolone (17). The authors reported a similar percentage of successful treatments in the two groups. At variance in another study, no significant changes in ocular involvement occurred in the majority of patients treated by this procedure (18).

Antioxidants

Oxygen free radicals have been shown in vitro to stimulate proliferation of orbital fibroblasts and their expression of 72 kDa heat shock protein. In a nonrandomized, comparative study, two groups of 11 patients with mild-to-moderately severe ophthalmopathy were given either allopurinol (300 mg daily) and nicotinamide (300 mg daily), given for 3 months, or placebo. Improvement of ocular conditions occurred in 9 of 11 (82%) antioxidant-treated patients but only in 3 of 11 (27%) placebo-treated patients ($p < 0.05$) (19). This is the only one available study on the use of antioxidants for GO, and therefore it is premature to draw conclusions on their effectiveness. Larger, prospective, randomized studies are warranted to investigate this issue.

Cytokine Antagonists

Cytokines play an important role in the pathogenesis of GO and blockade of the cascade of events involving cytokines might play an important role in the management of GO, particularly in the early stage of the disease.

The only available data on the effects of cytokine antagonists in vivo on GO were reported by Balazs et al. (20) using pentoxifylline, a drug with complex immunomodulatory effects on cytokine production. In a nonrandomized and uncontrolled study, these authors treated 10 patients with moderately severe GO with pentoxifylline (200 mg/day IV for 10 days, followed by 1800 mg/day orally for 4 weeks, and then reduced to 1200 mg/day until the end of a 3-month treatment) (20). Eight patients (80%) responded favorably. Soft tissue changes and proptosis were most responsive, whereas extraocular muscle involvement response was less impressive. Clearly, the results of this preliminary study must be interpreted with caution, and randomized and controlled studies are required to assess more accurately the true effectiveness of pentoxifylline.

Colchicine

Colchicine is an effective anti-inflammatory agent. A recent preliminary report on six GO patients has shown favorable results on soft tissue changes, and subjective symptoms (21). Since this study was uncontrolled, it is difficult to establish whether these changes are related to the natural history of the ophthalmopathy or to the effects of the drug.

REFERENCES

1. Bartalena L, Pinchera A, Marcocci C. Management of Graves' ophthalmopathy: reality and perspectives. Endocr Rev 2000; 21(2):168–199.

2. Gerding MN, Terwee CB, Dekker FW, Koornneef L, Prummel MF, Wiersinga WM. Quality of life in patients with Graves' ophthalmopathy is markedly decreased: measurement by the medical outcomes study instrument. Thyroid 1997; 7(6): 885–889.

3. Wiersinga WM. Immunosuppressive treatment of Graves' ophthalmopathy. Thyroid 1992; 2(3):229–233.

4. Bartalena L, Marcocci C, Pinchera A. Treating severe Graves' ophthalmopathy. Baillieres Clin Endocrinol Metab 1997; 11(3): 521–536.

5. Kahaly G, Schrezemeir J, Krause U, Schweikert B, Meuer S, Muller W. Cyclosporin and prednisone vs. prednisone in treat-

ment of Graves' ophthalmopathy: a controlled, randomized and prospective study. Eur J Clin Invest 1986; 16:415–422.

6. Marcocci C, Bartalena L, Tanda ML, Manetti L, Dell'Unto E, Rocchi R, Barbesino G, Mazzi B, Bartolomei MP, Lepri P, Cartei F, Nardi M, Pinchera A. Comparison of the effectiveness and tolerability of intravenous and oral glucocorticoids associated with orbital radiotherapy in the management of severe Graves' ophthalmopathy: results of a prospective, single-blind, randomized study. J Clin Endocrinol Metab 2001; 86:3562–3567.

7. Marcocci C, Bartalena L, Panicucci M, Marconcini C, Cartei F, Cavallacci G, Laddaga M, Campobasso G, Baschieri L, Pinchera A. Orbital cobalt irradiation combined with retrobulbar or systemic corticosteroids for Graves' ophthalmopathy: a comparative study. Clin Endocrinol (Oxf) 1987; 27: 33–42.

8. Bartalena L, Marcocci C, Manetti L, Tanda ML, Dell'Unto E, Rocchi R, Cartei F, Pinchera A. Orbital radiotherapy for Graves' ophthalmopathy. Thyroid 1998; 8:439–441.

9. Kahaly G, Roesler HP, Pitz S, Hommel G. Low- versus high-dose radiotherapy for Graves' ophthalmopathy: a randomized, single blind trial. J Clin Endocrinol Metab 2000; 85:102–108.

10. Mourits MP, van Kempen-Harteveld ML, Garcia MBG, Koppeschaar HPF, Tick L, Terwee CB. Radiotherapy for Graves' orbitopathy: randomised placebo-controlled study. Lancet 2000; 355(9214):1505–1509.

11. Gorman CA, Garrity JA, Fatourechi V, Bahn RS, Petersen IA, Stafford SL, Earle JD, Forbes GS, Kline RW, Bergstrahl EJ, Offord KP, Rademacher DM, Stanley NM, Bartley GB. A prospective, randomized, double-blind, placebo-controlled study of orbital radiotherapy for Graves' ophthalmopathy. Ophthalmology 2001; 108(9):1523–1534.

12. Prummel MF, Wiersinga WM. Immunomodulatory treatment of Graves' ophthalmopathy. Thyroid 1998; 8:543–546.

13. Prummel MF, Mourits MP, Berghout A, Krenning EP, van der Gaag R, Koornneef L, Wiersinga WM. Prednisone and cyclosporine in the treatment of severe Graves' ophthalmopathy. N Engl J Med 1989; 321(20):1353–1359.

14. Krenning EP, Kwekkeboom DJ, Bakker WH, Breeman WAP, Kooij PPM, Oei HY, van Hagen M, Postema PTE, deJong M, Reubi JC, Visser TJ, Reijs AEM, Hofland LJ, Koper JW, Lamberts SWJ. Somatostatin receptor scintigraphy with [^{111}InDTPA-D-Phe^1]- and [^{123}I-Tyr^3]-octreotide: the Rotterdam experience with more than 1000 patients. Eur J Nucl Med 1993; 20:716–731.

15. Krassas GE. Somatostatin analogues in the treatment of thyroid eye disease. Thyroid 1998; 8:443–445.

16. Antonelli A, Saracino A, Alberti B, Canapicchi R, Cartei F, Lepri A, Laddaga M, Baschieri L. High-dose intravenous immunoglobulin treatment in Graves' ophthalmopathy. Acta Endocrinol (Copenh) 1992; 126:13–23.

17. Kahaly G, Pitz S, Muller-Forell W, Hommel G. Randomized trial of intravenous immunoglobulins versus prednisolone in Graves' ophthalmopathy. Clin Exp Immunol 1996; 106: 197–202.

18. Seppel T, Schlaghecke R, Beker A, Engelbrecht V, Feldkamp J, Kornely E. High-dose intravenous therapy with 7S immuno-globulins in autoimmune endocrine ophthalmopathy. Clin Exp Rheumatol 1996; 14(suppl 15):S109–S114.

19. Bouzas EA, Karadimas P, Mastrorakos G, Koutras DA. Anti-oxidant agents in the treatment of Graves' ophthalmopathy. Am J Ophthalmol 2000; 129:618–622.

20. Balazs C, Kiss E, Vamos A, Molnar I, Farid NR. Beneficial effect of pentoxifylline on thyroid-associated ophthalmopathy. J Clin Endocrinol Metab 1998; 82:1999–2002.

21. Stamato FJC, Manso PG, Maciel JR, Wolosker AMB, Maciel RMB, Furlanetto RP. Colchicine as a new option for the clinical treatment of Graves' ophthalmopathy. VIth International Symposium on Graves' Ophthalmopathy, Amsterdam, Nov 27–28, 1998.

24

Surgical Paradigms in the Management of Thyroid Orbitopathy

JACK ROOTMAN

Department of Ophthalmology and Visual
Sciences, and Department of Pathology,
University of British Columbia,
Vancouver General Hospital, Vancouver,
British Columbia, Canada

INTRODUCTION

The overall management paradigm for thyroid orbitopathy involves careful assessment of prognostic factors and degree of disease activity prior to intervening surgically (1–3). We prefer to try to achieve medical stabilization of activity before surgery. Having said this, however, there are indications for surgical intervention during active disease vs. the more common intervention when there is nonprogressive, stable orbitopathy (Fig. 1).

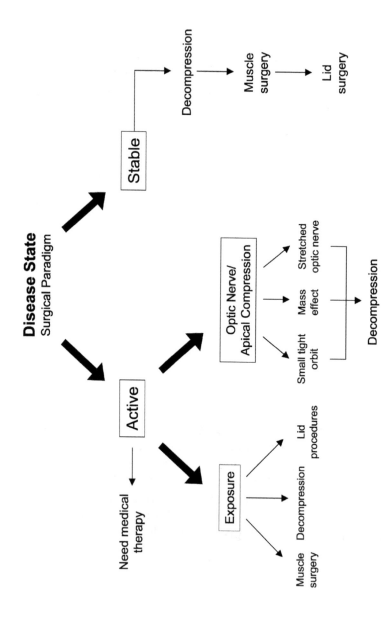

Figure 1 Indications for surgical intervention in thyroid orbitopathy.

SURGICAL INTERVENTION DURING ACTIVE ORBITOPATHY

It is our practice to intervene in active disease only if there is significant exposure of the globe that will not respond to medical interventions, or if there is significant optic neuropathy. The three components of exposure that might require surgical intervention are severe proptosis, lid retraction (both upper and lower), and involvement of the inferior recti leading to a loss of normal Bell's phenomenon. The graded surgical approach would suggest first trying to do simple lid surgeries to cover the cornea, starting with a temporal tarsorrhaphy and moving to upper and lower lid relaxing procedures (4,5). If, however, the orbit appears extremely tense and very chemotic, it might be appropriate to proceed to decompression with or without lid procedures in order to relieve both the proptosis and the congestive element associated with the crowded orbit. There are some circumstances when it is appropriate to release the inferior rectus, for example, when the eye is not only displaced downward by mass effect but hypotropic due to significant inferior rectus involvement.

There are three instances during the active phase of Graves' orbitopathy when early decompression is appropriate for the management of optic neuropathy. All relate to physical and imaging evidence of effect on the optic nerve, either compression or stretching. With regard to apical compression, there are two sets of circumstances, one related to significant mass effect at the apex with secondary congestive features and the other is the anatomically small tight orbit syndrome. In both, the patients are suffering from the crowded orbital apex syndrome and we would normally intervene first with pulsed corticosteroids, to see whether the orbitopathy could be modified enough to improve the optic neuropathy, and delay surgery (until the orbit has "quieted" down). Usually this can be assessed within 1 week to 10 days of high-dose corticosteroids. Failing that, patients having significant proptosis with imaging evidence of enlarged muscles, dilated superior ophthalmic vein, dilated proximal end of the optic nerve sheath, and profound proptosis may require decompression (6). Our choice of decompression method would be governed by the amount of decompression we wish to achieve (roughly 2 mm per wall) and the location of the disease within the orbit. Generally, these cases show quite profound relief of the clinical congestive features immediately after surgery; however, their outcome with regard to secondary strabismus is worse than the group that is either stable (nonactive) or are having decompression for cosmetic or reconstructive reasons (7). This correlates with both severity and activity of disease at the time of decompression.

The second instance in which decompression for optic neuropathy might be a primary choice is in the case of the small, tight orbit syndrome. This is usually seen in Asians or individuals who have evidence of relatively large marrow space at the junction of the lateral orbital wall and sphenoid wing, producing an anatomically tight apex (8,9). These patients respond dramatically to decompression, particularly if it takes advantage of expanding the greater wing of sphenoid in the posterolateral orbit as well as the medial orbit.

The final instance when surgery is appropriate for managing optic neuropathy is in the presence of significant proptosis with stretching of the optic nerve, which may cause globe tenting and optic neuropathy. This is an uncommon occurrence but would require active, early surgical intervention.

In the case of optic neuropathy, the key issue is to decompress the orbital apex and we tailor our procedure to focus on this as an outcome based on the preoperative anatomy. In addition, we consider other factors, such as the degree of desired reduction of exophthalmos or volume change (10,11).

STABLE ORBITOPATHY

The majority of patients with Graves' orbitopathy who undergo surgery do so after the disease has been stable and nonprogressive for at least 6 months. It is the accepted paradigm that if a patient is to undergo surgery for thyroid orbitopathy that the order of management should be decompression followed by muscle surgery followed by lid surgery, since decompression can affect motility and muscle surgery can affect the position of the lid (5). The general principles in managing these patients consist of a careful evaluation and individualization of approach, medical control to abate activity, patient education with regard to the risks and benefits of surgery, and the repair of mechanical and physical dysfunction in an orderly manner.

The decision making for the specific patient needs to take into consideration epidemiologic factors, such as age. The elderly usually require or prefer minimal intervention but are prone to more severe orbitopathy. Gender is also a factor in determining what the preferred outcome might be, which should be discussed and reviewed along with predisease photographs. Another epidemiologic factor is race, since in darker skinned people one would like to avoid or minimize skin incisions because of the potential for either pigmentation or depigmentation of the incision along with the possibility for hypertropic scarring. We have also noted that in patients with relatively tight lids, such as Asians, there is a tendency to lower lid epiblepharon and upper lid entropion brought about by the disease process, both of which need to be addressed by the surgical procedure.

Individual historical factors related to current and past surgical interventions as well as medical problems should be assessed prior to surgery. A review of the patient's past physical appearance is useful in guiding desired outcomes. There are, of course, a number of individual physical factors, such as specific facial contour, status of the sinuses, globe size, refractive error, contour and status of the lids, and condition of the cornea and tear film, which should be taken into consideration when designing the appropriate surgical procedure. For instance, patients who have evidence of midfacial hypoplasia may require augmentation or advancement of the orbital rim in order to achieve a reasonable outcome. The sinuses should be evaluated preoperatively in order to determine whether or not preexisting disease is present and to evaluate the contour, particularly of the ethmoid sinus roof and the thickness of the bony structures. Globe size may determine how much decompression can be logically achieved. As previously mentioned, lid contour and status need to be considered, particularly if there is evidence of in-turning of the lashes or significant scleral exposure. In some instances, patients with significant lower lid retraction who undergo decompression for their orbitopathy via a swinging eyelid approach can have lower lid lengthening procedures done at the same time. The need for lid position management may also relate to the state of the cornea and tear film.

There are a number of other disease-related factors that one should consider in surgical management of Graves' orbitopathy. These include the degree and nature of muscle involvement, degree of proptosis, amount of orbital compliance, presence or absence of apical crowding, imaging findings, disease severity, and disease activity. With regard to the degree and nature of muscle involvement, I have already noted that an absence of Bell's phenomenon associated with exposure may require muscle surgery at the time of decompression (inferior rectus recession). Sometimes, the surgeon may choose to avoid decompressing into the adjacent sinus if there is asymmetric and significant muscle involvement at that site. Degree of proptosis can affect the number of walls decompressed, which generally correlates with outcome insofar as one can achieve approximately 2 mm per wall decompressed and 0.7 mm for 1 cm^3 of fat resection. There is also a need to evaluate the degree of orbital compliance, especially as it relates to the orbital apex (governed by the bony configuration) and to the orbital septum (governed by the lid position and tension).

Imaging plays an important role in assessing disease-related factors with regard to defining old vs. new disease, amount of orbital fat, configuration of the orbital apex and sinuses, and ruling out sinus disease. Imaging also allows for evaluation of the depth of the orbit as well as its bony structure. New or active thyroid orbitopathy on imaging is characterized by relatively diffuse muscle swelling with a minor degree of heterogeneity, whereas old disease is characterized by fat replacement of the muscle (2). It also appears

that there are two types of orbitopathy, one with more significant muscle involvement and the other dominated by
expansion of the orbital fat (said to be more common amongst
Asians). Generally, patients with significant expansion of
orbital fat respond very well to decompressive techniques
and offer a greater opportunity for fat resection. Evaluation
of the orbital apex allows for determination of the roles of lateral, medial, and floor structures in potential decompression;
evaluation of the sinus configuration and presence/absence of
sinus disease may help in determining site and timing of
decompression or need for adjunctive surgery. Some patients
may have a particularly shallow orbit on imaging, implying
the need to advance orbital bones or utilize an onlay technique. The bony structure, particularly the size of the marrow
space and greater wing of sphenoid, may help in determining
the potential for decompressive effect.

I have already mentioned that surgery on active disease
may be associated with more complications and continued
progression of disease, thus requiring vigilant postsurgical
follow-up, continued medical care, and potentially repeat imaging. It is also worthy to note that inactive disease may
reactivate following decompression and although this is a
relatively rare event, we have seen it in a not insignificant
number of patients (12). It should also be remembered that
psychosocial factors may play an important role in determining the timing and nature of surgery for patients with Graves'
orbitopathy.

Preferred Decompression Techniques

There are multiple and variable technical options for decompression, which are listed in Table 1 (13). With regard to our
own preferences, we tend toward minimal incision approaches
using the medial caruncular incision with or without a lateral
canthal incision. If, however, we are considering fat resection,
we may utilize a swinging eyelid approach, which accesses the
lower lid fat as well as the inferolateral orbit. This also can be
augmented by a medial fat resection through the lid crease
superomedially as well as a medial caruncular approach for

Table 1 Technical Options in Decompression

A. Floor and medial wall
  1. Anterior
    Caruncular
    Medial skin
    Medial upper eyelid
  2. Sinus approach
    Ogura
    Transnasal endoscopic
B. Lateral wall ± floor ± roof ± augmentation or bony advancement
  1. Canthotomy
  2. Swinging eyelid approach
  3. Lateral upper eyelid approach
  4. Burke–Kronlein + medial approach
  5. Burke–Kronlein + Ogura or transnasal endoscopic
  6. Coronal approach
C. Soft tissue
  1. Orbital fat excision
  2. Blepharoplasty
    External
    Internal

Modified with permission from Ref. 2 (p. 199).

decompression (14). Earlier, I noted that there are instances where we might combine müllerectomy or upper lid lengthening at the beginning of a decompressive surgery. This would be under local anesthetic and would be followed by the decompression under general anesthetic. The addition of blepharoplasty is also an option. We also favor a more minimal approach laterally by simply exposing the lateral wall through a canthal incision that does not involve incising the lateral canthal tendon.

EYE MUSCLE SURGERY

In our opinion, the sine qua non of eye muscle surgery is the use of adjustable sutures to achieve the best outcomes (15). In principle, we prefer to use recessions vs. resections, since this is a cicatricial disease. The intraoperative rule of thumb is that one can achieve 2.5 diopters per mm of recession; however, the fewer the muscles involved, the more one can achieve per mm.

It is important to be aware of the potential for consecutive deviations in surgical management of strabismus related to Graves' orbitopathy. These tend to occur when the surgeon fails to recognize ipsilateral agonist involvement, leading to an overcorrection. This can be avoided by careful forced duction test as a primary aspect of corrective strabismus surgery.

LID PROCEDURES

The three major procedures for managing lid malpositions are müllerectomy, lower lid elevation, and blepharoplasty. As mentioned earlier, these are infrequently combined with decompressive surgery but usually are done subsequent to either decompression or strabismus surgery.

Müllerectomy can be achieved either through an internal conjunctival or an anterior approach (16–18). In both instances, relaxing both Müller's muscle and the levator aponeurosis is necessary. This is best achieved under local anesthetic, allowing for evaluation intraoperatively of lid position. Lower lid elevation is best achieved by placing a spacer between the lower lid retractors and the tarsal plate. Our general rule of thumb is that the choice of spacer should be increasingly rigid with increasing degrees of lower lid retraction. Finally, the principles we observe in blepharoplasty are aggressive fat resection and moderate skin resection to avoid tense lids. We will often add to the blepharoplasty, some resection of periorbital fat in the upper lid, particularly temporally overlying the bone, since this fat may have increased as a result of the orbitopathy.

The key issue in managing the surgical paradigm for thyroid orbitopathy is to recognize that this may be complex and must be individualized based on the activity and severity of disease. I have included a table describing the range of choices with regard to decompressive surgery in Graves' orbitopathy (Table 1).

REFERENCES

1. Marcocci C, Batalena L, Marino M, Rocchi R, Mazzi B, Menconi F, Morabito E, Pincera A. Current medical management of Graves' ophthalmopathy. Ophthal Plast Reconstr Surg 2002; 18(6):402–408.

2. Rootman J. Diseases of the Orbit: A Multidisciplinary Approach. 2nd ed. Philadelphia: Lippincott Williams & Wilkins, 2003.

3. Siracuse-Lee DE, Kazim M. Orbital decompression: current concepts. Curr Opin Ophthalmol 2002; 13(5):310–316.

4. Rootman J, Stewart B, Goldberg RA. Decompression for thyroid orbitopathy. In: Orbital Surgery: A Conceptual Approach. Philadelphia: Lippincott-Raven, 1995:353–384.

5. Shorr N, Neuhaus RW, Baylis HI. Ocular motility problems after orbital decompression for dysthyroid ophthalmopathy. Ophthalmology 1982; 89(4):323–328.

6. Nugent RA, Belkin RI, Neigel JM, Rootman J, Robertson WD, Spinelli J, Graeb DA. Graves' orbitopathy: correlation of CT and clinical findings. Radiology 1990; 177(3):675–682.

7. Nunery WR, Nunery CW, Martin RT, Truong TV, Osborn DR. The risk of diplopia following orbital floor and medial wall decompression in subtypes of ophthalmic Graves' disease. Ophthal Plast Reconstr Surg 2000; 13(3):153–160.

8. Rootman J. Aspects of current management of thyroid orbitopathy in Asians. Asia Pac J Ophthalmol 1998; 10(3):2–6.

9. Liao SL, Kao SCS, Hou PK, Chen MS. Results of orbital decompression in Taiwan. Orbit 2001; 20(4):267–274.

10. Rootman J. Decompression for thyroid orbitopathy: current concepts. Ophthalmic Pract 1997; 15(6):222–228.

11. Hurwitz JJ, Birt D. An individualized approach to orbital decompression in Graves' orbitopathy. Arch Ophthalmol 1985; 103(5):660–665.

12. Kalmann R, Mourits MP. Late recurrence of unilateral Graves' orbitopathy on the contralateral side. Am J Ophthalmol 2002; 133(5):727–729.

13. Goldberg RA. The evolving paradigm of orbital decompression surgery. Arch Ophthalmol 1998; 116(1):95–96.

14. Kazim M, Trokel SL, Acaroglu G, Elliott A. Reversal of dysthyroid optic neuropathy following orbital fat decompression. Br J Ophthalmol 2000; 84(6):600–605.

15. Lueder GT, Scott WE, Kutschke PJ, Keech RV. Long-term results of adjustable suture surgery for strabismus secondary to thyroid ophthalmopathy. Ophthalmology 1992; 99(6): 993–997.

16. Harvey JT, Anderson RL. The aponeurotic approach to eyelid retraction. Ophthalmology 1981; 88(6):513–524.

17. Mourits MP, Sasim IV. A single technique to correct various degrees of upper lid retraction in patients with Graves' orbitopathy. Br J Ophthalmol 1999; 83(1):81–84.

18. Thaller VT, Kaden K, Lane CM, Collin JRO. Thyroid lid surgery. Eye 1987; 1(Pt 5):609–614.

25

Graves' Orbitopathy: New and Future Treatment

MICHAEL KAZIM

Columbia University,
New York, New York, U.S.A.

Predicting the future is always risky business. While an advanced understanding of the cellular basis of Graves' orbitopathy holds great promise for a more rational therapeutic approach, often it is the unexpected development that fundamentally transforms the horizon. With this caveat, I will attempt to identify the more provocative recent reports and provide a view of the future, as flawed as it may prove to be.

For the most part, Graves' disease has been subject to descriptive clinical analysis for the 60 years following the first report by Robert Graves in 1834, followed shortly thereafter by Von Basedow. Identification of lid retraction, lid lag, and strabismus were all completed before the turn of the 19th century. Surgical maneuvers to reduce the resulting proptosis followed, as did procedures to reverse lid retraction and the diplopia. However, it was not until 1960 that modulation of the disease was attempted with the introduction of corticosteroids. While immunosuppression was effective at curbing the inflammatory phase, it failed to appreciably shorten the acute phase or the ultimate consequence of the inflammation, irreversible fibrosis. In 1973, computed tomograms (CT) provided the first noninvasive analysis of the disease. Identification of fusiform-enlargement of extraocular muscles became pathognomonic of the disease. However, the full spectrum and utility of the information available on the CT images was not appreciated until nearly 20 years later. Radiotherapy was at first, inadvertently applied to the orbit when used to treat the pituitary gland. Although the beneficial effects in the orbit were at first mistakenly attributed to treatment of the pituitary gland, ultimately in the early 1970s, protocols were developed to treat the orbit directly. With the advent of the linear accelerator and treatment planning that limited the total dose to the globe and in particular the lens, the risks of treatment were reduced considerably. Controversy still exists as to the indications, efficacy, and mechanism of orbital radiotherapy. Surgical approaches to bone decompression were modified most significantly in the 1980s, with a focus on the orbital approaches to the paraorbital sinuses and early efforts to quantitate the volumetric changes that occur with decompression of each of the orbital walls.

PATHOPHYSIOLOGY OF THE DISEASE

The most elusive area of investigation has proven to be a clearer understanding of the etiology of the orbital disease. While it is held that Graves' disease is an autoimmune process, definitive proof remains forthcoming (1–3). Unlike thyroiditis where a putative target of the immune system (TSH-receptor) and circulating antibodies against the target have been identified, in the case of the orbitopathy, neither has been defined. Considerable effort has been expended to identify the presence of the TSH-receptor (TSHr) in the orbit and pretibial tissues. Identification of a site-restricted, functioning receptor would support a common pathway of disease. TSHr mRNA has been identified in the orbital fat, extraocular muscles and skin from patients with thyroid-related orbitopathy (4–8). This however has required substantial gene amplification, suggesting that the gene may not be functional in vivo. In addition, TSHr mRNA can also be identified by PCR in other tissue sites not generally associated with Graves' disease and as well in patients without the disease (9). The findings suggest more generalized set of immunologic targets in Graves' disease and account for subtle previously unappreciated signs and symptoms. Alternatively, the work from Bahn's group (8) suggests that upregulation of the TSHr occurs in response to local cytokines. They have shown, in vitro, that orbital fibroblasts from patients with thyroid-associated orbitopathy increase expression of TSHr in response to IL-6.

While a specific orbital antigenic target has not been identified, the cell targeted by the immunologic attack has clearly shifted from the extraocular muscles to the orbital fibroblast. The behavior of orbital fibroblasts in vitro has been examined in detail (10). They express characteristic surface receptors, gangliosides, and inflammatory genes (11–13). Their unique phenotype suggest that they may play an active role in tissue remodeling and modulation of local inflammatory responses. Unlike many other fibroblasts, those from the orbit display cell-surface CD40, a receptor initially found on B-lymphocytes and important to the activation of those cells. CD40 is activated by CD154, which is displayed on the surface of T lymphocytes. When CD40 on orbital fibroblasts is engaged by CD154, several inflammatory fibroblast genes are activated. IL-6 and IL-8 expression is dramatically upregulated, which in turn can result in enhanced chemotaxis of bone-marrow derived inflammatory cells to the orbit (14). PGHS-2, the inflammatory cyclooxygenase, is induced by CD40 ligation on orbital fibroblasts (15). This induction results in substantial increases in the production of PGE_2. Synthesis of glycosaminoglycans is also increased by CD40 ligation (15). Many of the consequences of CD40 ligation in human fibroblasts are mediated through the activation of

NF-κB and can be attenuated with physiological concentrations of glucocorticoids (15). This finding is entirely consistent with the therapeutic benefit associated with these steroids in acute thyroid-associated orbitopathy. The actions of other proinflammatory cytokines, such as IL-1, and the T-lymphocyte derived molecule, leukoregulin, also result in exaggerated orbital fibroblast gene inductions, which may have important roles in the orbital inflammatory response (16–18). A subpopulation of orbital fibroblasts appears capable of undergoing adipocyte differentiation in vitro (19). This may account for the orbital soft-tissue expansion that predominates in some patients.

What are we lacking in the treatment of Graves orbitopathy? At present, there is a great deal known about the stable phase of the disease as the majority of histopathologic specimens are derived from patients in this phase of the disease. There is no reason to believe a priori that the histologic or cellular events occurring in the stable phase of the disease parallel those that exist in the acute inflammatory phase. The events occurring in the acute phase of disease remain under-represented in studies to date. New interest exists in the earliest events of the inflammatory phase of the disease. It may be this period in which a cascade of events is established that defines the disease. If this proves to be the case, specific therapy may be effective at blunting or eliminating the downstream events associated with a protracted inflammatory episode, and ultimately the fibrotic stable phase.

Why has the acute phase of the orbitopathy remained elusive? Primarily, it is difficult to identify. Acute phase disease may be present for weeks to months before it is identified by the patient, the primary treating physician and ultimately the orbital disease specialist. By that time, the truly early events may have passed and a reactive inflammatory cascade established. Were we able to identify patients earlier would we be better off? If so, what evaluations would be of value? Serologic testing would be helpful if the disease process is initiated by circulating cellular or humoral factors. If, conversely, the most critical events occur locally in the orbit, then tissue from that site will be required for investigation. Unfortunately, access to this tissue is limited by the generally held impression that surgery upon the soft-tissue of an acutely inflamed orbit can exacerbate the inflammation.

As an alternative to human tissue, an animal model of Graves' orbitopathy remains the "Holy Grail." First attempts at producing an animal model came from George Smelser's lab. The guinea pig harderian gland was thought to swell in response to a chemically induced hyperthyroid state. Unfortunately, the model failed to hold up under close scrutiny. While animal models of the autoimmune hyperthyroidism and pharmacologically induced proptosis exist (20–24), no convincing animal model of immune related orbitopathy has been produced. Some recent animal studies may provide an understanding of some subset of the pathophysiology of the human orbitopathy. Feldon's group (25) has produced a cat model of orbital congestion by ligating the superior ophthalmic vein. The congestion results in enlargement of the rectus muscles in a pattern and configuration typical of Graves' orbitopathy. Histologically, they identified lymphocytic infiltration of the rectus muscles (25). This model may provide an understanding of how orbital congestion potentiates the acute phase inflammation in Graves' orbitopathy (26). Another study has identified a mouse line that can be induced to proliferate orbital fat in response to T-cell knock-out (22). A more representative animal model would provide the vehicle for identifying the earliest features of the disease and testing of new therapeutic modalities.

MEDICAL THERAPY

The single most effective treatment for acute phase Graves' orbitopathy is the full spectrum immunosuppression and blockade of the inflammatory cascade achieved by the administration of between 0.5 and 1.0 mg/kg of prednisone. Unfortunately, the associated adverse effects resulting from this daily dose make long-term use impractical in most cases. Several small studies have examined the efficacy of pulsed high-dose intravenous corticosteroids administered at extended intervals. The results have been mixed but suggest an alternative to daily dosing.

Nonsteroidal anti-inflammatory drugs have found a place in the treatment of mild early-phase inflammation and the associated pain. The effect of these drugs on the inflammatory cascade is modest and is unlikely to provide much relief in the treatment of more severe orbitopathy.

How might future medical treatments be directed? A more complete understanding of the acute phase of the disease could be instrumental. If the disease results from a generalized upregulation of the immune system, then restoring the immune function to normal levels would be preferred to the current approach of generalized immunosuppression. Alternatively, if a specific trigger for the disease (i.e., infectious agent) were identified, it would be the specific target.

Selective immunomodulation has been considered. To date, results have been generally disappointing with other immunosuppressor agents when compared to corticosteroid agents. Included in this group are cyclophosphamide, azathioprine, methotrexate, cyclosporine, plasmapheresis, IV immunoglobins, and more recently octreotide and lanreotide. Why do these drugs fail to provide the beneficial effect that is desired? To begin, we may be treating too late in the course of the disease. In the later stages, the disease process may be so generalized in the cascade as to require the broad-spectrum relief of immune system over-action that is provided by corticosteroid therapy. Alternatively, the newer agents may have a mechanism of action that is too specific. In place of a single drug used at maximum tolerated levels, a combination of the drugs acting synergistically may be more effective and produce less toxicity. The model for this therapeutic approach exists in the treatment of other autoimmune diseases (i.e., rheumatoid arthritis, lupus, Wegener's disease).

New classes of anti-inflammatory agents have been introduced. Monoclonal antibodies have been developed to TNFα, and IL-2 receptors, and blocking cytokines exist to IL-1 receptors. Certainly the monoclonal antibody library will grow exponentially over the next several years. Some have suggested targeting the T-cell population with newly developed agents including the monoclonal antibody Rituxamab. This approach is appealing as the agents are more specific than corticosteroids; however, their safety profile needs to be established. Careful consideration should be given to the use of this new class of drugs. There is a report of a patient treated for multiple sclerosis with anti-CD52 (T-cell specific antibody) that induced a reactivation of thyroid-associated orbitopathy (27,28).

Anti-fibrotic agents such as pirfenidone act at a post-transcriptional level to down regulate proinflammatory cytokine (TNF-α and interferon-γ) production, which in turn limits fibroblast proliferation and collagen matrix synthesis while upregulating IL-10 that is an anti-inflammatory cytokine. This class of drugs holds promise for the treatment of any inflammatory condition that results in fibrosis.

If an agent is developed with greater therapeutic value, which patients should be treated? A strong argument can be made that the majority of patients with Graves' orbitopathy require no treatment. By most accounts, 80% of patients with clinically measurable orbital disease have a self-limited course that results in no residual measure disease. Of the 10% of patients that will have more significant pathology, 80% have sufficiently mild disease that no surgical rehabilitation is required. In the more severely affected group is the even smaller group of patients that requires intervention to treat optic neuropathy. It is the most severely effected group that would be best suited to therapeutic trials. Predicting which patients will ultimately progress to this degree remains elusive. At present, there is no serologic or imaging technology to identify this group. It has been suggested by Rootman that the patient's historical account of the progression of orbitopathy can identify those most likely to be severely affected. In our experience, the accuracy of the patients' accounts can vary. We agree that early in the course of disease some patients will exhibit an exaggerated rate of disease progression that is prognostic of bad outcome. To determine the rate of progression of the disease, we will examine the patients twice within a 4–6 week interval. If there is significant measurable change in the proptosis or worsening of the ocular rotations, consideration to medical intervention will be given. Otherwise, observation intervals will be extended to 3–4 months.

Until recently, quantification of the orbitopathy has depended on some modification of the original classification scheme devised by Werner in 1963. While NOSPECS is a helpful pneumonic to remember the clinical manifestations of the disease, it fails to indicate either the severity or activity of the orbitopathy. All current scoring systems suffer from the same shortcoming. When used to evaluate patients for activity of disease or response to treatment, a numerical sum of severity will obscure the relative contribution of each subset of the disease. From a therapeutic standpoint, optic neuropathy should be weighted more heavily than lid retraction. A more recent attempt has been made by the EUGOGO group to establish a grading system in order to apply it to clinical trials (29). It remains to be put to the test of routine clinical practice as it may prove to be prohibitively comprehensive. What is needed is a simple and reproducible testing parameter for each of the orbital manifestations of the disease. Activity is then established by change in the measurements over time.

Nonclinical parameters, which have been explored, include MRI. The presence of contrast enhancement or bright T2 relaxation of the extraocular muscles has been shown to correlate with disease activity (30–35). Octreotide uptake in the orbital tissues has been shown to be of equal predictive value (36,37).

Orbital radiotherapy has appreciated recent reconsideration in the literature. It was reassuring that a long-term follow-up study of patents, dating from 1977, treated with orbital radiotherapy for Graves' orbitopathy did not experience an increased risk of cancer death (38). More controversial was the first prospective study of radiotherapy for Graves' orbitopathy (39,40). The Mayo study clearly demonstrated that radiotherapy fails to significantly alter the outcome for those patients with stable phase or mild orbitopathy. Their study excluded those patients in the acute phase with compressive optic neuropathy or rapidly progressive congestive orbitopathy. In the latter two groups, data continue to indicate the beneficial effects of orbital radiotherapy (41,42).

IMPROVEMENTS IN ORBITAL DECOMPRESSION

Orbital decompression surgery will be required until our understanding and medical therapy of the inflammatory process is sufficiently advanced to eliminate the subgroup of patients in which the soft-tissue volume expansion has resulted in either clinically significant proptosis or compressive optic neuropathy. Over the past decade, several trends have evolved in the area of orbital decompression. Most important has been the concept of graded orbital decompression. The notion of graded decompression is predicated on the concept that surgery should be designed to reverse the soft-tissue to bony disparity caused by the disease, while limiting the adverse effects of the surgery. Preoperative planning should include a neuro-ophthalmic examination to identify the presence and etiology of optic neuropathy. Noninvasive imaging identifies the relative contribution of extraocular muscle and orbital fat expansion. Examination of pre-morbid facial photographs will help to estimate the degree of proptosis reduction that will be required and thereby the amount of either bony expansion of soft-tissue reduction that is needed. Using this strategy, function and appearance can be restored while limiting the associated risks.

Orbital fat decompression was a critical addition to the surgical armamentarium (43–45). While initially difficult to predict the effect of the surgery, most recent results have clearly related the degree of decompression to two factors: preoperative Hertel measurements and the degree of extraocular muscle volume enlargement as determined by preoperative imaging. When segregated in this fashion, patients with normal rectus muscle volume and preoperative Hertel measurements of greater than 25 mm can be expected to average 5 mm reduction in proptosis. Fat decompression can also be performed in conjunction with standard bone decompression techniques in order to augment the resultant decompressive effect.

Bone decompression has benefited from the use of endo-scopic transnasal approaches that provide improved visualization of the orbital walls and more reliable postoperative sinus drainage. The latter results in a lower rate of sinusitis and thereby limits the occurrence of orbital cellulitis postoperatively (46,47). There has been a general trend toward avoiding the orbi-tal floor as a decompressive space, as most surgeons have found it to produce higher rates of diplopia, globe ptosis, infraorbital anesthesia, and lid retraction. Finally the approach to the medial wall if not endoscopic has been made easier with the trans-caruncular approach (48).

IMPROVEMENTS IN EYELID SURGERY

Surgical repair of lid retraction in patients with Graves' orbi-topathy remains frustrating due to its degree of unpredict-ability. Recent attention has been taken to the importance of upper lid Mueller's muscle as a site of the inflammatory process (49).

A transverse anterior blepharotomy as described by Korneff and reported by Elner holds promise to both simplify the procedure and improve the outcome of upper eyelid retraction repair (50).

The sole surgical modification introduced for lower lid retraction repair has been new allograft and xenograft materials to be used as spacer grafts. Both the thin wafers of Medpor (51) and the sheets of Alloderm (52) have been reported to support lower eyelid retraction repair. Medpor is the most technique-dependent, and has been associated with extrusions that might be expected with a stiff material in this location.

STRABISMUS SURGERY

Correction of diplopia resulting from restrictive strabismus achieves greatest success in the stable phase of the disease, when the surgical target is not shifting. While the vast majority of cases succeed with muscle recession, there are some cases of large angle deviation (greater than 60 prism diopters) that fail to respond to maximal bilateral recessions. In those cases, Nardi has described (personal communication) a tendon lengthening procedure that utilizes Tutoplast to improve the length–tendon relationship of the fibrotic muscles. For the remainder, Prendiville et al. (53) have suggested that the intraoperative goal of producing a balanced set of forced duction tests produces single binocular vision in primary and reading gaze in 70% of cases. We agree that intraoperative forced duction testing is an important factor to consider. However, we feel that formal orthoptics measurements remain a critical adjunct to treatment. They provide the most reliable indicator of stabilization of the orbitopathy and are vital to preoperative planning. Careful orthoptic analysis will identify subtle muscle involvement that is often responsible for surgical failure. Using these assessments in combination, we have appreciated a near 80% success rate.

REFERENCES

1. Erdei I, Fazakas S, Kiss B, Szegedi G, Petranyi G. The autoimmune status in Graves' disease. Acta Med Acad Sci Hung 1974; 31:173–179.

2. Kendall-Taylor P. The pathogenesis of Graves' ophthalmopathy. Clin Endocrinol Metab 1985; 14:331–349.

3. Bahn RS. Understanding the immunology of Graves' ophthalmopathy. Is it an autoimmune disease?Endocrinol Metab Clin North Am 2000; 29:287–296

4. Heufelder AE, Bahn RS. Evidence for the presence of a functional TSH-receptor in retroocular fibroblasts from patients with Graves' ophthalmopathy. Exp Clin Endocrinol 1992; 100:62–67.

5. Heufelder AE, Dutton CM, Sarkar G, Donovan KA, Bahn RS. Detection of TSH receptor RNA in cultured fibroblasts from patients with Graves' ophthalmopathy and pretibial dermopathy. Thyroid 1993; 3:297–300.

6. Dutton CM, Joba W, Spitzweg C, Heufelder AE, Bahn RS. Thyrotropin receptor expression in adrenal, kidney, and thymus. Thyroid 1997; 7:879–884.

7. Bahn RS, Dutton CM, Joba W, Heufelder AE. Thyrotropin receptor expression in cultured Graves' orbital preadipocyte fibroblasts is stimulated by thyrotropin. Thyroid 1998; 8:193–196.

8. Bahn RS. Thyrotropin receptor expression in orbital adipose/connective tissues from patients with thyroid-associated ophthalmopathy. Thyroid 2002; 12:193–195.

9. Agretti P, Chiovato L, De Marco G, et al. Real-time PCR provides evidence for thyrotropin receptor mRNA expression in orbital as well as in extraorbital tissues. Eur J Endocrinol 2002; 147:733–739.

10. Smith TJ, Wang HS, Hogg MG, Henrikson RC, Keese CR, Giaever I. Prostaglandin E2 elicits a morphological change in cultured orbital fibroblasts from patients with Graves' ophthalmopathy. Proc Nat Acad Sci USA 1994; 91:5094–5098.

11. Wang HS, Cao HJ, Winn VD, et al. Leukoregulin induction of prostaglandin-endoperoxide H synthase-2 in human orbital fibroblasts. An in vitro model for connective tissue inflammation. J Biol Chem 1996; 271:22718–22728.

12. Smith TJ, Sempowski GD, Wang HS, Del Vecchio PJ, Lippe SD, Phipps RP. Evidence for cellular heterogeneity in primary cultures of human orbital fibroblasts. J Clin Endocrinol Metab 1995; 80:2620–2625.

13. Berenson CS, Smith TJ. Human orbital fibroblasts in culture express ganglioside profiles distinct from those in dermal fibroblasts. J Clin Endocrinol Metab 1995; 80:2668–2674.

14. Sempowski GD, Rozenblit J, Smith TJ, Phipps RP. Human orbital fibroblasts are activated through CD40 to induce proinflammatory cytokine production. Am J Physiol 1998; 274:C707–C714.

15. Cao HJ, Wang HS, Zhang Y, Lin HY, Phipps RP, Smith TJ. Activation of human orbital fibroblasts through CD40 engagement results in a dramatic induction of hyaluronan synthesis and prostaglandin endoperoxide H synthase-2

expression. Insights into potential pathogenic mechanisms of thyroid-associated ophthalmopathy. J Biol Chem 1998; 273:29615–29625.

16. Young DA, Evans CH, Smith TJ. Leukoregulin induction of protein expression in human orbital fibroblasts: evidence for anatomical site-restricted cytokine–target cell interactions. Proc Nat Acad Sci USA 1998; 95:8904–8909.

17. Cao HJ, Smith TJ. Leukoregulin upregulation of prostaglandin endoperoxide H synthase-2 expression in human orbital fibroblasts. Am J Physiol 1999; 277:C1075–C1085.

18. Smith TJ, Wang HS, Evans CH. Leukoregulin is a potent inducer of hyaluronan synthesis in cultured human orbital fibroblasts. Am J Physiol 1995; 268:C382–C388.

19. Sorisky A, Pardasani D, Gagnon A, Smith TJ. Evidence of adipocyte differentiation in human orbital fibroblasts in primary culture. J Clin Endocrinol Metab 1996; 81:3428–3431.

20. Dayan CM, Londei M, Corcoran AE, et al. Autoantigen recognition by thyroid-infiltrating T cells in Graves' disease. Proc Nat Acad Sci USA 1991; 88:7415–7419.

21. Kohn LD, Shimojo N, Kohno Y, Suzuki K. An animal model of Graves' disease: understanding the cause of autoimmune hyperthyroidism. Rev Endocr Metab Disord 2000; 1:59–67.

22. Ludgate ME. Animal models of thyroid-associated ophthalmopathy. Thyroid 2002; 12:205–208.

23. Kim-Saijo M, Akamizu T, Ikuta K, et al. Generation of a transgenic animal model of hyperthyroid Graves' disease. Eur J Immunol 2003; 33:2531–2538.

24. Yamada M, Li AW, West KA, Chang CH, Wall JR. Experimental model for ophthalmopathy in BALB/c and outbred (CD-1) mice genetically immunized with G2s and the thyrotropin receptor. Autoimmunity 2002; 35:403–413.

25. Saber E, McDonnell J, Zimmermann KM, Yugar JE, Feldon SE. Extraocular muscle changes in experimental orbital venous stasis: some similarities to Graves' orbitopathy. Graefes Arch Clin Exp Ophthalmol 1996; 234:331–336.

26. Hudson HL, Levin L, Feldon SE. Graves exophthalmos unrelated to extraocular muscle enlargement. Superior rectus muscle inflammation may induce venous obstruction [see comment]. Ophthalmology 1991; 98:1495–1499.

27. Rotondi M, Mazziotti G, Biondi B, et al. Long-term treatment with interferon-beta therapy for multiple sclerosis and occurrence of Graves' disease. J Endocrinol Invest 2000; 23:321–324.

28. Coles AJ, Wing M, Smith S, et al. Pulsed monoclonal antibody treatment and autoimmune thyroid disease in multiple sclerosis. Lancet 1999; 354:1691–1695.

29. Prummel MF, Bakker A, Wiersinga WM, et al. Multi-center study on the characteristics and treatment strategies of patients with Graves' orbitopathy: the first European Group on Graves' Orbitopathy experience. Eur J Endocrinol 2003; 148:491–495.

30. Ott M, Breiter N, Albrecht CF, Pradier O, Hess CF, Schmidberger H. Can contrast enhanced MRI predict the response of Graves' ophthalmopathy to orbital radiotherapy? Br J Radiol 2002; 75:514–517

31. Yokoyama N, Nagataki S, Uetani M, Ashizawa K, Eguchi K. Role of magnetic resonance imaging in the assessment of disease activity in thyroid-associated ophthalmopathy. Thyroid 2002; 12:223–227.

32. Mayer E, Herdman G, Burnett C, Kabala J, Goddard P, Potts MJ. Serial STIR magnetic resonance imaging correlates with clinical score of activity in thyroid disease. Eye 2001; 15:313–318.

33. Bailey CC, Kabala J, Laitt R, et al. Magnetic resonance imaging in thyroid eye disease. Eye 1996; 10:617–619.

34. Hoh HB, Laitt RD, Wakeley C, et al. The STIR sequence MRI in the assessment of extraocular muscles in thyroid eye disease. Eye 1994; 8:506–510.

35. Laitt RD, Hoh B, Wakeley C, et al. The value of the short tau inversion recovery sequence in magnetic resonance imaging of thyroid eye disease. Br J Radiol 1994; 67:244–247.

36. Gerding MN, van der Zant FM, van Royen EA, et al. Octreotide-scintigraphy is a disease-activity parameter in Graves' ophthalmopathy. Clin Endocrinol 1999; 50:373–379.

37. Krassas GE. Somatostatin analogues in the treatment of thyroid eye disease. Thyroid 1998; 8:443–445.

38. Marcocci C, Bartalena L, Rocchi R, et al. Long-term safety of orbital radiotherapy for Graves' ophthalmopathy. J Clin Endocrinol Metab 2003; 88:3561–3566.

39. Gorman CA, Garrity JA, Fatourechi V, et al. A prospective, randomized, double-blind, placebo-controlled study of orbital radiotherapy for Graves' ophthalmopathy [see comment]. Ophthalmology 2001; 108:1523–1534.

40. Gorman CA. Radiotherapy for Graves' ophthalmopathy: results at one year. Thyroid 2002; 12:251–255.

41. Kazim M. Perspective—part II: radiotherapy for Graves orbitopathy: the Columbia University experience. Ophthal Plast Reconstr Surg 2002; 18:173–174.

42. Feldon SE. Radiation therapy for Graves' ophthalmopathy: trick or treat? [comment]. Ophthalmology 2001; 108: 1521–1522.

43. Trokel S, Kazim M, Moore S. Orbital fat removal. Decompression for Graves orbitopathy. Ophthalmology 1993; 100: 674–682.

44. Olivari N. Thyroid-associated orbitopathy: transpalpebral decompression by removal of intraorbital fat. Experience with 1362 orbits in 697 patients over 13 years. Exp Clin Endocrinol Diabetes 1999; 107(suppl 5):S208–S211.

45. Olivari N. Transpalpebral decompression of endocrine ophthalmopathy (Graves' disease) by removal of intraorbital fat: experience with 147 operations over 5 years [see comment]. Plast Reconstr Surg 1991; 87:627–641. Discussion 642–643.

46. Kennedy DW, Goodstein ML, Miller NR, Zinreich SJ. Endoscopic transnasal orbital decompression. Arch Otolaryngol Head Neck Surg 1990; 116:275–282.

47. Kacker A, Kazim M, Murphy M, Trokel S, Close LG. "Balanced" orbital decompression for severe Graves' orbitopathy: technique with treatment algorithm. Otolaryngol Head Neck Surg 2003; 128:228–235.

48. Shorr N, Baylis HI, Goldberg RA, Perry JD. Transcaruncular approach to the medial orbit and orbital apex. Ophthalmology 2000; 107:1459–1463.

49. Cockerham KP, Hidayat AA, Brown HG, Cockerham GC, Graner SR. Clinicopathologic evaluation of the Mueller muscle in thyroid-associated orbitopathy. Ophthal Plast Reconstr Surg 2002; 18:11–17.

50. Elner VM, Hassan AS, Frueh BR. Graded full-thickness anterior blepharotomy for upper eyelid retraction. Trans Am Ophthalmol Soc 2003; 101:67–73. Discussion 73–75.

51. Morton AD, Nelson C, Ikada Y, Elner VM. Porous polyethylene as a spacer graft in the treatment of lower eyelid retraction. Ophthal Plast Reconstr Surg 2000; 16:146–155.

52. Shorr N, Perry JD, Goldberg RA, Hoenig J, Shorr J. The safety and applications of acellular human dermal allograft in ophthalmic plastic and reconstructive surgery: a preliminary report. Ophthal Plast Reconstr Surg 2000; 16:223–230.

53. Prendiville P, Chopra M, Gauderman WJ, Feldon SE. The role of restricted motility in determining outcomes for vertical strabismus surgery in Graves' ophthalmology [see comment]. Ophthalmology 2000; 107:545–549.

26

Management Controversies and Preferences in Thyroid Orbitopathy: Panel Discussion and Question Period*

JACK ROOTMAN and FRANK BUFFAM[†]

Department of Ophthalmology and Visual
Sciences, and Department of Pathology,
University of British Columbia and the Vancouver
General Hospital, Vancover, British Columbia,
Canada

In a session moderated by Frank Buffam, four endocrinologists—Colum Gorman, Daphne Khoo, Claudio Marcocci, and Wilmar Wiersinga—and three orbital specialists—Michael Kazim, John Kennerdell, and Jack Rootman with significant

---

* Panel members: Colum Gorman, Michael Kazim, John Kennerdell, Daphne Khoo, Claudio Marcocci, Jack Rootman, and Wilmar Wiersinga.
† Session moderator.

experience in the management of Graves' orbitopathy—were asked to discuss in 5 min how they would deal with both moderate and severe active Graves' orbitopathy as well as a third group of Grave's orbitopathy patients having optic neuropathy. This was followed by an open question period from the audience.

PANELISTS' PRESENTATIONS

Colum Gorman

From the perspective of his profession, that of endocrinology, Dr. Gorman first approaches patients with Graves' eye disease by placing the Graves' eye disease within the context of the whole person. In his practice, he has encountered Graves' patients with pancreatic cancer and small cell lung cancer, and he believes that the coexistence of other major morbidities certainly refines and defines what can be done for the ophthalmopathy. The next step in his approach is to determine what treatment has already been given, which can potentially limit the management options available to the clinician.

The patient's priorities are to be considered next as patients are often more concerned with their appearance rather than the degree of optic neuropathy they have, which is usually the focus of most clinicians. Following this, it is necessary to establish what the patient's expectations are for their outcome, which can at times be unrealistic. This is particularly true if one is dealing with persons who are very much in the public eye and for whom a very minor degree of lid alteration, for example, is a career modifying occurrence; for those persons, the expectations are sometimes quite unrealistic as to what can be accomplished and it is important at that point to try to reconcile patient expectations with what can actually be done.

Visual assessment by the orbital specialists in the Mayo Clinic follows, which establishes the disease's threat to vision. Once this has been assessed, the clinician determines whether protection vs. rehabilitation is required. If the patient's condition is rapidly progressive and assertive in its presentation, a protective stand is taken, whereas stable, long-term disease is indicative of a rehabilitative mode and the approaches for which are quite different.

As Dr. Gorman often plays the role of the coordinator of the patient's care, the next stage at this point is to outline from the beginning to end what are the expected sequential steps in the patient's total rehabilitation so that the patient has the entire perspective on what is required for total rehabilitation. The key element of this is free communication of a consistent message from the ophthalmologist and endocrinologist and a firm commitment to the patient that the team will be a part of this process.

Once these steps are in place, the approach to mild, moderate, and severe disease falls into place. If the disease is severe and vision threatening, it is typically a short course of steroids. Failure to respond to steroids leads to the offer of orbital decompression. If the disease is mild or moderate and stable, the approach is with the methods that have been described in this symposium, and that is primarily a surgical approach with muscle surgery first followed by lid surgery.

Michael Kazim

Dr. Kazim identified a few differences between his practice and that of Dr. Gorman, specifically the nature of the referral, which leads to a different type of patient being seen. He believed that his patients present very early in the course of their disease and therefore tend not to be stable-phase patients but rather acute-phase, which he considers to be a medical as opposed to a surgical condition.

Like Dr. Gorman, it is his opinion that the patient's first visit provides the specialist with the opportunity to set the tone for the rest of the patient encounter, which can last from 1 to 4 years. A typical first visit is about 1–1.5 hr—however long it takes—for Dr. Kazim to understand the patient's disease status and needs and for the patient to understand the complete approach he is offering. If patients somehow do not "buy into" his approach, they will have to convince him that their condition or their relationship to their condition, be it special functional or cosmetic needs, would alter the way he would normally proceed.

In his experience, the approach to mild, acute-phase disease is virtually 100 percent supportive. In the cases where it may be a little more congestive, some form of nonsteroidal anti-inflammatory drug may be used. At one point of time, he had studied nonsteroidal anti-inflammatories and based on particular characteristics of the drugs, chose Voltaren. (He notes that he did not study the outcome of treatment of the drugs.) Patients receive Voltaren 75 mg twice a day. Steroids are not routinely used, although occasionally a patient will present already on steroids but this happens less frequently. If patients are on steroids without compressive neuropathy, the steroids are withdrawn, since he does not believe that the drug will make a lot of difference in the long term. Only in cases of optic neuropathy will he proceed with surgical intervention, which is where his approach differs from that of Dr. Gorman's. Dr. Kazim's institution has a great deal of experience and success with a combination of radiation and steroids—radiation to limit the time frame of the disease and steroids to eliminate the optic neuropathy. They proceed surgically only where the steroids and/or radiotherapy are contraindicated or fail. All other patients fall into stable-phase disease and are treated surgically, as was described by other speakers.

John Kennerdell

Dr. Kennerdell noted that management of thyroid orbitopathy had been extensively covered during the symposium, most of which was in keeping with his approach. One important factor of management is to ensure that the approach was individualized to the patient. Another important factor is flexibility: individual treatment of the patient based on having available all the modalities. In his practice, all modalities are used, including, steroids, radiotherapy, chemotherapy, and various types of decompression. With muscle surgery, adjustable sutures are preferred, and a limbal approach is used, as in his opinion, there is a need to recess the conjunctiva but cover the insertion site. Another lid surgery technique is the upper and lower tarsal transplant, which is a simple procedure and the rejection rate is practically 0. It is a useful technique for resolving a 2.0–2.5 mm lower lid retraction. In his experience, he has only one buckle.

Muscle surgery is delayed for at least 6 months for stability, longer if possible. Lid surgery is delayed for a year. Both surgeries occur after the decompression has been done.

Like Dr. Gorman, most of his time is spent counseling the patient. This involves explaining in detail the whole course of the disease and what they may expect. Two brochures that summarize the disease are also provided. By and large, it is a counseling job with the exception of the more severe cases.

Thank you.

Daphne Khoo

Dr. Khoo is an endocrinologist in Singapore whose clinic sees a large number of Graves' disease patients. They see approximately 1500–2000 referrals of Graves' disease per year, and of these about 400 will have at least some form of thyroid eye disease. Very few of these cases actually end up with the ophthalmologist because of the volume, unfortunately. At one stage, a proposal had been put forth by the ophthalmologists that the thyroid eye disease patients be sent to them, but after 2 months they said they could not cope with the volume. Generally, about 10% the cases will eventually go to the ophthalmologists and obviously these will be the most symptomatic patients.

One unusual factor of their population base, relative to the Caucasian populations, is a very low prevalence of smoking. The majority of patients are Chinese females and of this group, only 8% are smokers, and this may be the reason why patients with far less severe ophthalmopathy are seen in their clinic. This has led to some question as to the applicability of data from Caucasian studies to their studies.

In terms of optic neuropathy, most patients end up with the ophthalmologist rather than with us, since they present most of the time with visual disturbances. With these patients, the management is quite clear-cut. High-dose pulsed methylprednisolone is administered for a couple of days and if there is no marked improvement, the patients undergo decompression surgery.

The other situations are more difficult because they have found that there is a great reluctance on the part of their patients to agree to decompression surgery for indications other than optic neuropathy. Despite careful explanation that the decompression is just the first of multiple surgeries, most patients do not give consent, which may explain the low numbers that were presented earlier by Dr. Seah, my colleague in ophthalmology from Singapore.

With regard to orbital irradiation, the problem there is a reluctance amongst the therapeutic radiologists in Singapore to give orbital radiation, largely because the incidence of nasopharyngeal carcinoma (NPC) is fairly high in the Chinese population. They have found with NPC that about 10 years after irradiation, it is very common to develop hypopituitarism, although patients may be fine for the first 10 years. Given the bad experiences with NPC, the therapeutic radiologists are very concerned with whether the shielding is currently adequate to prevent the onset of optic nerve damage or damage to other parts of the eye many years down the line. These fears of course may well be unfounded.

For the patients who have moderately severe disease but do not want either decompression or orbital irradiation, the course of management is often pulsed steroids, which is used frequently by their group. They have had good results with octreotide; unfortunately, the cost of this treatment modality is a big factor, as it is not subsidized by the government. Other treatments have been tried, including cyclosporine, pentoxyfylline and cox-2 inhibitors, all with varying degrees of success. In their experience, pulsed steroids and octreotide have been effective.

Claudio Marcocci

Dr. Marcocci's center is one of the major referral centers in Italy. They see a large number of patients with Graves' disease and Graves' ophthalmopathy and work side-by-side with the ophthalmologists. Once the patient has been evaluated, a great deal of time is spent discussing with the patient the natural history of the disease, what can be done for them, and what their expectations are.

For a patient with mild, active eye disease, they believe that it is important to restore and maintain euthyroidism with antithyroid drugs. Once the patient has reached euthyroidism, the choice of treatment for hyperthyroidism is not influenced by the presence of ophthalmopathy. Particular care is taken to avoid hypothyroidism that can be induced by excess in antithyroid therapy. They usually suggest the use of supporting measures until the disease becomes inactive, the so-called "wait-and-see" policy. Once the disease is inactive, rehabilitative surgery may be suggested if necessary.

In patients with moderate and active ophthalmopathy, it is necessary to have a rapid and permanent control of hyperthyroidism. For this purpose, once euthyroidism is reached with antithyroid drugs, the patient is treated with either radioiodine or thyroidectomy according to goiter size and sometimes at the request of the patient. When radioiodine is used, the patient also receives a shortened course of glucocorticoids. Particular attention is taken once again to avoid post-treatment hypothyroidism. Supportive measures are also suggested and once the disease is over in terms of activity, rehabilitative surgery is offered along with, in certain cases, orbital decompression.

For severe orbital disease, unless there is a risk of loss of vision, once control of thyrotoxicosis is obtained with permanent treatment through radioiodine or thyroidectomy, the use of total thyroid ablation is considered to get rid of all orbital antigens. Again, surgery is delayed until the disease is inactive.

In patients with sight-threatening ophthalmopathy, their approach differs according to whether the patient has already been treated elsewhere. Orbital decompression is usually offered as the initial treatment, if previous treatment from another institution has been noted. In cases where the patients have not had previous treatment elsewhere, they tend to use intravenous high-dose glucocorticoids, consisting of 1 g methyl prednisolone for 3 days repeated if necessary over the following weeks. If no response is noted, the patient is offered an orbital decompression, whereas if there is evidence of amelioration, we continue with the high-dose glucocorticosteroids along with orbital radiotherapy. Once stability has been achieved, decompression or rehabilitative surgery may be suggested if needed.

Jack Rootman

Dr. Rootman felt that the approach described by Dr. Marcocci mirrored to a large degree that of his practice.

With moderate disease, they attempt a disease modifying approach, if possible, and sometimes do a trial of steroids. Pulsed steroids are preferred and they will wait longer than 2 weeks before repeating the course. In some instances, the wait period has lasted 6 weeks, and they have found that quite a high proportion of the patients last longer than 2 weeks.

One caveat that Dr. Rootman noted was that diabetic patients with thyroid orbitopathy are a special population. Radiotherapy is certainly contraindicated in them. In this group of patients, he has had better results with pulsed steroids in combination with some sort of immunosuppressive drug to modify the disease. Alternatively, they may proceed earlier to surgery. If a small, tight orbital apex is encountered, the orbit specialist is usually forced to do surgery as a primary event for this population, high-dose steroids would also be administered.

He agreed whole heartedly with what the panels members had said, that the patients require a lot of patience and hand-holding and that they should have a very good prospective idea of what is going to happen to them, as it is disruptive to their lives. In his experience, many of the patients are very grateful for restoring them to as close to normal as possible, which should be the goal.

Dr. Rootman made one final remark with regard to nutrition and the issue of smoking. He agreed that these patients are better motivated to quit smoking, and many of them are interested in nutritional approaches. Indeed, the use of antioxidant therapy may not be inappropriate.

Wilmar Wiersinga

In all patients with Graves' ophthalmopathy, euthyroidism is restored using antithyroid drugs. Patients are held on a combination of antithyroid drugs plus thyroxine until treatment for their Graves' ophthalmopathy is complete, which may be in 2–3 years. Also, patients are asked to refrain from smoking and offered help to achieve this.

With regard to the specific treatment of Graves' ophthalmopathy within the three categories of very severe, moderately severe, and mild disease, the very severe cases are defined as those with optic neuropathy. In this group of patients, intravenous pulses of methyl prednisolone are given, 1 g daily for three successive days in the first week and repeated in the second week. After 2 weeks, visual functions are assessed and if no improvement noted, an urgent decompression is undertaken; otherwise, they continue with oral prednisone.

Management of patients with moderately severe Graves' ophthalmopathy is determined by the activity of the eye disease. If the eye disease is inactive in nature, a rehabilitative surgical program is initiated. If active eye disease is still present, the patients qualify for immunosuppressive treatment, and it is Dr. Wiersinga's opinion that the most effective treatment currently is a combination of intravenous pulses of methyl prednisolone plus radiotherapy.

Probably the most difficult cases, in a way, are the patients with mild Graves' ophthalmopathy. In a recent randomized clinical trial comparing retrobulbar irradiation with sham-irradiation in patients with mild Grave's ophthalmopathy, they found that radiotherapy was also an effective treatment, especially for diplopia and eye muscle motility, but the effect is limited. Radiotherapy did not prevent the worsening of the ophthalmopathy, which occurred in 30% of the irradiated patients and 30% of the sham-irradiated subjects. As a result of this study, his center continues to adopt the "wait-and-see" policy with the mild Graves' ophthalmopathy patients, despite the fact that the patients themselves do not perceive their eye disease as being mild. In another study, they developed a disease-specific quality of life questionnaire and applied it to this category of patients. One of the results of their study showed that these patients felt their quality of life was low, at the same level as patients with chronic inflammatory bowel disease or diabetic patients with their complications.

It is the practice in their center to see these patients with the orbital surgeon and also with a representative of the thyroid eye disease patient association. They have found that patients derive considerable help and support when they are able to talk to a fellow patient about the process they are about to enter.

Lastly, because many investigations are often needed, frequent visits to the hospital are not uncommon, which can be a problem for the patient. At their center, they have endeavored to change this by organizing the visits all into one day. Patients arrive early in the morning and blood tests are done. All the results of the thyroid function tests and thyroid antibodies are therefore complete and available by the end of the day. During the morning, the patient will first be seen by one of the endocrinology staffs and then by orbital surgeons. In the afternoon, imaging and all other required investigations are completed. By 4:30 in the afternoon, the patient is once again seen by the endocrinologist and orbital surgeon together and a diagnosis and management plan is then offered.

QUESTION AND ANSWER SESSION

Question 1 (from R. Goldberg)

"If all the experts agree that steroids are the mainstay treatment of medical Graves' orbitopathy, I, in my practice, find periorbital steroid injections absolutely indispensable. One cc of 40 mg per cc Kenalog—I find to be clinically about as effective as a 3-week course of oral prednisone and particularly in patients that are going to require a more extended course of steroids. It spares a lot of the systemic side effects of oral steroids. I was surprised that none of the speakers mentioned that. Is that not a popular treatment in other centers?"

Answer

John Kennerdell responded. He did not use steroid injections. He had tried them many years ago and got more complications than justification for the treatment. He also noted that in orbital disease, he preferred not to "put things in" and was very much against injections.

Question 1 (continued)

"I perhaps have given 500 or 800 injections and I really have not seen local complications related to the injection, but I am open-minded about it. At least my anecdotal experience is that they are safe and I think compared to the risk of continued oral steroids, the risks may favor injection, in my opinion. The injection can be periorbital with a small needle, just behind the septum or even right next to the septum. One cc of 40 mg per cc Kenalog—it does not have to be in the deep intraconal space to have a good effect."

Answer

Claudio Marcocci stated that his group performed a randomized trial a couple of years ago that compared the effectiveness of oral glucocorticoids and locally administered steroids. They found that the local treatment was much less effective than the general treatment. He then stated that currently they use the local injection in very, very selective cases with contraindication to systemic glucocorticoids as a treatment for ophthalmopathy.

Question 2 (from M. Potts)

"I have been interested in and committed to treating thyroid eye disease as an autoimmune disease for about 10 years and in the first few years, I tried radiotherapy and steroids. They worked but they are not enough by themselves and you need more. So in the last 6 years, and we are about to publish this, we have been using for our compressive optic neuropathy (our severe group) quadruple therapy. The quadruple therapy is you give them intravenous methyl prednisolone to recover their color vision and get their vision back. All you do is buy some time. Then you start them on azathioprine and low-dose oral steroids and orbital radiotherapy. If you give them quadruple therapy, you will find (when we produce our paper) that I have done no decompressions in the last 6 years. Also, because you return those muscles back to a normal size by immunosuppressing the disease that is going on in the muscles, we did only one squint operation in those 26 patients with dysthyroid optic neuropathy. So, if you hit them hard enough, early enough, you can reverse the process almost completely. We do end up doing a bit of lid lowering. We do a little bit of blepharoplasties, but if you use quadruple therapy, then you could switch the disease process off."

Answer

Jack Rootman commented that he would be interested in seeing these results as they differ from his experience. In his practice, the patients are usually not seen at an early stage of their disease but have had their "primary" immunologic event prior to presentation. He also expressed interest in seeing evidence of mechanical changes. In a recent study, they looked at over 200 patients treated with either corticosteroids, radiotherapy or observation and followed them for 5 years with CT imaging. Structurally, the muscles did not change in size; they may physically behave differently but they did not change in size.

Question 2 (continued)

"If you use MRI scanning, particularly STIR sequence scanning, you look at the amount of water in them and the water loading goes down; but you have to get these patients very early in their disease when there is mainly lymphocytes, before the fibroblasts proliferate. I think once the fibroblasts have proliferated, laid down the collagen, you have missed the boat. In the West Country, all the endocrinologists are very educated and send the patients very early to me. If you hit them very hard in that early sensitive phase, you can switch the whole disease process off."

Question 3

"I have got a three-part question. Dr. Wiersinga, am I to understand that when you are going to use steroids in patients with thyroid eye disease, your initial dose is IV pulsed? Is there a role for oral steroids at all in your treatment with thyroid eye disease, or I am getting an impression from the panel that everybody is going to IV pulsed steroids first. If you are going to use steroids, you might as well use them in big doses. Is that correct?"

Answer

In his opinion, Dr. Wiersinga felt that the efficacy of IV pulsed steroids is higher than that of oral steroids, and that the side effects of IV pulsed steroids are less than those of oral steroids. However, there have been two deaths reported from IV pulses, one from Vienna and the other from Pisa, with both patients dying from liver failure. Although it is a fairly rare event, severe liver function disorders can result from IV pulses. This has not been encountered in other diseases in which these IV pulses have been applied, such as rheumatoid arthritis, so some caution may be needed. The cumulative dose of glucocorticoids given by IV pulses is usually much higher than the cumulative dose of oral prednisone, so the question arises as to whether the difference in total glucocorticosteroid dose is factor. It is probably but there is also a suggestion from the Italians that if the total dose of IV glucocorticoids does not exceed 8 g, the severe side effects from the liver may be avoided.

Question 3 (continued)

"As a neuro-ophthalmologist, I use IV pulsed steroids constantly for patients with demyelinating disease and with reckless abandon. In fact, we have done quite well with it and now do it as home therapy, but the question really was what is the role for oral prednisone because many patients come to me from endocrinologists saying, 'I will start them on 40 mg or 60 mg and you can see them.' My answer is "to let me see them first and then possibly just do 1000 mg IV pulses. It makes better sense and I am not afraid to use that dose at all."

Answer

Jack Rootman commented that the biological difference between oral and IV steroids had not been brought forward. He has been very disillusioned with oral steroids because of the many side effects. As an ocular oncologist, he has had many discussions with pediatric oncologists about the use of oral steroids vs. IV pulsed steroids. In the treatment of lymphoma, a difference is noted. There is a lymphocytolysis that occurs with high-dose pulsed steroids that does not happen with oral corticosteroids, so there is something of a biologic rationale for that idea. There are a lot less of the other side effects with IV pulsed steroids so he is much more comfortable using it. In his practice, it is done as an outpatient procedure.

Question 3 (continued)

"I have also been impressed that we have not induced diabetes in patients who are diabetic, as sugar is not going up with IV pulses as opposed to oral. My second question is to Dr. Rootman. You alluded to the fact that you liked the transcaruncular approach to the medial orbital decompression. Is this to replace the endoscopic endonasal ENT approach, or which one do you like better?"

Answer

In response, Dr. Rootman felt that he could see the orbit better using the more direct orbital approaches, in fact, a lot better than looking up through the nose. He prefers it because it is a clear approach for him.

Question 3 (continued)

"The last question is for Dr. Kennerdell. I agree with you that in our institution also, I have had a great experience with radiotherapy, but had a recent very interesting experience with a call from an insurance company quoting the Mayo Clinic article saying, "But radiation does not work and you are asking me to approve a $12,000 therapy for your patient." I got around it by saying that it was not for severe ophthalmo-pathy and our patient had severe orbitopathy. They kind of believed me and approved it, but what is your indication to use radiation therapy and if you have had this problem with the insurance companies quoting the Mayo Clinic literature that says it does not work?"

Answer

John Kennerdell emphasized once again that they as a group believe that radiotherapy works in carefully selected patients. The carefully selected individualization of these patients is what is required. He believes that radiotherapy does not work in chronic patients and is not effective in patients that are subacute. However, radiotherapy does work in patients that are acute, with or without optic neuropathy.

Dr. Kennerdell made an additional comment with regard to the first question posed, regarding peribulbar steroid injections. The results of using of injected peribulbar steroids, in his experience, were variable and the complications high.

With regard to oral steroids, he generally uses steroids as a test for whether radiation therapy will work, but he tends to use oral steroids less and less. If steroids are used, usually in acute congestive patients whether they have optic neuropathy or corneal exposure, he tends to administer it in a high-dose fashion, as has been described, and will switch to oral steroids if they work and continue to work. Generally, if after a week the patient continues to have a good response, he will proceed with radiation therapy combined with oral steroids while the patient is receiving radiation. He has had good results with this method. If there is a poor response to high-dose steroids, he is inclined to be mechanical about the treatment.

Question 4 (from M. Mourits)

"From what I have heard today, I think we agree on many points nowadays. We agree about management of patients with mild orbitopathy. We generally agree about management of patients with vision-threatening disease. We agree about surgical approaches, although there are numerous different approaches. As long as they work, we do not mind. But the burning question is what do we do with active, moderately severe Graves' orbitopathy? I have not had an answer to that question yet. In these times of evidence-based medicine, we have demonstrated in two independent institutions that the efficacy of radiotherapy is very limited if at all present. Oral prednisone and IV prednisone, of which everybody is talking now, have never been tested in a controlled study. So my question is how do I treat these patients, which is the largest group of patients I see?"

Answer

Dr. Rootman's response was twofold. Firstly, the specialist needs to see the patients at an earlier stage of their disease to try and prevent it. Secondly, a more active approach to these studies needs to be taken to determine how to proceed with, or set guidelines for, these studies.

In return, Dr. Rootman asked that the audience consider the following question: why are orbital specialists discussing single-modality therapy for an "immunologically based disease" when virtually every other discipline has moved to multimodality therapies or sequential therapies based upon the biology of the disease process? Under present circumstances, there does not seem to be clear evidence agreed upon by all for the treatment of moderate to severe cases. He felt that the studies or reports done so far were anecdotal and that the prospective, multitherapy studies needed to be done. This seemed to be the path for the future.

Question 5 (from F. Buffam)

"Does anybody leave patients on moderate dose steroids for months?"

Answer

Dr. Rootman noted that he has had a bad experience with patients on long-term oral steroids, with side effects that ranged from perianal abscesses to psychotic episodes. He felt that the chronic use of oral steroids was really disappointing. He agreed with previous comments that there is much frustration in choosing the appropriate treatment but felt that oral administration was the worse way of using steroids.

Question 6 (from F. Buffam)

"What is the longest time period to leave a patient on steroids?"

Answer

Dr. Kennerdell indicated that, in his practice, the longest time he has left a patient on steroids was 3 months. He was very disappointed with oral steroids and leaves patients on them only as long as he absolutely has to use them; generally, he prefers their use in an acute manner only. It is more effective to find out what needs to be dealt with, whether this patient will respond or not, then turn to another modality.

Dr. Gorman commented that the course of treatment that one offers a patient is a negotiation between the patient on one hand explaining their discomforts and the physician on the other hand dispensing from a limited variety of therapies. Many times, it is a question for the patient of "I can put up with what I have wrong today but can you tell me when it will end?" If the patient is on the plateau phase of the illness, it is difficult to tell them when it will end but a general idea of when symptoms tend to ameliorate can be conveyed.

Dr. Rootman then noted that one could be more effective in prognosticating and allowing patients to know what is going to happen with their disease, which can be an enormous relief to a patient who has what used to be called "noninfiltrative disease." For example, a 30-year-old patient who is a non-smoker has good prognostic factors and therefore can be told that their disease will most likely not progress or worsen.

Dr. Kazim supported Dr. Rootman's remarks on giving patients a general, good, broad outlook at the initial visit. For patients who see him early in the course of their disease without a long history before they arrive, he tends to see them again in a month. If the patients proceed from not so bad to particularly bad over this 4-week period, it identifies for him those who will go through an acute congestive phase. This is generally a small number of patients but he prefers to identify them so that he can consider more aggressive intervention.

Dr. Wiersinga wished to comment on an earlier question, Question 4. He noted that much progress had been made over the last 10 years in this area, especially with carefully executed randomized trials, though research in Graves' management does lag behind other fields in this respect. New trials to research interventions are indeed the way forward. A member of the audience commented earlier on his "quadruple intervention" approach, which is probably a good approach; however, there are so many biases involved in this particular disease that Dr. Wiersinga could not accept his results without support from a prospective randomized clinical trial.

In order to make real progress, studies have to be completed faster and these studies should be multicenter. In Europe, the European Group on Graves' Ophthalmopathy (EUGOGO) was organized for this purpose, with participation from nine European centers. The main difficulty the group now faces is reaching inter-observer agreement, and once that is achieved, multicenter trials can begin. Then, more progress can be achieved in a shorter period of time.

Question 7 (from P. Dolman)

"I am a little confused about the classification of mild, moderate and severe as different panelists describe it. I think some panelists are saying that severe ophthalmopathy means there is optic neuropathy and in my mind, that is a separate category and has a different management strategy. I think some are saying that mild disease is what we would categorize as already quiescent; these patients have surgical problems with lid retraction, and perhaps proptosis and will need surgery for that. Therefore, I believe that if we are to discuss mild, moderate, and severe disease, we should really refer to inflammatory activity or progress or whatever term one wants to use to prove that something can be medically responsive. I still feel a bit muddy when the broad terms, moderate or severe, are applied to different aspects. Because of this, our group proposed the "VISA" (vision, inflammation, strabismus, and appearance) classification to define the medical features of inflammation."

Answer

Dr. Rootman responded by noting that he was the one who initially posed the question to the panel and that it was in the context of active, moderate disease. He had hoped the panel would divide management into the categories of what was going to be done for soft tissue components (inflammation), strabismus, and appearance. He noted that optic neuropathy patients are a different category, since they can present with variable activity or soft-tissue or inflammatory features associated with their optic neuropathy and will need to be managed on an individual basis. The use of the categories proposed by the VISA classification allowed for defining the character of the disease and appropriate management.

27

A New Technique in Managing Distensible Venous Vascular Malformations of the Orbit

**THOMAS R. MAROTTA and
DOUGLAS A. GRAEB**
Diagnostic and Therapeutic
Neuroradiology, St. Michael's Hospital,
University of Toronto, Toronto,
Ontario, Canada

JACK ROOTMAN
Department of Ophthalmology and
Visual Sciences, and Department of
Pathology, University of British
Columbia, Vancouver General
Hospital, Vancouver,
British Columbia, Canada

INTRODUCTION

Multidisciplinary approaches to human diseases arise out of limitations in treating complex disorders with methods that fall into single areas of expertise. With combined expertise, otherwise difficult lesions become more easily managed. We have been able to apply interventional neuroradiologic techniques to a variety of vascular lesions of the orbit (1,2) to successfully treat what might otherwise be considered untreatable.

321

This presentation will outline the technique that we use in treating selected patients with distensible venous vascular malformations (DVVMs) of the orbit (orbital varices).

CLASSIFICATION OF ORBITAL VASCULAR LESIONS

An exhaustive discussion of this classification is beyond the scope of this presentation but is discussed in detail elsewhere (2,3). The overall concept distinguishes "new growth" from "malformation" and emphasizes the difference between an acquired arteriovenous shunt or fistula (i.e., carotid-cavernous fistula) and other vascular malformations. Vascular malformations can then be subdivided based at least in part on flow into no-flow, venous flow, and arterial flow lesions. A lymphatic vascular malformation would typify the no-flow lesion, and arteriovenous malformation the arterial flow lesion. Venous flow lesions include distensible venous, nondistensible venous, and combined nondistensible venous–lymphatic vascular malformations. It is the DVVMs that enlarge with Valsalva maneuver or bending for which the combined technique of direct puncture embolization followed by surgical excision has been used.

DVVMs may be superficial, deep (posterior to the globe), or a combination of these. Their involvement may extend beyond the boundaries of the orbit to include the face, paranasal sinuses, or intracranially; these are called complex venous malformations (Fig. 1).

ANATOMY OF ORBITAL REGION VENOUS STRUCTURES AND RELATIONSHIP WITH DVVMs

The orbital venous system has a significant outflow connection via the superior and inferior orbital veins to the cavernous sinus, venous plexus of the pterygopalatine fossa, and supratrochlear and angular veins of the face.

The relationship of DVVMs to normal veins of the orbit and its neighboring structures is variable but at least in part

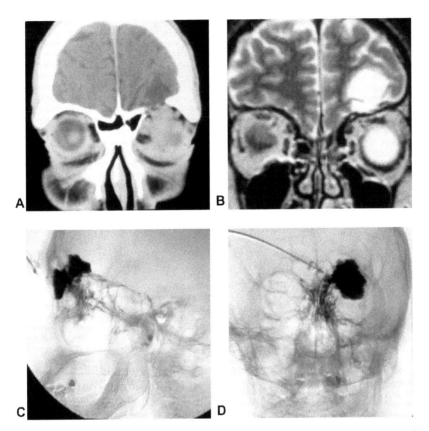

Figure 1 Coronal CT (A) and MR (B) imaging and lateral (C) and frontal (D) views from a direct injection show a complex DVVM extending from superficial to deep in the orbit and also intracranially through a bony defect in the roof of the orbit. (Borrowed with permission from Ref. 2.)

predictable by the location of the malformation. The distensibility of these lesions indicates relatively large functioning connections with the normal venous system. When the pressure in the venous system is elevated, it is reflected back stream into the malformation, which distends. Depending on venous connections, these DVVMs can on occasion be visualized by indirect orbital venographic techniques. Those connected to the superior ophthalmic vein may be seen this way (Fig. 2). However, the best means to delineate specific

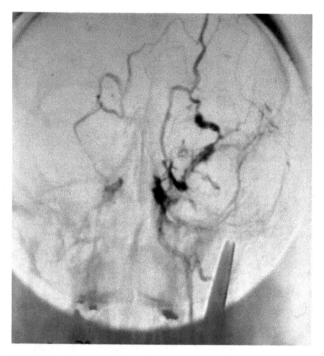

Figure 2 Direct venogram demonstrates a venous orbital malformation. This is characterized by an ectatic venous outflow channel that is part of the superior ophthalmic vein. (Borrowed with permission from Ref. 3.)

features of a DVVM and its connections is by direct intralesional injection. The DVVMs can be relatively simple ectatic areas that merge with adjacent normal orbital veins (Fig. 3B), or more complex malformations with multiple channels and saccular areas that flow into dysplastic venous networks to the pterygopalatine fossa or the superior or inferior ophthalmic venous systems (Figs. 3 and 4).

CLINICAL MANIFESTATIONS OF DVVMs

Generally, DVVMs do not warrant treatment. Superficial lesions might be seen as dark, tortuous epibulbar varices or as subcutaneous lid masses (Fig. 5). Deep lesions will be less obvious at rest but cause intermittent proptosis when the patient strains (Valsalva maneuver), bends, or exerts physical effort. At rest, these patients may have enophthalmos because of fat atrophy and orbital expansion associated with the DVVM. Occasionally, a deep lesion will present with some surface bruising related to a hemorrhage that has tracked forward. Combined lesions will have some combination of the above findings, and complex lesions will extend outside the orbit to involve the venous system of the face and intracranial areas. Facial lesions might have some surface discoloration and may become problematic from a cosmetic point of view.

Our indications for treating selected patients with DVVMs of the orbit are intermittent or unrelenting pain, progressive expansion, and cosmesis. Only one of our patients has presented with reduced vision in addition to discomfort and esotropia. Symptoms of distensible lesions are summarized in Table 1.

INVESTIGATION OF DVVMs

Initial investigation is with computed tomographic (CT) scanning or magnetic resonance imaging (MRI), both of which are usually done with and without contrast enhancement. The CT scanning is performed with the patient lying flat on the table at rest for the axial imaging plane and then somewhat strained with the head hanging over the back of the table to attain the coronal plane. This positioning effectively produces a Valsalva maneuver and the lesions are usually distended and more conspicuous on the coronal images (Fig. 6). For MRI, the patient remains flat and quiet throughout with the various imaging planes being provided computationally. Thus, when MRI is used, it is important to ask the patient to strain during at least one of the acquisitions in order to "bring out" the lesion (Fig. 7). The CT and MRI will delineate the primary focus of the orbital lesion and should reveal any involvement beyond the orbit into the face, skull base, paranasal sinuses, and intracranial areas. Dynamic ultrasound and the use of Doppler may aid in confirming the hemodynamics of the DVVMs.

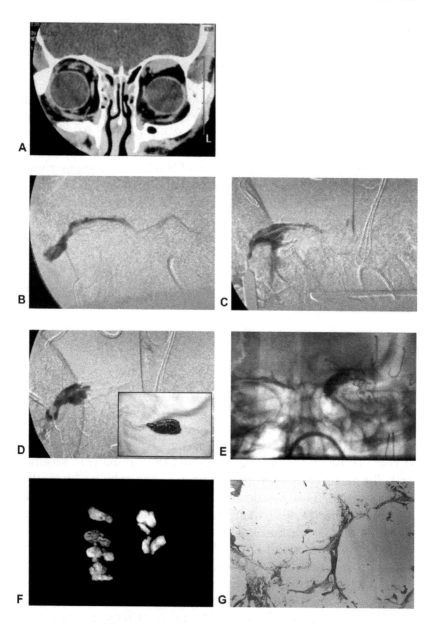

Figure 3 (*Caption on facing page*)

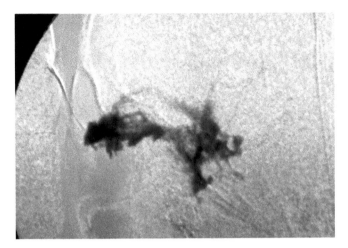

Figure 4 Direct injection lateral view with multiple channels and saccular areas extending beyond the orbit into the anterior cranial fossa and pterygopalatine region. (Borrowed with permission from Ref. 2.)

Venography is also used for investigation. Indirect venography is done by accessing the venous system via a vein, usually in the frontal scalp, and directing contrast injection toward the orbit by placing a tourniquet around the head

---

Figure 3 (*Facing page*) Enchanced CT scan (A) reveals the presence of a venous malformation affecting the left superior orbit. The patient underwent excision of his lesion via left lateral orbitotomy. A direct intralesional lateral view venogram performed intraoperatively revealed an ectatic area draining straight back through the superior ophthalmic vein to the cavernous sinus (B, C). With pressure applied at the superior orbital fissure, control of outflow is confirmed venographically before injection of the cyanoacrylate mixture. The glue cast is seen in situ following embolization (D) and following excision (D-inset). An intraoperative fluoroscopic anterior–posterior view (E) confirmed the presence of the glue cast within the superior orbital venous malformation, correlating well with CT findings. The excised cast itself is demonstrated on x-ray (F). The histology of thin-walled vessels after the casting material has been removed is shown in (G). (Fig. 3A–E borrowed with permission from Ref. 2.)

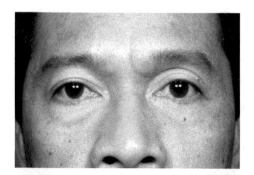

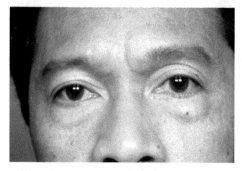

Figure 5 The left lower lids show some fullness when the patient strains. (Borrowed with permission from Ref. 2.)

below the orbits or by asking the patient to compress the angular veins. As noted, visualization is somewhat limited by this technique because of anomalous connections. Direct puncture with contrast injection into the lesion is the best

Table 1 Symptoms of Distensible Lesions

Symptom	%
Pain/discomfort	43
Periorbital swelling	40
Abnormal prominence of eye	33
Periorbital hemorrhage	20
Abnormal ocular motility	10
Enophthalmos	7
Subconjunctival hemorrhage	7
Compressive optic neuropathy	3

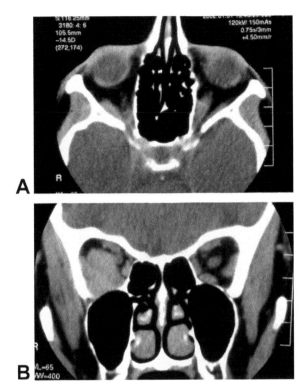

Figure 6 Axial (A) and coronal (B) CT scans demonstrate an inferior orbital DVVM, which is more conspicuous on the coronal view.

technique to understand their features and most importantly, their connections to the normal venous system. For access to superficial lesions, using a small butterfly needle is relatively straightforward and can be done in the angiography suite prior to making a decision to proceed to the operating room for treatment. For combined and complex lesions with superficial components, access into the superficial component allows visualization of deeper lesions by demonstrating connecting channels. Lesions that are deep will usually require surgical exposure to allow controlled access for venography. For such deep lesions, the intention to treat is established preoperatively with a relatively high level of certainty that the venographic findings will be appropriate for subsequent

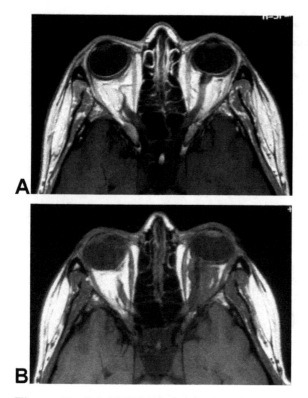

Figure 7 Axial MRI (A) shows that the lesion in the superior orbit is more distended with Valsalva maneuver (B).

controlled injection of glue mixture prior to surgical removal of the DVVM and that there is a low risk of shared circulation to normal structures. For these, a mobile C-arm angiography unit with digital subtraction and road mapping capability is available for our use in the operating room.

OPTIONS FOR TREATMENT WITH EMPHASIS ON NEW TECHNIQUE

Surgical treatment of DVVMs of the orbit is difficult, since varices are tortuous tangles of fragile, thin walled, malformed vessels with a tendency to rupture and bleed easily during surgery. There are also multiple and complex relationships with venous drainage pathways within the orbit and out into the face, pterygopalatine fossa, paranasal sinuses, bones, and intracranial space. The exact margins of the lesion are difficult to see and separate from surrounding structures at surgery. Surgery requires meticulous control of bleeding, identification, cauterization, clipping, or obstruction of out-flow and inflow channels.

Several strategies have been used to treat DVVMs of the orbit. These include intralesional thrombosis using thermo-electric desiccation (4) and retrograde venous catheterization and embolization with platinum microcoils (5,6). We had concerns pursuing these techniques based on numerous direct puncture venographic studies, which showed that many of the lesions have complex anatomy consisting of, or draining through, multiple thin walled channels that would be at significant risk for rupture by either antegrade or retrograde catheterization.

Our goal was to find a technique that would reduce vascularity and define the margins of the lesion for easier surgical excision. We felt that controlled injection via direct puncture of a liquid embolic agent could accomplish this. There is a long experience of using cyanoacrylate (glue) for devascu-larizing brain arteriovenous malformations. Neurosurgeons have noted that resecting what remains of a brain arteriove-nous malformation after glue embolization is not impeded by the presence of glue. The glue-casted part of the nidus can be handled and retracted for resection like a tumor mass, allowing for removal with little blood loss.

For treatment of selected DVVMs of the orbit, the proce-dure is done in the operating room with a mobile digital C-arm angiography unit. Puncture into the lesion allows for venography to identify the extent and drainage pathway. For lesions with intracranial communication (i.e., into the cavernous sinus), surgical exposure allows for control of the venous outflow (and glue) by appropriately placed pressure (either direct or indirect). When potential dangerous commu-nications are seen to be controlled by repeat venography, injection of the cyanoacrylate glue mixture is performed under live subtracted fluoroscopy to form a cast of the lesion.

The vascular lesion and its cast are then surgically excised in a relatively blood-free field (Fig. 3).

RESULTS AND COMPLICATIONS OF TREATMENT

We have published the results of this treatment technique in a select group of six patients out of a larger series of 30 patients with DVVMs of the orbit (2). Four additional patients, of 23 seen since the study series, have been treated successfully but not formally reported. All patients have done well except two. One patient had a superficial lesion treated by glue injection from a direct percutaneous access point without surgical exposure. It was decided not to resect the casted lesion at that time, as it was reasonably flat in contour and no longer distending with ventilator-induced Valsalva maneuver. However, a foreign body reaction developed with localized swelling and tenderness, requiring subsequent surgical excision of the lesion. The other patient with a complication was our first on whom this technique was tried. She was suffering from severe pain and proptosis, and at the outset was accepting the possibility of visual loss if it meant her pain would be gone. Analysis of her treatment indicates that her malformation was not completely excised after embolization. Understanding the hemodynamics and venous outflow is important for success and complication avoidance. Occlusion of the drainage pathway of a lesion or lesions with glue might lead to enlargement or stasis within remaining portions if these are not completely excised. This situation may also lead to thrombosis or hemorrhage with potential risk to vision from pressure effect, which we believe was the mechanism that caused partial visual loss in this patient. The thrombosed portion of her lesion regressed and she was left completely free from pain and without proptosis.

FUTURE CONSIDERATIONS

Other embolic agents besides glue have been used to devascularize lesions in areas of the body outside the orbit. Among these are polyvinyl alcohol particles, microfibrillar collagen, and ethanol (7). These agents could be directly injected into DVVMs to produce thrombosis but this may be complicated by acute and significant swelling (particularly with ethanol), leading to more profound secondary effects such as visual loss. There is also concern that lesions treated with such agents can overtime recanalize and therefore recur. Because of this, such agents are not likely to be very useful.

The goal will be to find an agent that can be injected directly into these lesions to bring about closure and permanent regression, precluding the need for intraoperative maneuvers with wide exposures and resection.

CONCLUSION

We have reviewed the features of DVVMs of the orbit and provide a look at a new technique for treating these lesions using the combined expertise of interventional neuroradiology and orbital surgery.

REFERENCES

1. Marotta TR, Lingawi SS, Katz SE, Woodhurst WB, Rootman J. Intraorbital rupture of a cavernous internal carotid aneurysm. Ophth Plast Reconstr Surg 2001; 17(1):67–72.

2. Lacey B, Rootman J, Marotta TR. Distensible venous malformations of the orbit. Clinical and hemodynamic features and a new technique of management. Ophthalmology 1999; 106(6): 1197–1209.

3. Rootman J, Marotta TR, Graeb DA. Vascular lesions. Rootman JDiseases of The Orbit: A Multidisciplinary Approach. 2nd ed. Philadelphia: Lippincott Williams and Wilkins, 2002:507–553.

4. Handa H, Mori K. Large varix of the superior ophthalmic veins: demonstration by angular phlebography and removal by electrically induced thrombosis. Case report. J Neurosurg 1968; 29: 202–205.

5. Mavilio N, Pau A, Pisani R, Casasco A, Rosa M. Embolisation of orbital varix via superficial temporal vein. Interventional Neuroradiol 2000; 6:137–140.

6. Marotta TR. Letter to the Editor. Embolisation of orbital varix via superficial temporal vein. Interventional Neuroradiol 2000; 6:353.

7. Schweitzer JS, Chang BS, Madsen P, Vinuela F, Martin NA, Marroquin CE, Vinters HV. The pathology of arteriovenous malformations of the brain treated by embolotherapy. II. Results of embolization with multiple agents. Neuroradiology 1993; 35:468–474.

28

Vascular Intervention: Current and Future Opportunities

ALAN A. McNab

Orbit, Plastic and Lacrimal Clinic, Royal Victorian
Eye and Ear Hospital, Victoria,
Melbourne, Australia

INTRODUCTION

Interventional radiological techniques have assisted the orbital surgeon in the management of some orbital vascular lesions and a variety of other lesions with a significant blood supply. It has also expanded the spectrum of vascular lesions that can be managed by either the radiologist alone or in combination with orbital and other surgeons. This presentation will summarize the techniques currently available and touch on future possibilities. It will not describe methods such as computed tomography or ultrasound guided biopsy, or the potential for stereotactic techniques, which are now used widely in neurosurgery and probably have a place in the management of a small proportion of lesions affecting the orbit. Specifically, the following disorders will be discussed: carotid-cavernous sinus fistulas, arteriovenous malformations, distensible venous anomalies, preoperative embolization of tumors, and aneurysms.

CAROTID-CAVERNOUS SINUS FISTULAS

Carotid-cavernous fistulas (CCF) are the commonest lesions encountered by the orbital specialist that lend themselves to interventional radiological techniques. These fistulas (CCF) have been classified in several ways, and this classification has some bearing on the therapeutic approach employed (if treatment is required). The most useful classification in terms of interventional radiological techniques employed is that of Barrow et al. (1), who organizes CCFs into four types.

> Type A: direct shunts between the internal carotid artery (ICA) and the cavernous sinus (often traumatic in origin, sometimes the result of rupture of an ICA, and of high flow).
> Type B: a shunt between meningeal branches of the ICA and the cavernous sinus.
> Type C: a shunt between the meningeal branches of the external carotid artery (ECA) and the cavernous sinus.
> Type D: a shunt between meningeal branches of both the ICA and ECA.

Type B, C, and D fistulas (often called dural fistulas) are often "spontaneous" and more often low flow. Type D tends to be more frequent than the purer forms of B and C. Additionally, a fistula may be supplied by meningeal branches of the ICA and ECA from one or both sides. The clinical signs may be (a) ipsilateral to the meningeal branches that supply the fistula; (b) contralateral, usually when the superior ophthalmic vein on the side of the fistula has thrombosed and the fistula drains to the opposite side of the cavernous sinus via intercavernous connections, or (c) bilateral, depending on the anatomy of the intercavernous sinus and the meningeal branches of supply.

The anatomy of the fistula is important in planning the therapeutic approach to each patient, and the only way to get an accurate assessment of the anatomy is with selective bilateral internal and external carotid angiography. The patient may be treated during the same angiography session provided the anatomy allows for occlusion of the fistula by endovascular techniques.

The majority of Type A fistulas occur in the setting of trauma. Interventional radiological techniques have been successful in the majority of these cases, without the need for neurosurgical or orbital surgical approaches. The aim is to close the fistulous connection whilst maintaining the patency of the ICA. This is usually achieved with detachable balloons, which are floated into the fistula via a catheter in the ICA, filled to occlude the fistula, and then detached from the catheter (Fig. 1). If an arterial approach is not possible, a transvenous approach is an alternative, usually via the inferior petrosal sinus reached via the internal jugular vein. For transvenous approaches, thrombogenic coils (Fig. 2) are most commonly employed to fill and thrombose the cavernous sinus and thereby obliterate the fistula.

Type C and D fistulas may be treated by trans arterial embolization of the external carotid artery branches of supply. Liquid or particulate matter may be used. In Type D fistulas, this may be enough to reduce the flow in the fistula and thrombose it without direct closure of the ICA branches, although often the fistula will persist. Selective embolization of meningeal branches of the ICA is usually not possible.

The transvenous approach to CCFs via the superior ophthalmic vein (SOV) is now well established and involves the orbital surgeon directly in the management of these patients. Patients benefiting from this approach are those where other trans arterial and transvenous approaches have failed. Some have suggested the technique be employed primarily, but where a fistula can be successfully treated by the radiologist alone, without the need for a surgical procedure, it would seem sensible to use that approach first.

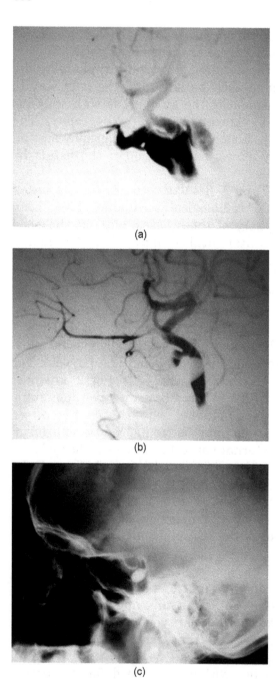

(a)

(b)

(c)

Figure 1 (*Caption on facing page*)

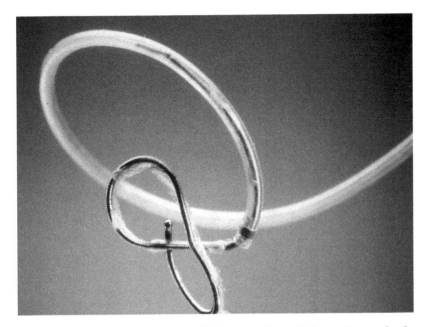

Figure 2 A thrombogenic coil being released from the end of a catheter.

The SOV approach was first described in the literature by our institution, the Royal Melbourne Hospital, in 1983 (2). A patient with a longstanding high flow Type D carotid-cavernous fistula had a direct approach made to it via exposure of an enlarged SOV in the anterior-superior orbit, using stainless steel coils to thrombose the fistula. Since that time, we and others have used the technique and published a series of patients successfully treated this way (3–7).

Exposure of the SOV is usually readily accomplished via an upper eyelid crease or sub-brow incision (Fig. 3a). The SOV

Figure 1 (*Facing page*) A left lateral internal carotid angiogram demonstrates rapid filling of a carotid cavernous fistula. (b) After placement of a detachable balloon (partially obscuring the ICA), the fistula no longer fills the cavernous sinus with dye. (c) Left lateral plain skull x-ray shows the balloon in the cavernous sinus filled with contrast medium.

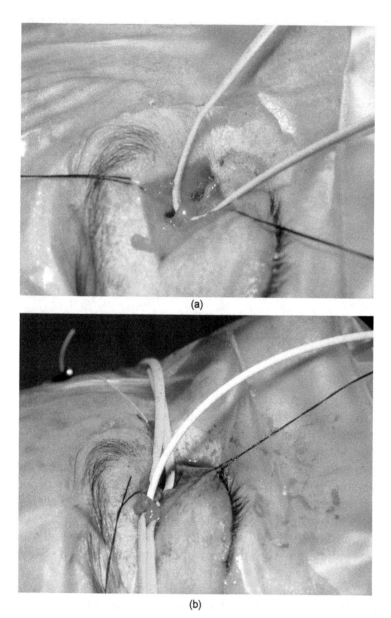

(a)

(b)

Figure 3 (a) The superior ophthalmic vein has been isolated in the right anterior orbit via a sub-brow incision. (b) The superior ophthalmic vein has been controlled with two vascular loops (blue) and a catheter inserted into the vein (white).

anastomoses usually with the angular and supraorbital veins in the superomedial lid and anterior orbit, and the best place to find the SOV is just below the trochlea of the superior oblique. In longstanding and high flow fistulas, there may be very large veins in the eyelid itself and these may be very tortuous. It may be difficult to tell which direction is towards the cavernous sinus in these cases. Once the vein is isolated, vascular tape or loops are passed beneath it to help control the blood flow while a venotomy is made and a catheter fed into the vein (Fig. 3b). A guide wire is then passed along the SOV to the cavernous sinus, a catheter passed over it, and an injection of dye made to ascertain the exact position of the catheter. Thrombogenic coils are then deposited in the cavernous sinus, starting posteriorly and moving anteriorly. A check carotid angiogram is made to determine if there is still any flow in the fistula. The catheter is removed and the SOV may be ligated.

For fistulas with bilateral drainage (through both SOVs), one SOV may be used to access both sides of the cavernous sinus, provided that the intercavernous sinus(es) is large enough to negotiate from one to the other side. Both sides may then be embolized (Fig. 4).

This technique may be limited by aberrant anatomy of the SOV. In some cases, the SOV may not extend to the anterior orbit, presumably because of prior partial thrombosis, or variant anatomy (Fig. 5). The entire SOV may thrombose prior to the technique being employed. We have managed a patient whose predominant drainage of the fistula via cerebral veins was thought to be a risk; however, prior to the patient reaching the procedure room, the SOV had thrombosed, thus protecting the eye but making access via the SOV impossible.

Some authors have preferred to perform this technique in the operating room rather than the angiography suite, arguing the need for all the equipment available in the operating room. We have found it quite feasible to have all the necessary equipment moved to the angiography suite, which has the advantage of having available, all the sophisticated angiography equipment and avoids dependence on less

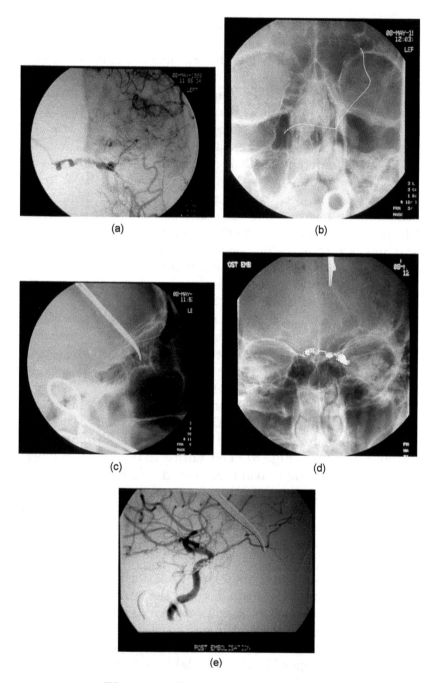

(a)

(b)

(c)

(d)

(e)

Figure 4 (*Caption on facing page*)

sophisticated portable angiographic equipment. One exceptional case of ours had to be treated in the operating room because of extreme obesity. The patient's weight exceeded that allowable on the angiography table and direct puncture of the femoral vessels could not be achieved, so that the carotid and jugular vessels had to be exposed in the neck, as well as exposing the SOV in the anterior orbit. His fistula was successfully treated.

Many patients will temporarily worsen after embolization of their CCF. This same worsening is seen in spontaneous thrombosis of the SOV in some cases of CCF (8). In the majority of these treated and spontaneously resolving cases, the signs resolve over days to weeks.

In patients who cannot be adequately treated in these ways, neurosurgical approaches remain an option. Direct puncture of the cavernous sinus at craniotomy may be used to gain access for embolization, and techniques to reach the cavernous sinus using cerebral veins have also been described. Closure of the ICA above and below the feeding vessels may be a last resort, and interventional radiological techniques may be used for this, using trial occlusions to assess the adequacy of the circle of Willis before permanently occluding the ICA.

There have also been reports of transcutaneous puncture of the deep SOV (9) or even cavernous sinus via the orbit where other techniques have failed. Clearly, there is a significant risk of hemorrhage within the orbit or cranial cavity.

Figure 4 *(Facing page)* (a) An anterior venous phase carotid angiogram of a patient with a bilateral Type D carotid-cavernous sinus fistula. There is filling of both superior ophthalmic veins via the cavernous sinuses, connected by a prominent intercavernous sinus. (b) A guide wire has been placed via the left superior ophthalmic vein into the left cavernous sinus and then across into the right cavernous sinus via an intercavernous sinus. (c) Lateral view of the guide wire seen in (b). (d) An antero-posterior view after placement of thrombogenic coils in the right and left cavernous sinuses. (e) Right lateral internal carotid angiogram shows no filling of either superior ophthalmic vein after successful embolization.

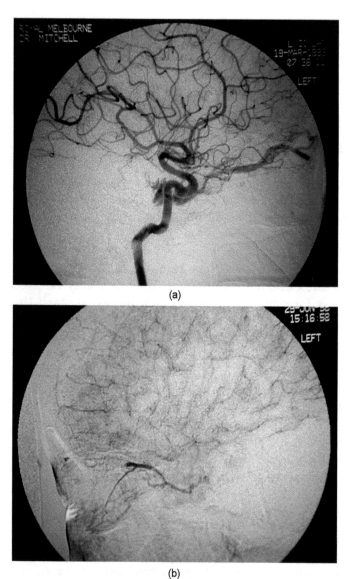

Figure 5   (a) A right lateral view of an internal carotid angiogram
shows a patient with early filling of the superior ophthalmic veins
by a Type D carotid-cavernous sinus fistula. (b) Left lateral late
venous phase carotid angiogram of the same patient taken several
weeks later shows termination of the superior ophthalmic vein in
the mid-orbit.

ARTERIOVENOUS MALFORMATIONS

Arteriovenous malformations (AVMs) of the orbit are rare lesions and have been notoriously difficult to treat. They are distinct from CCFs and are usually congenital lesions where there is direct high flow from arterial feeding vessels through a central nidus of low resistance, bypassing the normal capillary bed, to numerous draining veins. They tend to enlarge over time and may be clinically unapparent until later in life. Closure of draining veins is pointless, as others are recruited, and unless all feeding arteries can be obliterated, new arterial supply will also be recruited. One method of treatment is complete surgical excision alone, which of course in the orbit is extremely difficult because of likely hemorrhage and damage to surrounding structures.

A better technique employs preoperative embolization of as much of the arterial supply as possible, then surgical excision (10–12) (Fig. 6). The time between embolization and surgery should be 1–3 days, so that advantage can be taken of the reduced or obliterated blood supply before new arterial supply is recruited.

DISTENSIBLE VENOUS ANOMALIES

Interventional radiological techniques have a part to play in the management of these lesions, which are characterized by abnormal venous channels in the orbit with a clear connection to the venous side of the circulation. When the venous pressure rises with changes in posture, straining, or Valsalva maneuver, the veins expand, producing increased proptosis, fullness, feelings of pressure behind the eye, and sometimes pain.

In some cases, single dilated veins (a varix) may be safely surgically excised but all too often, these lesions are complex, with multiple channels, and often thin-walled vessels that bleed readily.

Interventional radiological techniques have expanded the therapeutic possibilities for these often-difficult lesions.

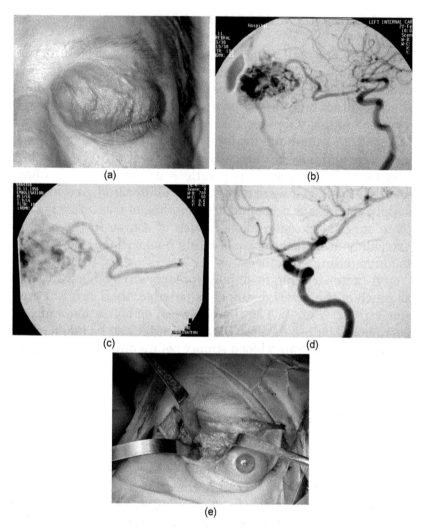

Figure 6 (a) An external view of a man with a large left orbital arteriovenous malformation (AVM). (b) A left lateral internal carotid angiogram shows brisk filling of the AVM. (c) Selective left ophthalmic artery angiogram fills the AVM rapidly, and (d) postembolization angiogram shows no filling of the AVM. (e) An intraoperative view of the AVM in the superomedial orbit exposed via an upper lid split orbitotomy.

Cases of simple orbital varices treated by standard endovascular embolization have been described. If the anatomy of the venous anomaly is suitable, it may be possible to reach it via a femoral venous approach to the internal jugular vein, the inferior petrosal sinus, cavernous sinus, and thence to the venous anomaly itself where thrombogenic coils may be deposited (13). Alternatively, a direct surgical exposure of the venous anomaly, catheterization, and placement of thrombogenic coils can be performed (14).

A novel multidisciplinary approach to distensible venous anomalies has been described by Lacey et al. (15). The lesion is surgically exposed and defined by direct injection of contrast. After defining the draining veins posteriorly at the superior and/or inferior orbital fissures, direct or indirect pressure is applied at these sites to close these communications and then a cyanoacrylate glue mixture injected into the lesion to form a cast. The lesion and its cast are then excised with less bleeding than would otherwise be encountered.

We have used a modification of this technique, leaving the cast in the venous anomaly without adverse effect and avoiding surgical excision. A further difficulty encountered in our case was incomplete closure of other anteriorly draining veins, allowing glue to migrate anteriorly and resulting in incomplete filling of the orbital venous anomaly. Rootman has recommended excision after glue injection because of foreign body reaction in one of their cases where glue remained (15).

PREOPERATIVE EMBOLIZATION OF TUMORS

Some orbital neoplasms have a high blood flow (Fig. 7), making surgical excision in the confines of the orbit more difficult and dangerous. Hemangiopericytomas are a case in point.

If the lesion is suspected of having a high blood flow, this may be confirmed by Doppler ultrasound, CT angiography, MR angiography, or by direct angiography. If the arterial supply of the lesion can be clearly identified on angiography, and some or all of the feeding vessels embolized, this will greatly

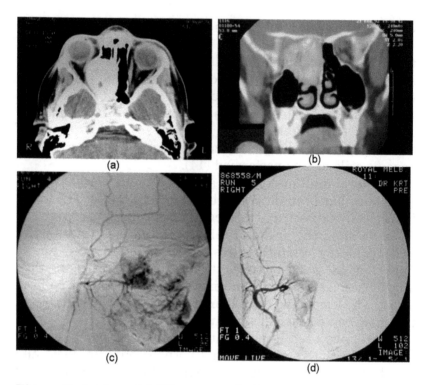

Figure 7 (a) An axial CT scan on soft-tissue window with contrast shows a large cavernous hemangioma of bone arising in the ethmoids and involving the posterior orbit. (b) Coronal CT scan on bone window setting shows the lesion in the ethmoids and posterior orbit. (c) A pre-embolization right lateral external carotid angiogram shows a tumor blush with pooling of contrast in some of the cavernous spaces of the cavernous hemangioma of bone, while an anterior pre-embolization external carotid angiogram (d) shows the tumor blush due to moderately brisk circulation within a cavernous hemangioma of bone.

facilitate its surgical removal by reducing blood loss and making the surgical field easier to work.

There has been a reluctance to embolize the ophthalmic artery or its branches because of the risk to vision. However, many lesions that would benefit from preoperative embolization obtain much of their blood supply from the ophthalmic artery. By careful case selection, judicious use of embolic agents, and the use of provocative testing, embolization of the ophthalmic artery can be safely accomplished without visual loss in a significant number of cases (16). These authors used direct injection of lignocaine and amytal as the provocative agents to assess the dependence of the retina and optic nerve on the ophthalmic artery circulation.

ANEURYSMS

Aneurysms have largely neuro-ophthalmic manifestations and are therefore outside the confines of this presentation. However, the techniques used in the management of aneurysms may have spin-offs for cases with orbital vascular lesions and a large impetus to the development of newer techniques has been the possibility of treating aneurysms using minimally invasive or interventional radiological techniques.

FUTURE DIRECTIONS

It is certain there will be continued development in the basic materials used by interventional radiologists with smaller and more maneuverable catheters and guide wires, and novel embolic agents. Additionally, the combined use of techniques to allow embolization of lesions whilst protecting the normal circulation continues to expand. Examples include temporary balloon occlusion above broad-necked aneurysms to allow safer embolization of the aneurysm, and the placement of stents with the mesh of the stent acting as a barrier to the passage of detachable balloons back into the ICA during occlusion of broad-necked aneurysms.

Advances in imaging technology will allow three-dimensional imaging and virtual trips down blood vessels and into vascular lesions. This will allow better definition of complex vascular anomalies and safer treatments. Guidance systems for catheters are also likely to be improved, with less reliance on the manipulative skills of the radiologist. Such systems may ultimately lead to "hands-free" interventional techniques.

REFERENCES

1. Barrow DL, Sector RH, Braun IF, Landman JA, Tindall SC, Tindall GT. Classification and treatment of spontaneous carotid cavernous fistula. J Neurosurg 1985; 62:248–256.

2. Tress BM, Thomson KR, Klug GL, Crawford B. Management of carotid-cavernous fistulas by surgery with combined interventional radiology. J Neurosurg 1983; 59:1076–1081.

3. Hanneken AM, Miller NR, Debrun GM, Nauta HJ. Treatment of carotid-cavernous sinus fistulas using a detachable balloon catheter through the superior ophthalmic vein. Arch Ophthalmol 1989; 107(1):87–92.

4. Monsein LH, Debrun GM, Miller NR, Nauta HJ, Chazaly JR. Treatment of dural carotid-cavernous sinus fistulas via the superior ophthalmic vein. Am J Neuroradiol 1991; 12(3): 435–439.

5. Miller NR, Monsein LH, Debrun GM, Tamargo RJ, Nauta HJ. Treatment of carotid-cavernous sinus fistulas using a superior ophthalmic vein approach. J Neurosurg 1995; 83(5):838–842.

6. Quinones D, Duckwiler G, Gobin PY, Goldberg RA, Vinuela F. Embolization of dural cavernous sinus fistulas via superior ophthalmic vein approach. Am J Neuroradiol 1997; 18(5):921–928.

7. Gioulekas J, Mitchell P, Tress B, McNab AA. Embolization of carotid cavernous fistulas via the superior ophthalmic vein. Aust N Z J Ophthalmol 1997; 25(1):47–54.

8. Sergott RC, Grossman RI, Savino PJ, Bosley TM, Schatz NJ. The syndrome of paradoxical worsening of dural-cavernous sinus arteriovenous malformations. Ophthalmology 1987; 94(3):205–212.

9. Benndorf G, Bender A, Campi A, Menneking H, Lanksch WR. Treatment of a cavernous sinus dural arteriovenous fistula by deep orbital puncture of the superior ophthalmic vein. Neuroradiology 2001; 43(6):499–502.

10. Rootman J, Kao SCS, Graeb DA. Multidisciplinary approaches to complicated vascular lesions of the orbit. Ophthalmology 1992; 99(9):1440–1446.

11. Goldberg RA, Garcia GH, Duckwiler GR. Combined embolization and surgical treatment of arteriovenous malformation of the orbit. Am J Ophthalmol 1993; 116(1):17–25.

12. Hayes BH, Shore JW, Westfall CT, Harris GJ. Management of orbital and periorbital arteriovenous malformations. Ophthal Surg 1995; 26(2):145–152.

13. Takechi A, Uozumi T, Kiya K, Yano T, Sumida M, Yoshikawa S, Pant B. Embolisation of orbital varix. Neuroradiology 1994; 36(6):487–489.

14. Weill A, Cognard C, Castaings L, Robert G, Moret J. Embolization of an orbital varix after surgical exposure. Am J Neuroradiol 1998; 19(5):921–923.

15. Lacey B, Rootman J, Marotta TR. Distensible venous malformations of the orbit: clinical and hemodynamic features and a new technique of management. Ophthalmology 1999; 106(6):1197–1209.

16. Lefkowitz M, Giannotta SL, Hieshima G, Higashida R, Halbach V, Dowd C, Teitelbaum GP. Embolization of neurosurgical lesions involving the ophthalmic artery. Neurosurgery 1998; 43(6):1298–1303.

29

The Future of Imaging in Orbital Disease

WIESLAW L. NOWINSKI

Biomedical Imaging Laboratory,
Agency for Science, Technology and Research
(ASTAR), Singapore

ABSTRACT

Technology is one of the major driving forces in diagnosis and treatment. This paper gives a short overview of the state-of-the-art in technological advancements covering visualization, registration, modeling, virtual reality, surgical simulators, and surgical robotics. Examples illustrating how these advances impact ophthalmic and brain surgery are given. We also provide our vision about future orbital surgery.

INTRODUCTION

Advances in computers, diagnostic imaging, medical physics, biomedical engineering, and applied mathematics have enabled continual growth in minimally invasive surgical techniques. Computer-aided surgical systems enable surgeons to treat patients faster, with greater precision and without the significant trauma formerly experienced. In addition, the advent, growth, and development of computer-aided technologies as adjunctive educational, training, and certification methods in surgery will likely affect the surgical practice in ways that are difficult to predict. The advances impact also orbital surgery as well and open new avenues.

This review gives a short overview of the state-of-the-art in technological advances in surgery, including Internet use, visualization, registration, modeling, stereoscopic perception, three-dimensional (3D) interaction, virtual reality, surgical simulators, and surgical robotics.

TECHNOLOGICAL ADVANCEMENTS

In diagnosis and treatment in particular, the patient-specific data have to be easily accessed, visualized, quantified and, most importantly, interacted with. The Internet allows the data to be accessed from anywhere at anytime by anyone authorized. In addition to the multimodal scan transfer, video, audio, human body models, model manipulation parameters, and control data can be transmitted. The wide acceptance of Internet standards and technologies, such as HTML, XML and Java, is instrumental in building global computer networks which, within the next few years, will penetrate our society more than any previous network. High-speed networks combined with medical imaging, surgical simulation, and surgical robotics enable tele-consultation, tele-presence, tele-monitoring, tele-education, and remote collaboration.

Advances in Medical Imaging

Traditionally, radiological scans have been displayed as cross-sectional images; however, their effective interpretation requires the use of volume visualization (1). The developments of faster magnetic resonance imaging acquisition techniques, multidetector computed tomography, and rotational x-ray angiography result in the routine acquisition of large, high-resolution volumetric datasets of human anatomy, function, and disease. Three-dimensional visualization of the territory into which the surgeon will be going is critical to successful orbital surgery (2). Numerous techniques have been developed for fast volume visualization, including multiplanar reformatting, maximum intensity projection, virtual endoscopy, surface rendering (3), and volume rendering (4) (Figs. 1 and 2). In surface rendering, the surface of the structure of interest is extracted from the data and it is represented as numerous small polygons that are shaded and lighted for realistic display. Volume rendering uses the complete dataset and treats it as semitransparent gel.

Some visualization techniques, such as surface rendering, may require segmentation prior to visualization. Image segmentation (5) is partitioning of the processed image into

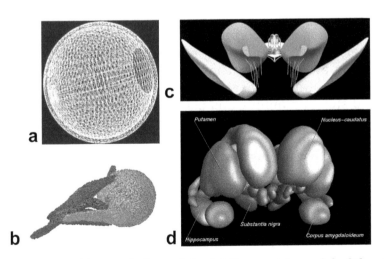

Figure 1 Human body models. (a) Parametric model of the globe. (b) Volumetric model of the globe and muscles. (c) Surface model of the oculomotor nuclear complex, fascicles, and surrounding structures. (d) Surface model of subcortical structures.

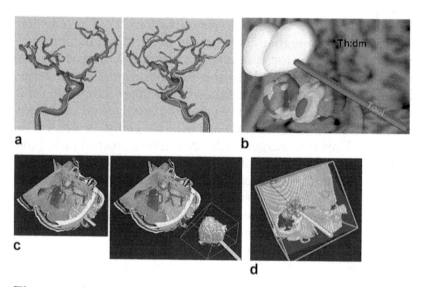

Figure 2 Surgery simulation. (a) Catheter navigation within a 3D cerebral model. (b) Picking a structure of interest (the dorso-medial thalamic nuclei). (c) Removing a skull base tumor. (d) Performing CT craniotomy.

components homogeneous with respect to some feature(s). Segmentation is an important initial step also in image analysis, registration, compression, and computer-aided surgery. As therapy evolves toward minimally invasive approaches, visualization of multimodal volumetric datasets is becoming a critical step in planning and performing therapeutic procedures. Multiple imaging modalities, in order to be displayed together, have to be registered first.

Registration (or matching or alignment) (6) is finding a spatial transformation mapping location in one image to their corresponding locations in another image or model (Fig. 3a and b). Registration in its simpler form is rigid and in a more complex form deformable. Registration techniques also allow human body models to be adapted to the individual anatomy of the patient. Then, information inherent in these models is automatically mapped to the patient-specific data (Fig. 3c).

Multimodal imaging has proved extremely useful in orbital surgery. Computed tomography (CT) and magnetic reso-

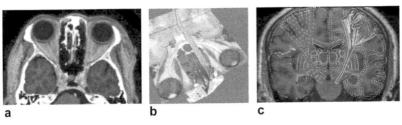

a   b   c

Figure 3 Registration. (a) Multimodal in two dimensions—CT and MRI axial images are fused together. (b) Multimodal in three dimensions—cadaveric section images and CT of the Visible Human Data are registered. (c) Model-to-data—a brain atlas in contour representation is superimposed on a coronal brain scan.

nance imaging (MRI) provide excellent morphological detail of the eye and orbit. These modalities are used to diagnose and determine the extent of ocular or periocular tumors, diagnose inflammatory conditions of the orbital region, and determine the severity and extent of ocular trauma. Magnetic resonance angiography (MRA) and color Doppler ultrasonography provide detailed information regarding vascular lesions and flow. To diagnose corneal disorders, various types of microscopy are used, such as specular, confocal, and ultrasound biomicroscopy. Other forms of multimodal registration in ophthalmology exist, such as the development of computer-aided geometric models of the eye, which we describe later in this review (7,8).

Modeling focuses on the construction and use of human body models. These models encapsulate anatomical knowledge and provide means to predict, simulate, validate, and enhance the outcomes of diagnostic and surgical procedures. The models can also incorporate certain age, gender, or racial characteristics that may affect surgical decision making.

Geometric modeling deals with geometrical properties of structures to be rendered and manipulated. Physical modeling captures physical properties of modeled structures, which usually requires complicated mathematical and numerical models. By changing the parameters of a biomedical model, various physiological and pathological situations can be simulated.

Surgical procedures involve 3D stereoscopic perception and 3D manipulation with six degrees of freedom (i.e., three translations and three rotations). To fully exploit the potential of (multimodal) medical images in computer-aided surgery, these images should be perceived stereoscopically and explore using 3D interaction.

There are several technologies for achieving 3D perception in surgical simulation, including stereoscopic glasses, head-mounted display (HMD), digital holography, virtual retinal display, and virtual reality projectors (9). Stereoscopic glasses containing shutters over each eye are one of the most frequently used. The glasses are synchronized to a computer monitor, which is able to generate left- and right-eye images. The HMD is a visual display system worn on the user's head usually as goggles. Limitations of the HMD include size and weight producing encumbrance and fatigue, limited picture resolution, stereopsis, and the time lag and smoothness of the servo-mechanism that drives the remote camera to follow head movements.

To achieve 3D interaction with stereoscopic multimodal images, we have developed a device called *Dextroscope* (10,11). It consists of a mirror-based display, 3D input devices, and graphics workstation. A stereo virtual image is seen reflected in a mirror allowing the user wearing shuttered glasses to reach into the virtual space below this mirror. The *Dextroscope* provides compatibility of the physical space and the visual virtual space, so that physical tools manipulate virtual objects in a hand–eye coordinated manner.

Virtual Reality Surgical Simulation

The term *virtual reality* (VR) refers to a human–computer interface simulating realistic environment while enabling user interaction. Surgeon–computer interaction may be multimodal including speech, touch, and gesture recognition and synthesis. The surgeon may also see the real world with computer-generated images superimposed on the natural viewing field, so-called *augmented reality*. Augmented reality systems allow the surgeon to have real structures and anatomy as visual landmarks, while supplementing them with useful clinical information such as presurgical scans and human body models.

Advances in more realistic physical models, ultrahigh-resolution displays, intuitive two-handed 3D interaction, rapid and accurate mapping of the human body models into patient-specific data, and more sensitive haptic devices increase the usefulness of virtual and augmented reality in clinical practice.

The successful use of flight simulators has inspired their application to surgical training. A virtual reality surgical simulator typically consists of five components, human body models (virtual patient), physical modeler, pathology modeler, virtual surgical instruments, and VR interface. Before performing a surgical procedure on a real patient, the surgeon will be able to practice and plan on a high-fidelity computer model of patient-specific data to simulate the intervention. In this way, the safest and most effective surgical approach can be planned and evaluated requiring less time in an operating room and improving human performance. Careful planning will minimize the amount of surgical trauma and maximize the outcome to the patient (2).

Computer-based surgical simulation is useful not only for preoperative planning but also for education, training, and skill assessment. Requirements for surgical simulator include realism to accurately represent the detailed shape of patient's organs, real-time interaction, quantitative deformation, haptic feedback, and simulation of various surgical operations such as drilling (including vibration and sound), cutting, grasping, sucking, pushing, pinching, picking, suturing, vaporizing, coagulating, clipping, and knot tying.

The sense of touch is an integral part of surgery and simulating it is an essential component of the surgical simulator. Forces and torques are produced via a haptic device. For this purpose, knowledge of the characteristics of the simulated living tissues is required (12). When an object is palpated with a haptic device, several components influence its feel including stiffness, damping, and static and dynamic friction. The quality of feel is determined both by the realism of the biomedical model and human perception.

Surgical Robotics

Robotic systems, introduced to surgery from the early 1980s, are able to increase the accuracy and dexterity of surgeon, reduce the tremor of human hand, and amplify or reduce the movements and/or forces applied by the surgeon (13).

The scale of operations in today's surgical practice is becoming so small that even skilled surgeons are reaching the limits of their dexterity. The accuracy of manual intervention is limited by physiological tremor at the instrument tip, which can be as large as 50 μm peak to peak at the hand-held instrument tip. On the other hand, vitreoretinal microsurgery, for instance, involves removing membranes as thin as 20 μm from the retina. In addition, new treatments, such as cell implants, will require accuracy of 10 μm or better, which can only be achieved with robotic teleoperators.

In microsurgery, the robot scales small motions and forces to the optimal range of human perception, enabling improved performance and new microsurgical procedures. Several robotics systems have been developed to support microsurgery. A six-degree-of-freedom manipulator for vascular microsurgery in the retina has been described by Jensen et al. (14), and a teleoperated microsurgical robot for eye surgery is presented by Hunter et al. (15). A telemanipulator, robot assisted microsurgery (*RAMS*) (14), scales down the surgeon's hand motion and filters tremor. RAMS assists surgeons in manipulating surgical instruments more precisely than it is possible manually. In addition, forces sensed at the surgical instrument can be amplified. Urban et al. (17) have reported a system for microsurgery with kinesthetic feedback. Using a hexapod robot produces a repeatable positioning accuracy of better than 2 μm. The system scales movements and senses forces at instruments. The surgeon controls the robot from the operating cockpit. Taylor et al. (18) describe a steady-hand robotic system for microsurgical augmentation that provides smooth, tremor-free precise positional control, and force scaling.

There are numerous other technologies that enhance computer-aided surgery, including sensing, miniaturization, intelligent instruments, smart- and biomaterials, MEMS, optics, and wireless communication.

HUMAN BODY MODELS

Deformable body models along with warping techniques provide means for analysis of medical images. Examples of practically useful deformable models are electronic brain atlases (19,20) that are applicable to several areas including functional neurosurgery (21–23), human brain mapping (24), neuroradiology (20), and neuroeducation (25).

The material used for building a human body model may originate from various sources, such as radiological images or photographs of cadaveric sections. Alternatively, a model can be based on human and/or animal studies or derived from mathematical formulas, and subsequently constructed by using computer-aided design (CAD) tools.

The construction of electronic orbital anatomy models is in its infancy despite the fact that critical neurovascular structures are limited to a 30-cm^3 space only. Preliminary efforts typically do not use in vivo data but the modeled structures are rather approximated by simplified geometrical primitives like spheres and arcs (7,26), generated from mathematical models (15,27), based on literature studies (28), or derived from cadaveric sections (8). The ophthalmic model described by Parshall (7) has two components, the eyeball and orbit. The eyeball model was obtained from statistical norms based on the assumption that the eye had radially symmetrical outer walls. Nonsymmetrical components were then obtained by using CAD tools. To capture the irregular structures of the orbit, images of frozen cadaveric orbital sections were manually digitized, segmented, and registered. Both models were then manually registered to produce the final eye model. The model described by Hunter et al. (15) and Sagar et al. (27) is constructed from a parametric representation that can be displayed with varying degrees of detail. The corneal surface is obtained from confocal laser microscopy and the retinal vasculature from a fractal tree. In addition, a finite element method is used to produce a physical model suitable for telesurgical simulation. A realistic and accurate simulation of physical properties of the eye is a complicated process that requires the use of a supercomputer (29).

Our initial work, to develop a deformable eye model for ophthalmic surgery planning, uses multimodal data (8). The model of the cornea is obtained from Scheimpflug images and some of the external orbital structures, including the rectus muscles, optic nerve and sclera, are derived from the segmented cadaveric images of the Visible Human Female Data (Fig. 1b). Another model constructed in our laboratory contains the oculomotor nuclear complex and fascicles (28). This model facilitates an understanding of spatial relationships in the region and hypothesizes on the possible concentration of neurons involved in convergence. The model is based on the published studies in nonhuman primates and patients, and the 3D structures are constructed using CAD tools (Fig. 1c).

PRESENT COMPUTER-AIDED SURGERY AND SIMULATION

Simulators developed for ophthalmic surgery are able to support various procedures such as retinal coagulation (30), cataract surgery (27,31), and vitrectomy (32,33). *SOPHOCLE* is a training simulator for retinal photocoagulation (17). Its objective is to teach laser retinal photocoagulation in different disorders using a virtual eye. The simulator uses a real slit-lamp but the fundus and retinal photocoagulation impacts are virtual.

The eye surgery simulator (31) generates images of the eye and surgical instruments through the stereo-operating system and controls the position and orientation of the chosen instrument by moving the stylus. Four instruments are simulated, scalpel, forceps, scissors, and phacoemulsifier. This enables simulated cutting of the sclera and insertion of a phacoemulsifier to remove a cataract. During the instrument–tissue interactions, three feedback motors generate component force feedback along three orthogonal axes. The procedures can be recorded for subsequent playback and analysis.

A virtual reality vitrectomy simulator (32) assists in correcting retinal detachment. The VR interface consists of a 3D mouse and stereo glasses but has no tactile feedback. The simulator contains a deformable eye model and the simulated instruments include pick, blade, suction, cutter, laser, and drainage needle.

EyeSi (33) simulates vitrectomy in a more realistic way. Developed for training and rehearsal, *EyeSi* contains a mechanical eye providing a tactile feedback. Two physical instruments are inserted into this physical eye. One instrument simulates a lamp and the other can serve as a picker, cutter, or vitrector. The movements of the physical instruments are tracked by cameras and their corresponding virtual movements within the computer eye model are displayed in a stereoscopic viewer that emulates the surgical microscope.

Much more effort has been spent in developing systems for brain surgery, and we will briefly illustrate state-of-the-art example systems developed in our laboratory for brain intervention. Several diseases can be treated endovascularly. The development of a computer simulator for endovascular intervention, however, is a challenging task. This type of simulator shall have standard generic features (discussed in the section on Virtual reality surgical simulation) as well as provide advanced methods for segmentation of vasculature, geometric modeling and meshing of vasculature, physical modeling of interventional devices and vasculature, hemodynamic analysis, and device–vessel interaction analysis. It also shall contain a large database of interventional devices. In addition, specific clinical procedures have to be simulated including angioplasty, stent placement, and aneurysm coiling. An example in Fig. 2a shows catheter navigation within a 3D cerebral model using our interventional neuroradiology simulator *NeuroCath* (34).

The endovascular simulator shall provide hybrid visualization, including simulated fluoroscopy, surface and volume rendering, and virtual endoscopy. The latter type of display can also be useful when simulating endoscopic procedures such as approaching the orbit through the paranasal sinuses.

Useful tools empowering a computer-aided surgery system may facilitate segmentation, registration, visualization, mensuration, and surgery simulation. Several of these tools are available in our computer-aided neurosurgery systems, *BrainBench* (11) and *VIVIAN* (10). The patient-specific multimodal data along with individualized human body model can be visualized and manipulated, allowing the surgeon to pick a structure of interest (Fig. 2b) or remove a tumor (Fig. 2c) and look at it from any viewpoint, while its surrounding structures are revealed. A simulator should be able to support a wide range of cutting and drilling accessories for bony dissection and reconstruction. An example in Fig. 2d illustrates craniotomy simulated by a virtual drill removing bone and tissue in a volumetric CT image.

FUTURE COMPUTER-AIDED ORBITAL SURGERY

Based on the current trends and advances in underlying component technologies, we predict that the future computer-aided surgical systems will:

- becoming robust, safe, versatile, more intelligent and autonomous, and hopefully less expensive;
- be highly miniaturized and use MEMS and nanotechnology;
- be voice- and gesture-enabled with extensive vocabularies; and
- have vision, touch, smell, and locomotion.

The future computer-aided orbital surgery system must also support multiple surgical approaches (2) as well as different types of interventions including microsurgery, endoscopy, endovascular procedures, and telepresence. In addition, the system should provide skill assessment by comparing the actual intervention with the database of accepted and unaccepted surgical approaches.

Technological advancements keep minimizing trauma to the patient and maximizing surgical outcome. The surgeon is equipped today with a growing arsenal of instruments and multiple sources of information. At the same time, this powerful instrumentarium and vast amount of information impose new constraints and increase the surgeon's physical and mental workload. Therefore, we envisage that this current phase of exploiting dramatic technological advancements will be succeeded by a new phase focused more on conceptual changes. These changes will be needed to preserve the central role of the surgeon while freeing him or her from the technology-oriented overload.

To achieve this goal, we have proposed an integrated and intelligent environment for future neurosurgery (13), and we envisage that a similar kind of environment will also be suitable for treatment of orbital disease. In our opinion, the surgeon of the future will need a single assistant integrating all necessary instrumentation and sources of information. This intelligent assistant should perform two major functions: 1) DO it and 2) TELL or SHOW me. We therefore call this yet-to-be-built tool, DOTELL (13). The dotell controls all pre-, intra-, and postoperative information; performs all routine operations; makes technology transparent to the surgeon; and controls all instruments used in the operating room. It is an intelligent tool with robotic capabilities that integrates information infrastructure, knowledge-based decision support, imaging systems, and therapeutic modalities as well as provides monitoring and advice and performs actions.

The dotell has three major units, input, digital central nervous system, and output. The input unit interfaces with the patient, data, instruments, human body models, operating room, network, and surgeon. The output unit is linked to the patient, instruments, operating room, network, and surgeon and contains three main modules (DO, TELL, and SHOW). The digital central nervous system controls all inputs and outputs, and processes information.

The dotell is voice- and gesture-enabled, and contains a natural speech recognition analyzer and a feature-based gesture analyzer. This allows the surgeon to control the dotell in a natural and intuitive way.

The dotell accesses all preoperative data, including morphological, functional, pathological, and vascular scans, and registers them mutually providing a single, multimodal volumetric image. During the procedure, the preoperative scans are actualized with the intraoperative scans and the surgical situation is monitored. The dotell has access to deformable models integrating anatomical, functional, and biophysical maps of the human body. It registers these models with the patient-specific data and plans the procedure.

The DO module of the dotell's output unit is a robotic system dealing with the patient and a variety of surgical instruments. It contains multiple robotic synchronized arms, each with arbitrary motion, precise force control, and a wide range of motion and force scaling. The robotic system can operate on the patient autonomously under the surgeon's supervision or guidance. The TELL module contains a voice generator and generates replies to the surgeon's queries. The SHOW module, which provides stereoscopic display, may use techniques as discussed earlier. To free the surgeon from wearing any devices, we equip the dotell with digital holography and voice recognition capabilities. Dotell, as a surgeon's personal assistant, is highly customizable. A personalized dotell can be customized to know a surgeon's protocols and preferred settings, recognize his or her speech patterns and gesture preferences, and collect cases and prepare studies.

SUMMARY

The current technological breakthroughs mark just the beginning of dramatic changes forthcoming to computer-aided surgery. They will further be accelerated by introducing new computer technologies such as molecular computing, making computers of orders of magnitude more powerful and far cheaper than today's machines.

Extensive efforts of multidisciplinary teams with active involvement of clinicians and researchers are necessary to develop and validate realistic modeling techniques, build accurate orbital models, and develop and test suitable orbital simulators. New conceptual solutions will be needed to exploit technology benefits and preserve the central role of the surgeon while at the same time freeing him or her from the technology overload.

ACKNOWLEDGMENTS

Several staff from my laboratory contributed to this work, among many others—Yu Chun Pong, Chui Chee Kong, Xu Meihe, Ng Hern, Luis Serra, Ralf Kockro, and Anthony Fang.

REFERENCES

1. Solaiyappan M. Visualization pathways in biomedicine. In: Bankman IN, ed. Handbook of Medical Imaging. Processing and Analysis. San Diego: Academic Press, 2000:659–684.

2. Rootman J, Stewart B, Goldberg RA. Orbital Surgery: A Conceptual Approach. Philadelphia: Lippincott-Raven, 1995.

3. Lorensen W, Cline H. Marching cubes: a high resolution 3D surface construction algorithm. Comput Graph 1987; 21: 163–169.

4. Levoy M. Display of surfaces from volume data. IEEE Comput Graph Appl 1988; 8(5):29–37.

5. Pal NR, Pal SK. A review of image segmentation techniques. Pattern Recognit 1993; 26(9):1227–1249.

6. Hajnal JV, Hill DLG, Hawkes DJ, eds. Medical Image Registration. Boca Raton: CRC Press, 2001.

7. Parshall RF. Computer-aided geometric modeling of the human eye and orbit. J Biomed Comput 1991; 18(2):32–39.

8. Yu CP, Jagannathan L, Srinivasan R, Nowinski WL. Development of an eye model from multimodal data. In: Kim Y, Mun SK, eds. Proceedings of SPIE. Medical Imaging 1998: Image Display, San Diego, CA, 1998. San Diego: SPIE Press, 1998:3335:93–99.

9. John NW. Using stereoscopy in medical virtual reality. Stud Health Technol Inform 2002; 85:214–220.

10. Kockro RA, Serra L, Yeo TT, Chan C, Sitoh YY, Chua GG, Ng H, Lee E, Lee YH, Nowinski WL. Planning and simulation of neurosurgery in a virtual reality environment. Neurosurgery 2000; 46(1):118–137.

11. Serra L, Nowinski WL, Poston T, Hern N, Meng LC, Guan CG, Pillay PK. The Brain Bench: virtual tools for stereotactic frame neurosurgery. Med Image Anal 1997; 1(4):317–329.

12. Fung YC. Biomechanics. In: Mechanical Properties of Living Tissues. New York: Springer, 1993.

13. Benabid AL, Nowinski WL. Intraoperative robotics for the practice of neurosurgery: a surgeon's perspective. In: Apuzzo ML, ed. The Operating Room for the 21st Century. Neurosurgical Topics Series. American Association of Neurological Surgeons (AANS), Rolling Meadows, Illinois, 2003: 103–118.

14. Jensen PS, Grace KW, Attariwala R, Colgate JE, Glucksberg MR. Toward robot-assisted vascular microsurgery in the retina. Graefes Arch Clin Exp Ophthalmol 1997; 235(11):696–701.

15. Hunter IW, Doukoglou TD, Lafontaine SR, Charette PG, Jones LA, Sagar MA, Mallinson GD, Hunter PJ. A teleoperated microsurgical robot and associated virtual environment for eye surgery. Presence 1994; 2(4):265–280.

16. Das H, Zak H, Johnson J, Crouch J, Frambach D. Evaluation of a telerobotic system to assist surgeons in microsurgery. Comput Aided Surg 1999; 4(1):15–25.

17. Urban V, Wapler M, Neugebauer J, Hiller A, Stallkamp J, Weisener T. Robot-assisted surgery system with kinesthetic feedback. Comput Aided Surg 1998; 3(4):205–209.

18. Taylor RN, Jensen P, Whitcomb L, Barnes A, Kumar R, Stoianovici D, Gupta P, Wang ZX, deJuan E, Kavoussi L. A steady-hand robotic system for microsurgical augmentation. In: Taylor C, Colchester A, eds. Proceedings of the Medical Image Computing and Computer-Assisted Intervention—MICCAI '99. Lecture Notes in Computer Science. Berlin: Springer-Verlag, 1999:1679:1031–1041.

19. Nowinski WL, Fang A, Nguyen BT, Raphel JK, Jagannathan L, Raghavan R, Bryan RN, Miller G. Multiple brain atlas data-

base and atlas-based neuroimaging system. Comput Aided Surg 1997; 2(1):42–66.

20. Nowinski WL. Electronic brain atlases: features and applications. In: Caramella D, Bartolozzi C, eds. 3D Image Processing: Techniques and Clinical Applications. Medical Radiology Series. Berlin: Springer-Verlag, 2002:79–93.

21. Hardy TL, Deming LR, Harris-Collazo R. Computerized stereotactic atlases. In: Alexander E III, Maciunas RJ, eds. Advanced Neurosurgical Navigation. New York: Thieme, 1999:115–124.

22. Nowinski WL, Bryan RN, Raghavan R. The Electronic Clinical Brain Atlas. Multiplanar Navigation of the Human Brain. New York: Thieme, 1997.

23. Nowinski WL. Computerized atlases for surgery of movement disorders. Semin Neurosurg 2001; 12(2):183–194.

24. Nowinski WL, Thirunavuukarasuu A, Kennedy DN. Brain Atlas for Functional Imaging. Clinical and Research Applications. New York: Thieme, 2000.

25. Nowinski WL, Thirunavuukarasuu A, Bryan RN. The Cerefy Atlas of Brain Anatomy. New York: Thieme, 2002.

26. Peifer J. Virtual environment for eye surgery simulation. In: Medicine Meets Virtual Reality II: Interactive Technology and Healthcare, Proceedings, San Diego, 1994. Amsterdam: IOS Press, 1994:166–173.

27. Sagar MA, Bullivant D, Mallinson GD, Hunter PJ. A virtual environment and model of the eye for surgical simulation. In: SIGGRAPH '94 Conference Proceedings. New York: ACM Press, 1994:205–212.

28. Umapathi T, Siow WK, Mukkam RP, Loong SC, Tan CB, Tjia HTL, Nowinski WL. Insights into the three-dimensional structure of the oculomotor nuclear complex and fascicles. J Neuro-Ophthalmol 2000; 20(2):138–144.

29. Uchio E, Ohno S, Kudoh j, Aoki K, Kisielewicz LT. Simulation model of an eyeball based on finite element analysis on a supercomputer. Br J Ophthalmol 1999; 83:1106–1111.

30. Dubois P, Rouland JF, Meseure P, Karpf S, Chaillou C. Simulator for laser photocoagulation in ophthalmology. IEEE Trans Biomed Eng 1995; 42:688–693.

31. Sinclair MJ, Peifer JW, Haleblian R, Luxenberg MN, Green K, Hull DS. Computer-simulated eye surgery. A novel teaching method for residents and practitioners. Ophthalmology 1995; 102(3):517–521.

32. Neumann PF, Sadler LL, Gieser J. Virtual reality vitrectomy simulator. In: Wells WM, Colchester A, Delp S, eds. Proceedings of the Medical Image Computing and Computer-Assisted Intervention—MICCAI'98. Lecture Notes in Computer Science. Berlin: Springer-Verlag, 1998:1496:910–917.

33. Schill MA, Wagner C, Hennen M, Bender HJ, Maenner R. EyeSi—a simulator for intra-occular surgery. In: Taylor C, Colchester A, eds. Proceedings of the Medical Image Computing and Computer-Assisted Intervention—MICCAI'99. Lecture Notes in Computer Science. Berlin: Springer-Verlag, 1999:1679:1166–1174.

34. Nowinski WL, Chui CK. Simulation of interventional neuroradiology procedures. In: Proceedings of the International Workshop on Medical Imaging and Augmented Reality (MIAR '01), June 10–12, 2001, Hong Kong. Washington, DC: IEEE Computer Society Press, 2001:87–94.

30

The Future of Orbital Surgery

ROBERT ALAN GOLDBERG

Jules Stein Eye Institute
UCLA School of Medicine, Los Angeles,
California, U.S.A.

There is probably no surer way to make a fool of oneself than to try to predict the future. Had someone asked me 20 years ago, when I was a medical student, to forecast the advances that would affect the first half of my own practice I wonder if I could have possibly foreseen the sweeping changes that have made things so different now: effortless access to information and communication, decoding of the entire genome, paradigm shifts in the economics of medicine leading to limitation of resources, and my own progressive inability to work through the night and still be fresh the next day, to name just a few. I think the safest way to approach the delicate exercise of prognostication is to take a safe course. I cannot anticipate the insights, advances, and technology that will certainly make our current techniques fodder for amusing anecdotes one day, but I can identify areas that I hope will improve. In this monograph, I will review a bit of the history of orbital surgery that got us to where we are now. It is interesting to see which concepts and techniques were abandoned, and which ones stuck. We will look at the ideas and technologies that most significantly pushed our discipline along to the next level. Then, I will consider the areas in which our current concepts and techniques are still most wanting. By tracking the trajectory of the development of the discipline of orbital surgery, and assuming a certain amount of inertia, perhaps we can best imagine where it is going.

So many advances have allowed us to refine our ability to care for patients that it is hard to define the most important ones. In Table 1, I have listed the five advances that strike me as the critical steps in the evolution of orbital surgery. Physiology and histology underlie all of our decision making in orbital surgery, and as we understand more about the pathophysiology of disease (from an increasingly molecular and genetic perspective), it will drive all the upstream advances. I would include in this category advances that are anatomically based; I would not take anything away from the great historic anatomists (Fig. 1) who essentially described all of the gross structures as accurately as our best modern dissectors, but what has improved is continued imaginative application of anatomy to create new approaches. A perfect example of this in my opinion, and one of the great leaps in orbital surgery of all time, was the realization by Paul Tessier that the bony orbital and cranial skeleton could be taken apart and reconstructed.

Anesthesia and asepsis created the ability to perform safe surgery, and effective biologicals provided the means of

Table 1   The Five Big Steps Leading to Modern Orbital Surgery

---

1. Physiology and histology; the ability to construct a differential diagnosis
2. The development of anesthesia and asepsis, resulting in practical surgery
3. Effective biologicals: anti-inflammatories and antibiotics
4. Imaging technology: CT and MRI
5. Small incision surgical techniques

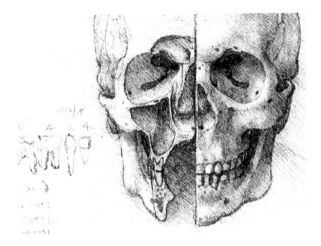

Figure 1 Five hundred years ago, Leonardo DaVinci drew with substantial accuracy many orbital anatomic relationships.

treating not only the medical arm of orbital disease, but also of treating some of the inevitable iatrogenic sequelae of surgery.

Imaging technology has powerfully changed our discipline. The orbit and cranial cavities are spectacular in the degree of critical delicate soft tissue structures packed intricately into a complex bony superstructure, and three-dimensional imaging has revolutionized orbitocranial diagnosis and surgical planning more, I suspect, than any other surgical specialty.

Finally, small incision surgical techniques and other minimally invasive or noninvasive technologies have advanced our ability to help our patients. We surgeons strut about proudly, bragging of our surgical successes, but cutting our patients is still a brutal process and every advance that minimizes the collateral damage to normal structures is a gift.

In Table 2, I have listed five limitations of modern orbital surgery that I believe most significantly attenuate our ability to help our patients. These limitations are both technical, relating to the gross nature of surgical instrumentation and technique compared to the extraordinary delicacy of tissues, and also biologic, reflecting our inability to diagnose and mod-

Table 2 Limitations of Modern Orbital Surgery

1. Surgery is still invasive: normal tissue is destroyed.
2. Surgery is not fine enough for infiltrative benign lesions such as lymphangioma and neurofibroma.
3. Surgical oncology fails because we cannot identify microscopic tumor margins preoperatively, so that we almost always remove too much or too little tissue.
4. Reconstructive and aesthetic surgeries fail because of poor control of wound healing; unpredictable fibrosis too often limits our best efforts.
5. Surgery fails because we cannot replace lost functioning parts.

ify the biologic processes that cause disease and that affect our surgical interventions in the postoperative period.

In Table 3, I have assembled a list of the five technologies that I believe have the best chance to help us overcome our current limitations. This is the riskiest part, of course, and if I am fortunate to be around in 20 or 30 years, I hope that I will get a smile from this monograph not only at my own expense for naivety and presumption, but also perhaps for some accurate guesses. It would be most disappointing of all to be correct on all five, because that would imply that our best evolving technologies were not eclipsed by some entirely new branch of science or intellectual pursuit.

Perhaps I can conclude with some illustrative cases (Cases 1–4) that point out some of the historic limitations, best current technologies, and hopes for the future. As I said

Table 3 Technologies That Will Help Us Defy These Limitations in the Future

1. Endovascular and nanotechnology leading to smaller and no incisions.
2. Better imaging including cellular level biological *in vivo* imaging.
3. Better control of surgical biology: premanufactured custom grafts, custom tissue implants, and better control of wound healing at a biological level.
4. Ability to control the immune system at a molecular level, so that there will be specific tests and treatments for Graves' and other autoimmune disease.
5. Detection and therapy of genetic alterations that are risk factors or proximate cause of disease.

CASE I. A 66-YEAR-OLD MAN PRESENTS WITH PROPTOSIS AND DECREASED VISION

Historic

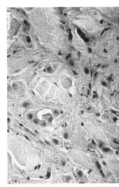

Imaging studies suggest Phlegmon of the orbit.

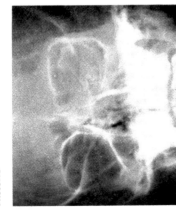

For pain, surgery is performed. Two-week hospital stay in netted bed to avoid infection.

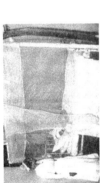

Two years later, phlegmon prostrate is noted with wasting and malaise, death occurs in 6 months.

Modern

Imaging studies show a destructive lesion of the greater wing of sphenoid. Differential diagnosis includes primary and metastatic neoplasia.

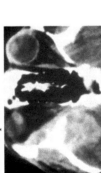

Systemic workshop reveals no obvious primary neoplasm. Fine needle aspiration shows adenocarcinoma, staining with PSA and demonstrating estrogen receptors.

Prostrate testing shows small nodule. Successful treatment with hormonal therapy, patient now in remission 10 years after diagnosis.

Future

Biologic noninvasive imaging shows neoplastic process involving greater wing of sphenoid, prostate, and small foci in ribs 3-4-5. Needle aspirate shows neoplastic cells; rapid cell phenotype stain confirms prostrate phenotype. Genetic analysis shows nonsense mutation on Codon M-4599, suggesting disinhibition of control of replication on growth segment KV-p. A custom antibody is made against the cell surface marker of the mutation and provides excellent control of the tumor, with minimal disease noted on whole body scan 5 years after diagnosis.

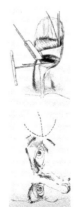

CASE 2. A 28-YEAR-OLD WOMAN WITH PROPTOSIS

Historic

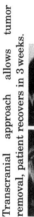

Roentogentography shows a vascular tumor.

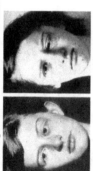

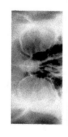
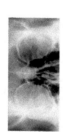

Transcranial approach allows tumor removal, patient recovers in 3 weeks.

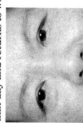

The tumor is removed through a hidden Baylis caruncular incision. The patient goes home that day and returns to work in one week.

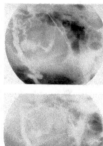

Modern

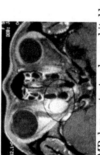

MR demonstrates deep orbital hemangioma.

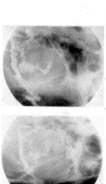

Future

Early diagnosis with biologic imaging. A nanodevice is inserted with image-guided needle, the device wraps around the tumor and focuses external microwave energy into the tumor, liquefying the contents. The liquefied contents are withdrawn and the needle is removed.

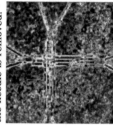
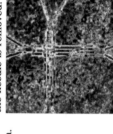

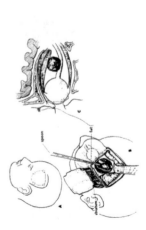

CASE 3. A 19-YEAR-OLD MAN FALLS OFF THE ROOF

Historic

Roentography shows fractures of the orbital floor and zygoma.

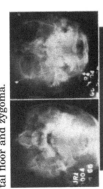

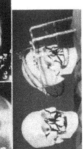

Through large cutaneous incisions, the fractures are explored to determine their nature. External fixation is applied during a 2-week hospitalization.

Modern

CT imaging elucidates the precise anatomy of bony features of the internal and external orbital skeleton.

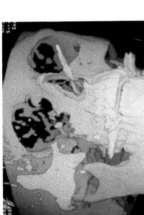

Through hidden incisions, the fractures are reduces using absorbable plates.

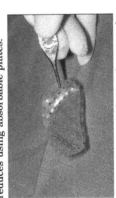

The patient goes home the next day and returns to work in 6 days.

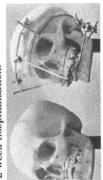

Future

Three-dimensional CT imaging defines the bony fractures. Biologic content is applied after the fractures are reduced through small incisions with intraoperative noninvasive real-time imaging to confirm alignment; the fractures quickly heal and the patient returns to work as a travel agent for intergalactic space travel.

However, after 3 weeks, he still has some double vision; dynamic imaging shows focal restriction of the connective tissues associated with the medial rectus. Ginacydin, a custom biologic agent, is injected into the area to focally modulate the fibroblast response; the diplopia quickly resolves.

CASE 4. A 60-YEAR-OLD WOMAN WITH A PAINFUL MASS IN THE LACRIMAL FOSSA

Historic

The tumor is approached surgically; because of bleeding, complete removal is not possible.

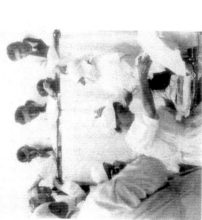

The tumor recurs in the orbit after 3 years, with pain, and exenteration is performed for pain control; the patient develops a postoperative infection which does not respond to heat treatments, becomes delirious, and expires.

Modern

Orbital imaging studies demonstrate an infiltrative tumor of the lacrimal gland.

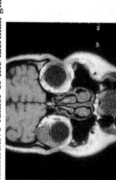

Bony orbitotomy allows complete removal of the tumor, developing a pane off the dura; histology shows adenoid cystic carcinoma with negative deep margins.

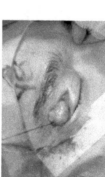

Despite radiotherapy, a deep orbital recurrence is noted 14 years later.

Future

Biologic tracer scan demonstrates suspected adenoid cystic carcinoma; micrometastasis demonstrated on cranial nerve 5 in one focal area only.

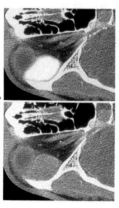

Ultrafine three-dimensional radiotherapy is applied to all microscopic areas of tumor cells, after specific biological preactivation. The main tumor mass is surgically removed using nanodevice directed fine dissection. The patient is alive 25 years later with no recurrence, still able to successfully work as a triporter manufacturer.

in my speech to Jack Rootman at the Vancouver Orbital Disease Seminar on March 16, 2002, Jack's greatest professional legacy is his family of devoted fellows, who filled up a substantial chunk of the auditorium when they walked up to honor him. Participating in the magical process of teaching and learning medicine, being fortunate to have mentors like Jack Rootman who have so powerfully shaped me, and accepting the responsibility of passing down not only the knowledge but also the tradition, has provided the most fulfilling experiences of my life.

REFERENCES

1. Troutman RC, Converse JM, Smith B. Plastic and Reconstructive Surgery of the Eye and Adnexa. Washington: Butterworths, 1962:77–91.

2. Spaeth EB. The Principles and Practice of Ophthalmic Surgery. Philadelphia: Lea & Febiger, 1941:30–34, 51–90.

3. The American Society of Ophthalmic Plastic and Reconstructive Surgery: The First Twenty-Five Years (1969–1994). In: Reifler DM, ed. History of Ophthalmic Plastic Surgery (2500 BC–AD 1994). San Francisco: Norman Publishing, 1994.

4. Clayton M, Philo R. . Leonardo Da Vinci: The Anatomy of Man. Boston: Bulfinch Press, 1992.

Index

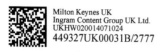

Milton Keynes UK
Ingram Content Group UK Ltd.
UKHW020014071024
449327UK00031B/2777